Animal Nursing
Assistar

For Elsevier:

Commissioning Editor: **Mary Seager, Rita Demetriou-Swanwick**
Development Editor: **Rebecca Nelemans**
Project Manager: **Emma Riley**
Designer: **Andy Chapman**
Illustrator: **Samantha Elmhurst**
Illustration Manager: **Merlyn Harvey**

Animal Nursing Assistant **Textbook**

Published in Association with BVNA

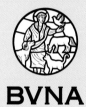

BVNA

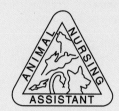

Edited by

Jo Masters CertEd VN
Practice Supervisor, Langport Veterinary Centre, Somerset, UK
Royal College of Veterinary Surgeons Examiner in Veterinary Nursing
Lead Examiner Certificate for Animal Nursing Assistants

Carole Martin VN DipAVN(Surg)
Head Nurse, Clifton Villa Veterinary Surgery, Cornwall, UK
Royal College of Veterinary Surgeons Examiner in Veterinary Nursing
Past President, British Veterinary Nursing Association

Foreword by

Dot Creighton DipAVN(Surg) VN
BVNA Past President and Honorary Member
RCVS VN Council Vice Chairman

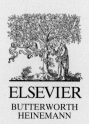

ELSEVIER
BUTTERWORTH
HEINEMANN

Edinburgh • London • New York • Oxford • Philadelphia • St Louis • Sydney • Toronto 2007

ELSEVIER
BUTTERWORTH
HEINEMANN

An imprint of Elsevier Limited

First published 2007
Reprinted 2009

ISBN-13 978 0 7506 8878 9

British Library Cataloguing in Publication Data
A catalogue record for this book is available from the British Library

Library of Congress Cataloging in Publication Data
A catalog record for this book is available from the Library of Congress

---

Note

Knowledge and best practice in this field are constantly changing. As new research and experience broaden our knowledge, changes in practice, treatment and drug therapy may become necessary or appropriate. Readers are advised to check the most current information provided (i) on procedures featured or (ii) by the manufacturer of each product to be administered, to verify the recommended dose or formula, the method and duration of administration, and contraindications. It is the responsibility of the practitioner, relying on their own experience and knowledge of the patient, to make diagnoses, to determine dosages and the best treatment for each individual patient, and to take all appropriate safety precautions.

To the fullest extent of the law, neither the publisher nor the authors assume any liability for any injury and/or damage.

The Publisher

Printed in China

Contents

Contributors

Victoria Aspinall BVSc MRCVS
Director, Abbeydale Vetlink Veterinary Training Ltd,
Gloucester, UK

Sally Bowden BSc(Hons) CertEd VN
Lecturer and Consultant in Veterinary Nursing,
Christchurch, New Zealand

Selena Burroughs BEd(Hons) VN
Lecturer in Veterinary Nursing, Bicton College, Devon, UK
RCVS VN Examiner, ANA Examiner

Helen Dingle CertEd VN
Curriculum Area Manager, Duchy College, Cornwall, UK
RCVS VN Examiner

Elizabeth Easter BSc CertEd VN
Lecturer and Consultant in Veterinary Nursing, Suffolk, UK

Caroline Gosden VN
Lecturer in Exotics, West Sussex, UK

Carole Martin Dip AVN(Surg) VN
Head Nurse, Clifton Villa Veterinary Surgery, Cornwall, UK
RCVS VN Examiner
Past President, British Veterinary Nursing Association

Jo Masters CertEd VN
Practice Supervisor, Langport Veterinary Centre,
Somerset, UK
RCVS VN Examiner, ANA Lead Examiner

Angela North MEd CertEd VN
Senior Curriculum Leader in Veterinary Nursing,
Warwickshire College, Warwick, UK

Karen Pitts VN
Lecturer in Veterinary Nursing, Nottingham, UK

Denise Prisk VN
Senior Theatre Nurse, Heathlands Veterinary Hospital,
Dorset, UK
RCVS VN Examiner

Amanda Rock BVSc MRCVS
Veterinary Surgeon, The Veterinary Hospital, Plymouth, UK

Jennifer Seymour CertEd VN
Lecturer in Veterinary Nursing, Penkridge, Stafford, UK
RCVS VN Examiner

Beverly Shingleton CertEd VN
Programme Manager, Plumpton College, West Sussex, UK

Jenny Smith Dip AVN(Surg) VN
Senior Theatre Nurse, Queens Veterinary School Hospital,
Cambridge, UK

Joy Venturi Rose MSc BAEd(Hons) VN
Freelance Consultant and Lecturer, Chichester College,
Chichester, UK

Ross D. White Dip AVN(Surg) VN
Teacher, Warwickshire College, Warwick, UK

Foreword

Animal Nursing Assistants (ANAs) continue to play a most valuable role in veterinary practice, hospital and referral settings. The importance of their work as an assistant to the veterinary nurse cannot be over-emphasised. Those that already fill this role will have gained valuable experience and often wish to progress further. Many employing practices encourage their staff to expand their knowledge and have traditionally used the ANA certificate. For both, this is an obvious pathway as the subjects covered – basic nursing, science, husbandry and reception skills – meet all their requirements. Trained ANAs are then able to assist members of the veterinary team more efficiently and can make their own mark in practice.

Literally hundreds of students have passed their ANA certificate (formerly Pre-VN) since the first enrolments in 1989. The qualification was first developed as a route into veterinary nurse training but was later recognised as a job role in its own right. Twelve years later, alterations were made to the Pre-VN qualification when it officially became the Animal Nursing Assistant certificate, in response to the changing needs within veterinary practice but also importantly the role of the veterinary nurse. At this time the syllabus was reviewed, taking into consideration feedback from students, Pre-VN holders and ANA tutors. The ANA entered the national qualifications framework and became a nationally recognised qualification. The RCVS Awarding Body had previously accepted the Pre-VN qualification as a direct route into veterinary nurse training. This continues to be the case with the ANA certificate, be it with the addition of key skills in the absence of the required GCSE results. Credit must be given to the few individuals who worked hard to produce this qualification and have since carried out its regular reviews on behalf of the BVNA.

The veterinary team are at the very front of animal welfare. Veterinary nurses clearly contribute to this, being heavily involved within all areas of the practice. The role of the VN is continually developing and by working alongside ANAs, VNs are able to dedicate more time to, for example, instigating nursing initiatives and increasing the standards of patient care. Recognising the importance of the ANA role in this context goes a long way to improving nursing standards and overall-practice standards.

As further proof of the qualifications success, in particular for those students moving up into VN training, the BVNA published statistics following the 2003 ANA survey. Nearly all respondents replied that their qualification will, or did, assist them with undertaking and passing their veterinary nursing qualification. It provided them with a good background knowledge, prepared them for their student veterinary nursing portfolio and when revising for their examinations. It also evidenced that the ANA firmly remained as the *pre-veterinary nurse* training of choice and allowed assistant staff to be trained while waiting for a vacant VN training position in their practice. Interestingly, many commented that having the ANA qualification assisted them in finding employment within a Veterinary Nurse Approved Centre (VNAC). In 2005 a similar ANA survey showed that this perception had not changed but also highlighted a lack of understanding when interpreting Schedule 3 of the Veterinary Surgeons Act 1966, as to the boundaries between the ANA role and that of a VN. At present the RCVS's advice as to these boundaries and the remit of VNs within the short RCVS Guide to Professional Conduct for Veterinary Nurses, is limited. This may change in the future, but both the ANA syllabus and VN syllabus can be referred to when looking to define the areas of practice for both groups.

Leaving veterinary nurses and ANAs aside, there continues to be interest in the role of the veterinary receptionist, who can be easily forgotten when it comes to training and CPD. Their role has developed over the years and to some employers individual receptionists have been referred to as reception managers due to the organisational skills required for someone on the frontline. Receptionists benefit greatly from a comprehensive basic knowledge directly related to their own practice setting. As stand alone module(s) or taking the full ANA certificate, gaps in their knowledge and skill can be filled. Receptionists provide a crucial link between the client and the veterinary nurse or veterinary surgeon and should also be able to work to a high standard, primarily in client care.

Traditionally the veterinary profession has respected the ANA certificate (and previously the Pre-VN qualification) and its high standards. Now the BVNA officially recognises successful ANAs with a personal badge and a separate membership category. The BVNA has also approved the use of the post-nominal letters -ANA – for all successful ANA candidates to use. The association may indeed progress past council discussions on the need for a conduct guide specifically written for ANAs, setting out minimum professional requirements, such as CPD.

Glancing through the pages of this textbook it is obvious that the revised syllabus for the ANA qualification has been taken into account. New areas such as basic radiographic positioning and the more recent reclassification of veterinary medicines have been included. ANA students will find this textbook invaluable. Equally this is a very useful reference tool, as a revision guide, for already qualified ANAs, student VNs, other members of the team such as veterinary receptionists and qualified veterinary nurses. Other courses focusing on animal or veterinary care will of course benefit greatly from its content.

Taking the above comments into account, this is by far the most valuable text for this position in practice. Few texts contain veterinary care or nursing assistant material in one concise book and I am in no doubt that this textbook will remain as popular as the qualification itself. As a book which has its place in my own library I will continue to use it as a source of reference as I know many of my colleagues do.

Dot Creighton

Introduction

It is hard to believe that it is five years since the Pre-Veterinary Nursing textbook was first published and we have been so pleased by its popularity and success. During these five years there have been many changes to the qualification, the most obvious being the name change from Pre-Veterinary Nurses to Animal Nursing Assistants (ANA).

The ANA qualification goes from strength to strength as its practical nature clearly depicts the role of support staff in general practice. Those who wish to train as veterinary nurses will find it a great stepping stone, others will benefit from its broad knowledge base and become useful practice members as a result.

We were delighted when BVNA council approached us to update the qualification's core textbook and all our previous contributors have reviewed and added to their chapters. The new syllabus update is reflected throughout the book and each chapter states its objectives and content in a clear manner. Multiple choice questions relating to each chapter are included to refresh knowledge and support students through the ABC/BVNA examinations.

Whilst this book is primarily intended for ANA students, it has been a widely used text in all animal care studies and all will benefit from its relevant yet scientific nature.

We are delighted with this new publication and wish you all the best with your studies.

Jo Masters CertEd VN
Carole Martin Dip AVN(Surg) VN

Acknowledgements

The editors would like to thank all the contributors who have taken the time and trouble to support the ANA qualification by providing this book with excellent chapters and knowledge base. Without the undying support of motivated and dedicated Veterinary Nurses publications such as this would not exist.

We would also like to thank BVNA Council for supporting this publication and our families, friends and colleagues who have supplied us with enough caffeine to get us through the editing!

This book is dedicated to all the Pre-VNs, ANAs and VNs whose drive and determination has got them where they are today – be proud of yourselves!

Jo Masters CertEd VN
Carole Martin Dip AVN(Surg) VN

Animal biological science

Basic biology

Amanda Rock

Chapter objectives

This chapter gives an introduction to:

- Basic atomic structure and characteristics of subatomic particles
- Cell biology – animal cell structure
- Osmosis and cell membranes
- Cell division
- Genetics
- Basic nutritional science

ATOMIC STRUCTURE

An atom is a particle, the smallest part of an element that can ever exist. The central nucleus is positively charged and contains protons and neutrons with electrons orbiting in its energy shells. If the whole atom was the size of Wembley stadium, the central nucleus would only be as big as the centre spot on the pitch. The great distance between the outer negatively charged electrons and the nucleus means that the attraction between them is weak and atoms can lose and gain electrons readily, allowing the atoms to become negatively or positively charged. Although they are too small to see with light microscopes and too small to be weighed, their relative atomic masses can be compared.

As the electrons weigh so little, virtually all the mass of an atom is concentrated in the nucleus. Therefore the mass number = the number of protons and neutrons.

The atomic number = the number of protons in the nucleus and identifies the atom.

Table 1.1 The subatomic particles, relative mass and relative charge		
The subatomic particles	**Relative mass**	**Relative charge**
Proton	1	+1
Neutron	1	0
Electron	1/1836	−1

A molecule is made from two or more atoms. Atoms share electrons so that each atom is normally surrounded by eight electrons. Metals are made up of atoms, non-metals are molecules, e.g. oxygen.

CELL BIOLOGY – ANIMAL CELL STRUCTURE

Introduction

Biology is about learning how living organisms function. The cell is the basic unit of life and an understanding of its structure and how it interacts with molecules is crucial to understanding the major body processes such as digestion and respiration.

Cell structures seen using a light microscope (Table 1.2)

You will see your first cells using a light microscope. The detail you see is limited by its resolving power, which is the minimum distance by which two points must be separated for them to be perceived as two

Table 1.2 Cell structures and their functions	
Structure	**Function**
Nucleus	Contains genetic material – the DNA
Mitochondria	Site of energy production
RER	Transports protein
SER	Synthesises fats and steroids
Ribosomes	Site of protein synthesis
Golgi body	Stores digestive enzymes
Lysosome	Digests waste materials
Vacuole	Collects end products of lysosome digestion
Centrioles	Cell division

separate points. The typical animal cell has a diameter of one-fiftieth of a millimetre. The cell is bounded by a thin cell membrane with a nucleus in the centre, surrounded by cytoplasm.

Cytoplasm contains granules, e.g. glycogen, a carbohydrate (CHO) food source. It is here that complex chemical reactions occur, providing energy for the cell's activities.

The nucleus is bounded by nuclear membrane. It contains all the hereditary material in the form of deoxyribonucleic acid (DNA) carried on structures called chromosomes.

Cell organelles seen with an electron microscope

The organisation in an individual cell is its ultrastructure. The entities making up this organisation are called organelles. Note that with a good quality microscope the Golgi body and mitochondria can be seen.

Endoplasmic reticulum (ER) – the cytoplasm consists of a matrix containing flattened parallel cavities, the lining membrane of which is continuous with the nuclear membrane.

Rough endoplasmic reticulum (RER) has granules called ribosomes attached to the lining membrane. Its

function is to transport proteins synthesised by the ribosomes.

Some ER is smooth (SER) as it has no ribosomes and is concerned with the synthesis and transport of lipids and steroids.

Golgi body – stacks of flattened cavities lined with SER containing secretory granules. The function is to add carbohydrate to newly synthesised proteins before leaving the cell.

Mitochondria – the power houses. The inner membrane is folded projecting into the interior (Figure 1.1). Most of the chemical reactions producing energy take place here. The folds of the inner membrane increase the surface area available for energy production.

Lysosomes – prominent dark bodies in the cytoplasm containing digestive enzymes to dispose of unwanted cell material. The lysosomes empty their contents into vacuoles.

The centrosome – lies near the nucleus and is made up of two centrioles. These are involved with cell divisions.

OSMOSIS AND THE CELL MEMBRANE
Cell membrane

The cell membrane surrounds each cell and is made up of lipids and proteins. One of its most important functions is to allow the transport of molecules into and out of the cell. Figure 1.2 shows the basic structure and examples of the ways substances pass through the membrane. There are two methods of transport:

■ **Passive** – where the cell does not expend any energy. Diffusion and osmosis are examples of this type of transport.

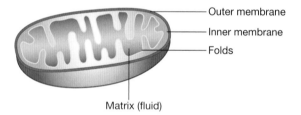

Outer membrane
Inner membrane
Folds
Matrix (fluid)

Figure 1.1 Cross-section of a mitochondrion.

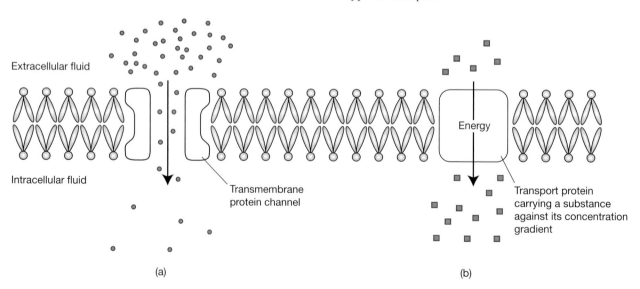

Extracellular fluid

Intracellular fluid

Transmembrane protein channel

Energy

Transport protein carrying a substance against its concentration gradient

(a)

(b)

Figure 1.2 Cell membrane showing passive diffusion (a) and active transport (b).

■ **Active** – where energy is required to move substances in and out of the cell. Examples of this type of transport include uptake of glucose and amino acids in the gut. Phagocytosis, endocytosis and exocytosis are all types of active transport.

Diffusion

The cell membrane is semi-permeable, i.e. it permits the passage of some substances and not others. Diffusion occurs when molecules move from a fluid of high concentration to a fluid of low concentration through the semi-permeable membrane. The protein channel in Figure 1.2 shows molecules diffusing from the extracellular fluid to the intracellular fluid.

Osmosis

Osmosis is a type of diffusion involving the movement of fluid from a low solute concentration (a weak solution) to a high solute concentration (a stronger solution) through the semi-permeable membrane (Figure 1.3).

Osmotic pressure

This is the pressure required to ensure fluid movement into and out of a cell is kept balanced. Osmotic pressure is measured against the osmotic pressure of plasma.

■ **Hypotonic solutions** have a lower osmotic pressure than plasma.
■ **Hypertonic solutions** have a higher osmotic pressure than plasma.
■ **Isotonic solutions** have an equal osmotic pressure to plasma.

Active transport

This is a process using energy to move substances in and out of the cell. An example of this type of transport is uptake of glucose and amino acids in the gut.

Phagocytosis

This is the process by which white blood cells (WBC) destroy invading bacteria and remove dead tissue from the body. The process is shown in Figure 1.4. The WBC wraps its cytoplasm around the particle and then releases the contents of its lysosomes to break down the invader or tissue. It is a form of endocytosis.

Endocytosis

This is the transport of large molecular weight proteins which are too large to pass through the membrane. The direction of transport is always inward.

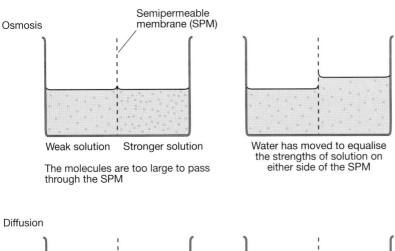

Osmosis

Semipermeable membrane (SPM)

Weak solution   Stronger solution

The molecules are too large to pass through the SPM

Water has moved to equalise the strengths of solution on either side of the SPM

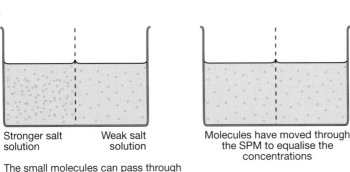

Diffusion

Stronger salt solution   Weak salt solution

The small molecules can pass through the SPM

Molecules have moved through the SPM to equalise the concentrations

Figure 1.3 Osmosis and diffusion.

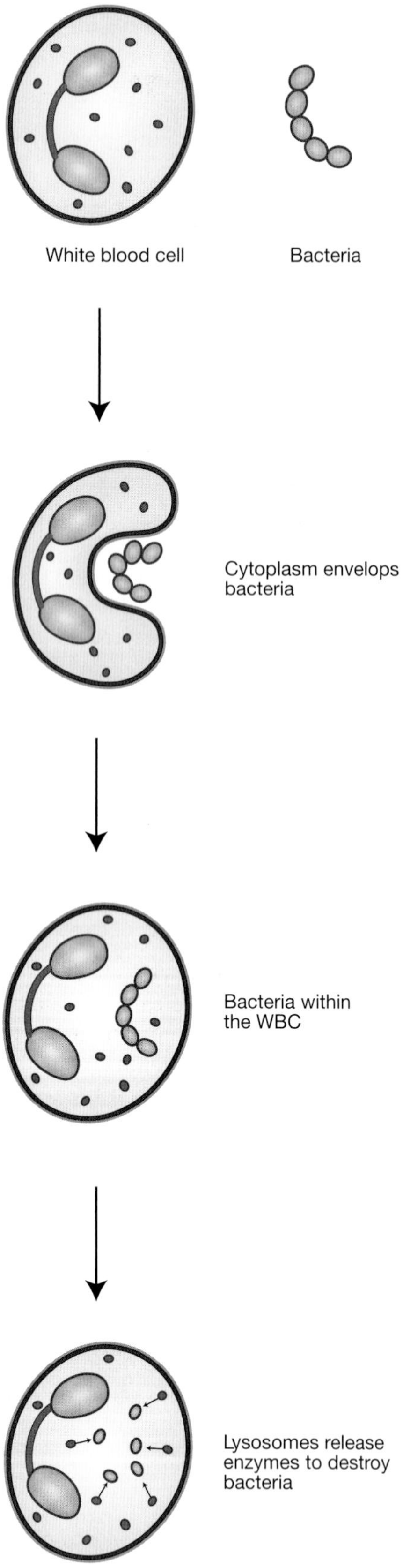

Figure 1.4 Phagocytosis.

Exocytosis

This is the transport of substances from the cell that are too large to pass through the cell membrane. The direction of transport is always outwards. Figure 1.5 shows the processes of endocytosis and exocytosis.

This is the process by which white blood cells (WBC) destroy invading bacteria, by releasing contents of lysosomes to ingest the invader.

Body fluids

■ **Extracellular fluid (ECF)** makes up about one-third of the total body fluid. The ECF bathes all the cells in the body and from this fluid, cells take up oxygen and nutrients and discharge waste products. The ECF is divided into two compartments in animals, one inside the vessels called the circulating blood plasma and one surrounding all the cells called the interstitial fluid.
■ **Intracellular fluid (ICF)** makes up the remaining two-thirds of total body fluid. This is the fluid found inside the cell.

Homeostasis

Fluid is continuously moving in and out of capillaries promoting the turnover of tissue fluid. Usually a balance is kept, but changes in pressure can lead to the accumulation of interstitial fluid in abnormally large amounts. This is called oedema.

Normal cell function depends upon normal fluid balance, homeostasis is the regulatory mechanism that controls this balance.

CELL DIVISION

Multicellular organisms begin life as a single cell and go on to become more complex by the process of cell division and differentiation (the process by which cells become specialised for a particular function). Even in adults, cell division continues to replace cells that die and need renewing, for example, hair and skin.

The most important structures in the cell during division are the chromosomes. They are responsible for passing on the genetic instructions from one generation to the next because they contain DNA, the blueprint of life. When a cell is not dividing each chromosome contains one DNA molecule, but prior to division the DNA duplicates so each chromosome has two parts, each called a chromatid, joined together at the centromere. Each species has a characteristic number of chromosomes. Cats have 38 and dogs 78. The nucleus of most cells contains two sets of chromosomes and therefore genetic material (Figure 1.6).

Labels for Figure 1.4: White blood cell; Bacteria; Cytoplasm envelops bacteria; Bacteria within the WBC; Lysosomes release enzymes to destroy bacteria

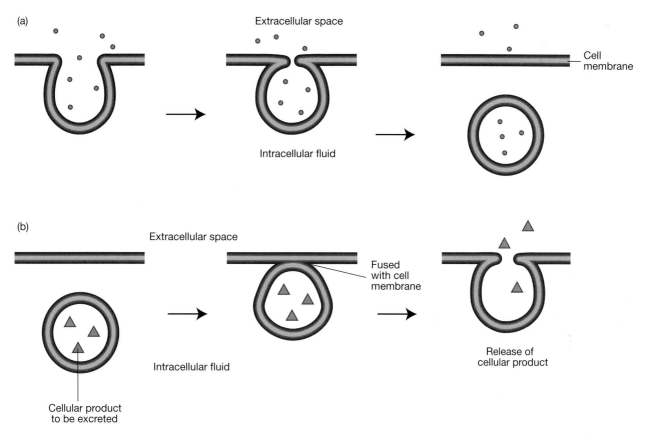

Figure 1.5   Endocytosis (a) and exocytosis (b).

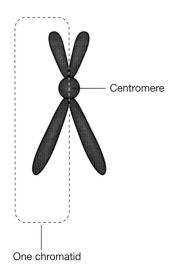

Figure 1.6   A chromosome.

Nuclear divisions are of two types depending on the number of chromosomes in the daughter cell. Mitosis results in identical daughter cells with the same number of chromosomes as the parent cell. Mitosis takes place when growth occurs, for example red blood cell production from bone marrow or skin cell production. Meiosis results in four daughter cells each containing half the number of chromosomes the parent cell had. For this reason meiosis is also called reductive division. This process occurs in the reproductive organs resulting in gamete (ova and sperm) production.

The cell cycle is the sequence of events in the life of a cell. The cell cycle starts and ends with cell division, and it consists of the stages of mitosis and interphase. Interphase is when the genes are being read to produce active proteins such as enzymes and the cell generally carries out its normal functions. Energy stores are replenished, new cell organelles are produced and the genetic material, the DNA, replicates. Cells that do not divide, such as those in muscle and nerve tissue, are always in interphase.

Mitosis

Mitosis is a continuous sequence of events, but they are described in four distinct stages: prophase, metaphase, anaphase and telophase (Figure 1.7).

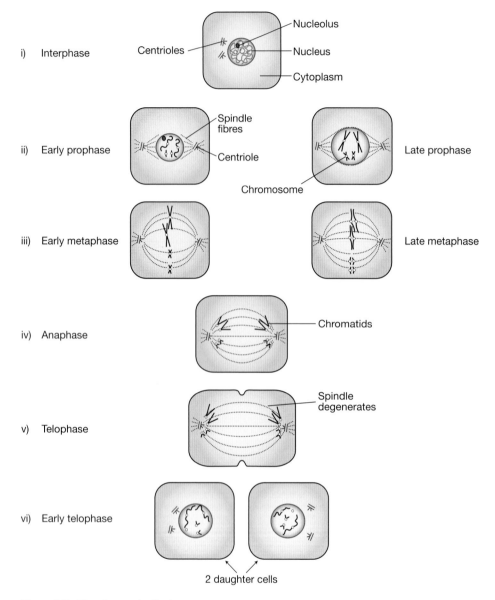

i)   Interphase

ii) Early prophase

Late prophase

iii) Early metaphase

Late metaphase

iv) Anaphase

v)   Telophase

vi) Early telophase

2 daughter cells

Figure 1.7   The stages of mitosis.

Prophase – at this stage the chromosomes have replicated and the two chromatids are identical. The normal activity of the cell stops and the nuclear membrane breaks down. The centrioles move to opposite sides of the nucleus, where they form the spindle. Here the cell is preparing for action.

Metaphase – the chromatid pairs attach themselves to individual spindle fibres and align themselves on the centre of the spindle. The chromosomes become attached at the centromeres and the chromatids separate slightly from each other. The chromosomes arrange themselves on the spindle completely independently, with no influence on each other.

Anaphase – the chromatids are pulled apart by the spindle fibres. The energy for this comes from the

mitochondria which gather around the spindle. The newly separated chromatids are now called chromosomes.

Telophase – the chromosomes reach the poles and become indistinct again. New nuclear membranes form and the cell divides into two. The daughter cells are now in interphase and ready for the next division.

Meiosis

In animals, meiosis occurs in the formation of gametes. These are the sex cells, the ova and sperm. The number of chromosomes, normally called the diploid number, is halved, resulting in a haploid number of chromosomes. This ensures that when the two gametes fuse

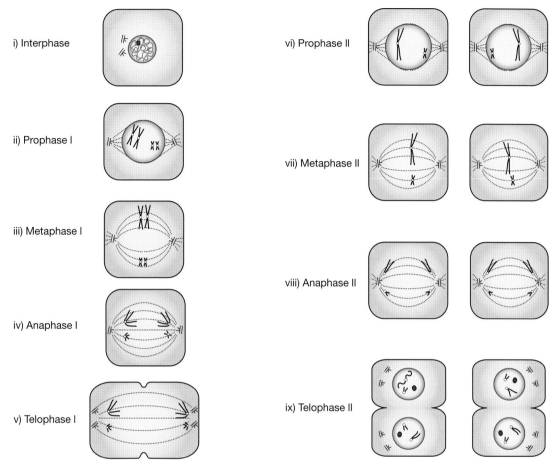

i) Interphase

ii) Prophase I

iii) Metaphase I

iv) Anaphase I

v) Telophase I

vi) Prophase II

vii) Metaphase II

viii) Anaphase II

ix) Telophase II

Figure 1.8 The stages of meiosis.

at fertilisation (the fusion of the sperm with the ova), there is the correct number of chromosomes in the offspring. The genes are also shuffled so that each gamete produced is genetically different.

Meiosis consists of two successive divisions. The basic difference between mitosis and meiosis is that in meiosis, the homologous chromosomes (those which are alike) pair up, whilst they stay apart in mitosis.

During the first part of meiosis, each homologous pair can swap parts of the DNA, called crossing over, allowing mixing up of the genetic code.

The stages are given the same names as in mitosis but are followed by a number I or II to indicate which of the two meiotic divisions it refers to.

Stages of meiosis (Figure 1.8)
Interphase – DNA replicates so there are four copies of each chromosome.
Prophase I – homologous pairs come together.
  Crossing over occurs to give genetic mix up.
Metaphase I – the homologous pairs arrange themselves on the centre of the spindle.

Anaphase I – the chromatids are pulled apart and move to opposite poles of the cell.
Telophase I – the division of cytoplasm begins.

There are now two cells, each with two copies of each chromosome that are genetically different from the parent cell.

Interphase
Prophase II – a new spindle forms.
Metaphase II – the chromosomes line up on the spindle.
Anaphase II – chromatids are pulled apart to opposite poles of the cell.
Telophase II – cytoplasm begins to divide.

There are now four cells, each with only a single chromosome, i.e. haploid.

Meiosis allows genetic variation so that offspring born to the same parents are different. This variation occurs in two ways. Firstly by the independent assortment of chromosomes to one pole or the other during cell division and secondly by the crossing over that occurs during prophase I.

GENETICS

Genetics is the science of heredity, the transmission of characteristics from one generation to the next. These characteristics could be eye colour, fur length or what sort of protein a cell produces.

Genes

The gene is the basic unit of inheritance for any characteristic. They are lengths of DNA that contain a specific code for any particular protein and each gene is located at a particular position on the chromosome called the gene locus.

Allele

An allele is one of a number of alternative forms of the same gene, occupying the same locus on the chromosome. For example, in a Labrador's coat colour, there is a yellow, chocolate and black allele – all of which are alleles for coat colour in alternative forms.

Homozygous

This is when both alleles of a particular gene are the same.

Heterozygous

This is when the alleles of a particular gene are different.

Genotype

This is the genetic make up of the animal, i.e. which alleles it carries.

Phenotype

This is what you see, the physical expression of the genotype.

Dominant

Genes that can be expressed in the phenotype even when only one copy of the allele is present are called dominant. These can suppress other alleles present. The dominant allele is represented by a capital letter, e.g. **B**.

Recessive

These alleles only show in the phenotype when both copies are present. They can only be expressed in the absence of a dominant gene and are represented by a lower case letter, e.g. **b**.

   Example – coat colour:
If **B** stands for black coat colour, and **b** represents brown coat colour:

BB = black
Bb = black (dominant masks recessive)
bb = brown (absence of dominant gene)

Zygote

When a sperm and ovum unite, the resultant cell is called a zygote and has a full diploid number of chromosomes, one half from the female parent and one half from the male.

Embryo

This is the new organism in its earliest stage of development, i.e. from the time that the fertilised ovum begins to develop, up to the time that the major structures appear.

Foetus

Once the major anatomical structures such as the limb buds appear, the developing young in the uterus is called a foetus.

Mendel's first law

Mendel was an Austrian monk alive in the nineteenth century. His study of the variation in the position of flowers on the plants in the monastery garden led him to the conclusion that the matings were not random, but could be predicted. He proved this and produced his first law which states that: the characteristics of an animal are determined by genes which occur in pairs, and that only one of a pair of genes can be represented in a single gamete (i.e. an ova or a sperm). To put this law in its simplest terms, **alleles separate to different gametes**.

   The experiment Mendel carried out to investigate this inheritance involved using only a single pair of characteristics.

   A black coat colour is represented by **BB** (two dominant alleles) and a brown coat colour is represented by **bb** (two recessive alleles). The result of this cross would be all heterozygous, expressing the dominant phenotype of black coat colour. If two of these offspring (known as the filial generation (FI)) were crossed the phenotypes shown would be three black coat colours and one brown. One is homozygous dominant (**BB**), two are heterozygous (**Bb**) and one is homozygous recessive (**bb**).

Genetic sex determination

One of the pair of chromosomes found in each cell are the sex chromosomes. These are the X and Y chromosomes and the genotype of the female is XX where that of the male is XY. These characteristic sex genotypes are found in most animals, but in the case of birds, the sex genotypes are reversed, females being XY and males XX.

In the production of the sperm and eggs, the sex chromosomes separate as Mendel predicted, one allele going to a different gamete. So all ova contain one copy of an X chromosome and sperm either contain an X or a Y. This means that it is the sperm that determines the sex of the offspring.

BASIC NUTRITIONAL SCIENCE
Introduction to nutrients

Feeding a pet is a challenge, with different diets required by different species, at different stages of their lives. Animals can be classified according to whether their diet is made up of plants, meat or both. Herbivores feed exclusively on plant materials, an example being the rabbit. Carnivores feed on other animals, for example the cat. Omnivores feed on both plant and animal matter, examples include the dog.

Inappropriate diet or malnutrition arises when an animal is under- or over-supplied with any of their required nutrients, this often leads to clinical disease.

Food is important for energy, growth, repair and reproduction. The components of food that fulfill these functions are called nutrients. Essential nutrients are those that must be eaten and cannot be synthesised by the body.

Nutrients are divided into six basic classes:

1. Water
2. Carbohydrates
3. Proteins
4. Fats
5. Minerals
6. Vitamins.

Water is the most important nutrient. The water requirement of a cat or dog in mL/day is roughly equivalent to the energy requirement in kcal/day, but this increases with heat, exercise, lactation, diarrhoea or anything that increases body water loss.

Energy gives cells the power to function and is obtained from fats, carbohydrates and proteins. Energy has no measurable dimension but can be converted to heat which can then be measured to work out the energy value of a food. An animal can not use all the energy in food, some being lost in the faeces, urine and the combustible gases produced during fermentation in the gut.

Carbohydrates contain the elements carbon, hydrogen and oxygen and can be divided into digestible sugars (e.g. glucose) and indigestible fibre (e.g. plant fibre).

Protein may come from plant and animal sources. Cereals, nuts, seeds, meat, fish and dairy products are all good sources of dietary protein. Protein consists of twenty different amino acids, many of which are essential in the diet. The higher the nutritional quality of the protein, the higher the proportion of essential amino acids it contains. Cats must eat meat to survive and have one of the highest protein requirements of all mammals. Taurine is an essential amino acid for cats, preventing retinal degeneration.

Fat gives palatability to food and is a great source of energy, providing twice as many calories per gram than either protein or carbohydrate. Fatty acids are described as saturated or unsaturated. Unsaturated fats contain essential fatty acids (EFAs) that are so important for healthy skin and coat, whilst fats in general are carriers of the fat-soluble vitamins A, D, E and K.

Minerals have many important functions in the body, a few of which are shown in Table 1.3. They are divided into two groups, macrominerals, such as calcium, phosphorus, sodium, potassium and magnesium and the microminerals. All of these are inorganic nutrients, sometimes referred to as the ash content of the food.

Vitamins are required in very small amounts and over-supplementation has no value and can be dangerous. Vitamins can be split into two categories; fat soluble (A, D, E and K) and water soluble (C and B complex vitamins). Most of the vitamins are essential in the diet. Vitamin A is found in liver and eggs and is needed for good vision, skin and bones.

- The vitamin B group includes thiamine, riboflavin, niacin, folic acid and cobalamin. They can be obtained from egg, liver and vegetables and are needed for metabolism.
- Vitamin C deficiencies affect wound healing.
- Vitamin D deficiencies affect teeth and bone.
- Vitamin E, which is also found in egg and liver, affects reproduction when deficient.
- Vitamin K is made by intestinal bacteria and is needed for blood coagulation.

Table 1.3 Minerals, food sources and functions

Mineral	Food source	Function
Calcium	Milk, cheese, bread	Bone and teeth development, blood clotting, nerve and muscle function
Iron	Most foods, especially meats	Required by blood cells
Phosphorus	Most foods	Bone and teeth development
Sodium, potassium and chloride	Most foods	Osmotic pressure, nerve and muscle function
Magnesium	Vegetables	Bone and teeth development
Copper	Shellfish and liver	Enzyme production
Chromium	Most foods	Metabolism of glucose
Manganese	Nuts, whole cereals	Enzyme production
Fluoride	Water	Bone and teeth development
Selenium	Meat, fish and cereals	Required by red blood cells
Iodine	Seafood	Thyroid hormone production
Zinc	Meat and dairy produce	Wound healing

Importance of a balanced diet

Home-made diets are often inadequate. It is often more expensive and certainly more time-consuming to cook a balanced diet for a dog or cat than to purchase a prepared pet food. Whether the food is dry, canned moist, or semi-moist all pet food manufacturers invest a lot of time and money into balancing their diets and label them as complete diets if they are suitable to be fed alone. Some foods are marketed as complementary diets and should be fed along with another diet to ensure all six groups of nutrients are supplied in the correct amounts.

Life-stage feeding is designed to give your pet the best possible food for its age and condition. Growing animals, pregnant or lactating animals need much higher energy levels and different vitamin and mineral levels at the correct ratios. Lifestyle is also a consideration, with sedentary animals requiring light diets and working dogs, performance diets. At every stage the nutrients must be balanced to the energy level of the food.

Nutritional support techniques

If the gut works, use it. Total parenteral nutrition means feeding intravenously and is rarely practised in veterinary medicine. Sometimes a little encouragement is needed to get a patient to eat, heating food to increase the aroma or hand feeding. Syringe feeding can be effective but stressful, and nasal feeding or gastrotomy tubes are alternatives.

Clinical nutrition

Dietary sensitivities are seen regularly in practice and most respond well to a bland diet such as of chicken and rice. Even itchy, food intolerant dogs can have their symptoms alleviated by a diet change. Obesity management is a growing area of veterinary medicine which occurs when energy intake exceeds expenditure. Many diseases are linked to obesity including arthritis and diabetes mellitus. Urolithiasis can also be managed in part by altering the balance of the nutrients in the diet.

Small mammal and exotic nutrition

Rabbits need roughage in their diets and are often obese due to sedentary lifestyles and overfeeding. Grass, hay and a variety of green foods should be fed every day. Pelleted rabbit food can be fed, but those where each pellet is a complete diet are preferable to the multi-coloured varieties to avoid selectiveness leading to an unbalanced diet. Cereal treats are not a good idea regularly as they contain sugar and contribute to the problem of obesity.

Guinea pigs need higher levels of vitamin C than rabbits and should be fed a proprietary guinea pig diet. Hay, grass and fresh fruit and vegetables are also good sources of nutrients.

Further reading
Lane, D.R., Cooper, B. (eds) (1999) Veterinary Nursing, 2nd edn. Butterworth-Heinemann, Oxford.

Body tissues and structures

Karen Pitts

Chapter objectives

This chapter gives an introduction to:

- Anatomical directions
- Tissues
- Body cavities
- Skeletal system
- Skin
- Special senses

Table 2.1 Common prefixes and suffixes

Prefix	Meaning	Suffix	Meaning
a/an	Lack of	-aemia	Blood
dys-	Difficult/ defective	-ectomy	Cut out
endo-	Within	-graphy	Recording
ex-	Out/ away from	-itis	Inflammation
haem-/haemo-	Blood	-logy	Study of
hydro-	Water	-oma	A swelling
hyper-	Above/ more than	-pathy	Any disease
hypo-	Below/ less than	-phagia	Eating
inter-	Between	-pnoea	Breathing
intra-	Within		
myo-	Muscle		
peri-	Around		
poly-	Many		
pyo-	Pus		
sub-	Beneath		

VETERINARY TERMINOLOGY

The use of correct veterinary terminology can pinpoint the exact location of an injury and give a clear description of an animal's symptoms. Most words can be split into two parts: the beginning and the ending, or prefix and suffix. By learning common prefixes and suffixes, you can often 'work out' an unknown complicated word for yourself. For example, for 'hypothermia': 'hypo' = low, below normal; 'thermi' = heat, temperature, so from this you can see that hypothermia means below normal body temperature.

Table 2.1 gives common prefixes and suffixes and Table 2.2 gives some commonly used words.

ANATOMICAL DIRECTIONS

To describe with confidence and clarity the relevant parts of an animal's body, we must be able accurately to describe the position of its various parts and the anatomical landmarks.

Figure 2.1 accompanies the following list of such words:

Cranial – towards the head
Caudal – towards the tail
Dorsal – towards the back (think of the dorsal fin of a shark)
Ventral – towards the belly

Head only: rostral = towards the nose; oral = towards the mouth.

Limbs

Proximal – closer to the body
Distal – further away (more distant) from the body

Proximal to carpus (forelimb) and hock (hindlimb)

Cranial – front of the limb
Caudal – rear of the limb

Distal to carpus (forelimb) only

Dorsal – front of the paw
Palmar – rear of the paw (think of the palm of your hand)

Table 2.2 Some commonly used veterinary terms	
Veterinary term	**Meaning**
Alopecia	Loss of hair
Anorexia	Loss of appetite
Anoxia or hypoxia	Lack of oxygen
Apnoea	Cessation of breathing
Bradycardia	Abnormally low heart rate
Cardiac	Relating to the heart
Cyanosis	Bluish colour of mucous membranes due to lack of oxygen
Dysphagia	Difficulty eating
Dyspnoea	Difficulty breathing
Emesis	Vomiting
Hypothermia	Abnormally low body temperature
Pyrexia	Fever
Tachycardia	Abnormally rapid heart beat
Tachypnoea	Rapid, shallow breathing
Tenesmus	Painful, unproductive straining

Distal to hock (hindlimb) only

Dorsal – front of the paw
Plantar – rear of the paw (think of planting your foot firmly on the ground)
Medial – closer to the middle of the body
Lateral – closer to the side of the body

TISSUES

When a group of cells together have a similar structure and function, they are known as tissue.

Tissues are classified into four basic types:

- epithelial
- connective
- muscle
- nervous.

Epithelial tissue

All epithelial tissue provides coverings and linings for the surfaces of the body – both inside and out. The main function of epithelium is to protect whatever it coats from wear and tear. It continually renews worn surfaces.

From this tissue glands are developed. Glandular epithelium either absorbs substances or secretes material made within the tissue.

Epithelium is classified according to the number of layers of cells, and cell shape (see Figure 2.2). Simple

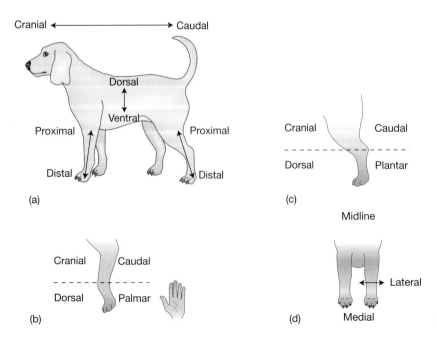

Figure 2.1 Anatomical directions.

epithelium is made up of a single layer of cells. Stratified epithelium is made up of more than one layer of cells. Cells immediately below stratified epithelium are continually dividing – pushing and flattening the outer layer, constantly replacing dead cells.

Shapes:

Squamous – flat
Cuboidal – cube-like
Columnar – tall and thin
Transitional – cube-like when relaxed and squamous when stretched.

Mostly, epithelial tissue is described using both the number of layers and the shape, e.g. simple squamous (see Table 2.3).

Connective tissue

Connective tissue supports. It holds cells and tissues together and transports substances. The cells of connective tissue are separated from each other by a substance called matrix. The structure of that matrix determines the function of that connective tissue.

Types:

- **Dense connective tissue** – has lots of collagen fibres (made by fibroblasts) in the matrix making it very flexible. Makes up tendons and ligaments.
- **Loose connective tissue** – 'loose packing' material. Found around glands, muscles and nerves filling spaces and holding organs in place.
- **Adipose tissue** – filled with lipids (fats) to store energy. Pads and protects parts of the body.
- **Yellow elastic tissue** – capable of expansion and recoil. Found in organs where shape alters, e.g. arteries and lungs.
- **Cartilage** – has a rigid, collagen-rich matrix that provides support. There are three types: Hyaline cartilage – covers ends of bone and helps joint movement. Yellow elastic cartilage – has yellow elastic fibres, and is more pliable. It is found in the ear and epiglottis. White fibrous cartilage – a bit like hyaline, and found between the vertebra.

Simple squamous

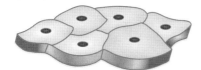

Single layer of thin, flat cells

Simple cuboidal

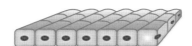

Single layer of cube-like cells

Simple columnar

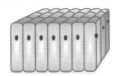

Single layer of tall, thin cells

Ciliated columnar

With small hairs

Figure 2.2   Types of epithelial tissue.

Table 2.3 Classification of epithelial tissue		
Epithelial	**Characteristics**	**Where found**
Simple squamous	Substances easily pass through	Capillaries, lungs, alveoli, lining blood vessels, heart, lymph vessels
Simple cuboidal	Greater volume than squamous, contains more organelles to perform more functions	Ovaries, kidneys
Simple columnar	As cuboidal	Stomach, small intestines, bronchioles, uterus
Ciliated	Has small hairs to move fluid or mucus	Nasal passage, trachea, bronchi
Transitional	These cells change shape from cuboidal when relaxed to squamous when stretched	Bladder, ureters, urethra, where lots of stretching may be required
Stratified squamous	Many layers, gives protection; outer layers constantly replaced by new cells from below	Epidermis, mouth, oesophagus, anus, vagina

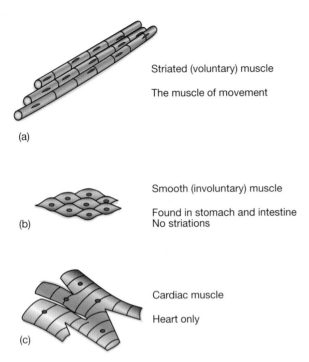

(a) Striated (voluntary) muscle

The muscle of movement

(b) Smooth (involuntary) muscle

Found in stomach and intestine
No striations

(c) Cardiac muscle

Heart only

Figure 2.3 Types of muscle tissue.

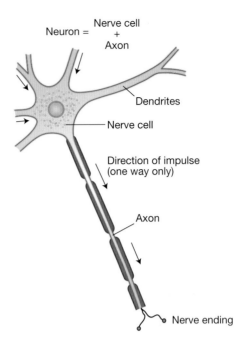

Neuron = Nerve cell + Axon

Dendrites

Nerve cell

Direction of impulse
(one way only)

Axon

Nerve ending

Figure 2.4 A neuron.

- **Bone** – hard mineral matrix to support and protect the body. The skeleton.
- **Blood** – liquid matrix, carries food, oxygen, waste products, etc. around the body.

Muscle tissue

The most important thing about muscle tissue is that it can contract (shorten). In fact, the only thing a muscle does when it is working is contract. There are three types:

1. **Skeletal muscle** – as the name suggests, this muscle attaches to the skeleton. It is normally under voluntary control. The cells are long, cylindrical and usually have several nuclei. Enclosed in a connective tissue fascia, and the cells are striped or striated (see Figure 2.3a).
2. **Smooth muscle** – this muscle cell has no striations, is tapered at each end and has a single nucleus. It forms the walls of hollow organs, helping with the movement of food through the digestive tract and the emptying of the bladder. Not under the animal's voluntary control, it is said to be involuntary (see Figure 2.3b).
3. **Cardiac muscle** – only found in the heart. Looks like striated muscle, but branches off frequently. Under involuntary control. Contracts rhythmically (see Figure 2.3c).

Nervous tissue

Responds to stimuli, controlling and co-ordinating many of the body's functions by producing a nerve impulse. It forms the brain, spinal cord and nerves.

The neurons which make up the nervous tissue are made up of three parts:

1. **Cell body** – where the general cell functions occur, and contains the nucleus.
2. **Dendrites** – a cell process or extension. They carry the nerve impulse toward the cell body. There are several per neuron.
3. **Axon** – a cell process that carries the nerve impulse away from the cell body. Only one per neuron (see Figure 2.4).

BODY CAVITIES

There are three main cavities in the body that contain viscera or organs. They are:

1. **Thoracic cavity** (chest)
2. **Abdominal cavity** (belly)
3. **Pelvic cavity** (within the pelvic bones).

Table 2.4 describes the boundaries of these cavities and the viscera found within them.

The thoracic cavity is divided into two parts by an area called the mediastinum. The lungs are on either side, and within the mediastinum are found the heart, trachea, oesophagus, major blood vessels and the thymus.

Table 2.4 Body cavity boundaries

Body cavity	Cranial boundary	Caudal boundary	Dorsal boundary	Ventral boundary	Viscera
Thoracic	First thoracic vertebra, first ribs, cranial sternum	Last thoracic vertebra, last ribs, caudal sternum, diaphragm	Thoracic vertebrae, dorsal part of ribs	Sternum, ventral part of ribs	Lungs, heart, major blood vessels, trachea, oesophagus
Abdominal	Diaphragm	Cranial pelvic cavity (no physical separation between abdominal and pelvic cavities)	Lumbar vertebrae and diaphragm	Abdominal muscles	Major blood vessels, kidneys, spleen, liver, stomach, pancreas, intestines
Pelvic	Cranial pelvic opening	Caudal pelvic opening	Sacrum, first coccygeal	Muscle, pelvic bone	Bladder reproductive organs

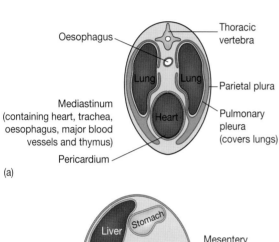

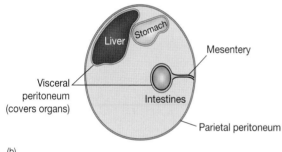

Figure 2.5 (a) Cross section of the thoracic cavity; (b) Cross section of the abdominal cavity.

Serosa

All of the body cavities are lined and all of the viscera are covered by a layer of membrane made up of epithelial and connective tissue. The epithelial cells produce small amounts of fluid called serous fluid and the membrane is called a serous membrane or serosa. The position of the serosa describes its exact name, i.e. pleura in the thoracic cavity, peritoneum in the abdominal and pelvic cavities (see Figure 2.5a).

The serosa lining the body cavity is called parietal and the serosa covering the viscera is called visceral (e.g. parietal pleura or visceral peritoneum) but it is all part of the same continuous membrane.

Abdominal serosa or peritoneum has areas between the parietal peritoneum and the visceral peritoneum that is also given a name. The part that connects the

intestines to the parietal peritoneum is called the mesentery (see Figure 2.5b).

To summarise:

Serosa – a large sheet of membrane, lining body cavities, covering viscera and producing a small amount of serous fluid.

Pleura – serosa lining the thoracic cavity.

Peritoneum – serosa lining the abdominal and pelvic cavities.

Parietal peritoneum – lines the wall of the abdominal cavity.

Parietal pleura – lines the wall of the thoracic cavity.

Pericardium – serosa surrounding the heart

Visceral peritoneum – covers the visceral organs.

Mesentery – specific part of the peritoneum that holds and connects the intestines to the parietal (wall) peritoneum.

The serosa acts to lubricate so that any movement of the organs does not cause damage.

SKELETAL SYSTEM

The skeletal system consists of bones, cartilage and ligaments; it allows body movement and provides support and protection as well as acting as a storage area, and a production site for red blood cells.

Functions:

- **Support** – rigid bone for weight-bearing, cartilage for flexible support, e.g. ear.
- **Protection** – hard bone protects underlying organs, e.g. brain.
- **Movement** – muscles are attached by tendons. Joints (where two or more bones come together) allow movement. Bones are attached to each other by ligaments.
- **Storage** – certain minerals (especially calcium and phosphorus) are stored in bone. When blood levels

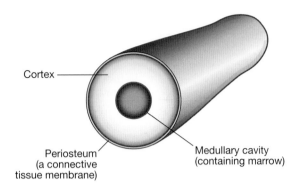

Cortex

Periosteum
(a connective
tissue membrane)

Medullary cavity
(containing marrow)

Figure 2.6   Cross-section through long bone.

fall, this triggers the release of minerals to help return the levels back to normal.

- **Blood cell production** – occurs in the cavities inside bone called marrow (see Figure 2.6).

The skeleton is divided into three sections:

1. **Axial skeleton** – forms a straight line down the body. Includes the vertebral column, skull and rib cage (see Figure 2.7a).
2. **Appendicular skeleton** – bones which are attached to the axial skeleton. Forelimbs, hindlimbs, pelvis (see Figure 2.7b).
3. **Splanchnic skeleton** – bony areas not attached to the framework of the skeleton but embedded in organs, e.g. os penis.

Figure 2.8 shows the complete skeleton of the dog and cat.

Bone types

Bones are made up of compact – very dense bone, and spongy bone – a framework with cavities within bone. Classification depends on bone shape. There are five types (see Table 2.5).

Long bone development

Bone cells are formed by special cells called osteoblasts. Bone formation is called ossification. There are two types:

- **Intramembranous ossification** – where bone is formed within connective tissue, e.g. in the bones of the skull.
- **Endochondral ossification** – occurs in long bone where cartilage is gradually replaced by bone.

Endochondral ossification

In the foetus, the skeleton is made up of cartilage. As the foetus develops the cartilage is replaced by bone tissue. When the shaft is all bone, ossification concentrates in the ends of bone.

Once the bone is formed, but the animal still has to grow, this centre of ossification is known as the growth plate (Figure 2.9a) where new layers of bone develop and add to the length of the bone, and so it grows. When the animal has finished growing, the growth plate fuses and forms a line of condensed bone tissue known as the epiphyseal line (Figure 2.9b).

Bone structure

A typical long bone is made up of a shaft or diaphysis and two ends or epiphyses. In joints the epiphysis is covered by articular cartilage and the rest of the bone is covered by a connective tissue membrane – the periosteum. The diaphysis has a cavity in the middle – the medullary cavity and an outer cortex (see Figure 2.10a,b).

It is in the medullary cavity that marrow is found. Yellow marrow is mostly fat and red marrow contains the blood-forming cells.

Blood vessels are connected with the marrow and pass through compact bone in little channels called nutrient foramen (a foramen always means a hole), and the blood vessels travel inside bone in Haversian canals (see Figure 2.10c,d).

In summary:

Epiphysis – head, ends of bone.
Diaphysis – shaft of bone.
Articulating cartilage – where movement occurs, protects the articulating surface (see synovial joints).
Medullary cavity – contains marrow.
Spongy bone – has hollow cavities, found in the epiphysis.
Compact bone – dense, gives strength, found in the diaphysis.
Periosteum – outer covering of bone.
Growth plate – where growth occurs.
Nutrient foramen – channels for blood vessels to enter.
Haversian canals – channels for blood vessels inside bone.

Figure 2.10b shows a cross-section of a long bone.

TENDONS AND LIGAMENTS

Both tendons and ligaments are made up of dense connective tissue. This is full of collagen, giving flexibility and strength.

- Tendons – attach muscle to bone (Figure 2.11).
- Ligaments – attach bone to bone (Figure 2.12) as in a joint.

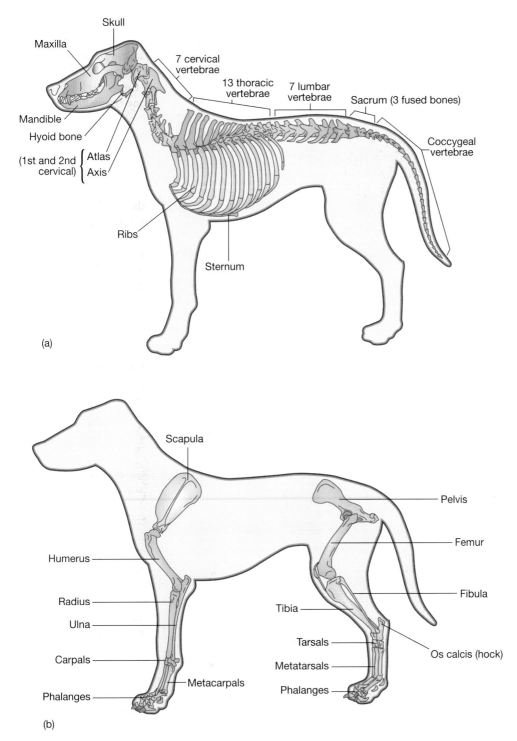

Figure 2.7   (a) Axial skeleton; (b) appendicular skeleton.

MUSCLES (Figure 2.13)

In order for the skeleton to move muscle power is required. The major muscles of the hind limb are quadriceps femoris, biceps femoris and gastrocnemius.

Another muscle that aids locomotion and helps give stability to the caudal part of the body is the lumbar expaxial; this is to be found along the lumbar vertebrae.

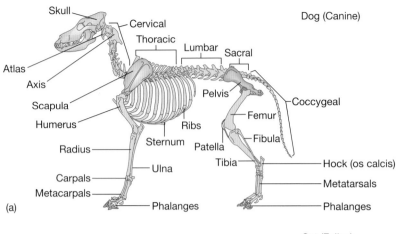

(a)

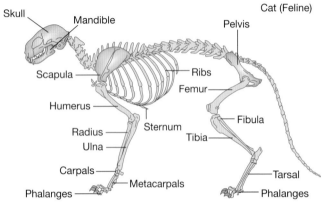

(b)

Figure 2.8   Skeletons of (a) dog and (b) cat.

Table 2.5	Bone types	
Bone type	**Structure**	**Position**
Long	Shaft of compact bone with spongy bone at either end	Femur, tibia, fibula, humerus, radius, ulna
Short	About as broad as long; spongy bone surrounded by compact	Carpals, tarsals, phalanges
Flat	Thin layers of compact bone separated by a small amount of spongy	Cranium, scapula, ribs
Irregular	Outer compact bone enclosing spongy; variety of shapes	Vertebrae – cervical, thoracic, lumbar, sacral, coccygeal
Sesamoid	Outer compact bone enclosing spongy; small bones, formed in muscle or tendon to assist passage over another bone	Patella, fabella

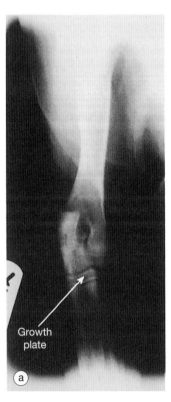

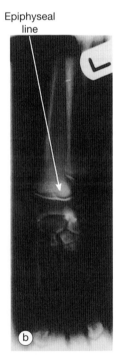

Figure 2.9   (a) The growth plate and (b) epiphyseal line.

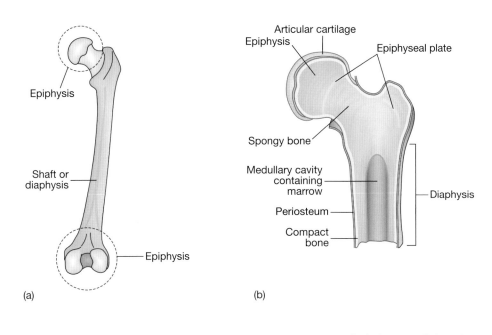

Figure 2.10   A long bone. (a) Right femur, (b) section through long bone, (c) spongy bone, (d) compact bone.

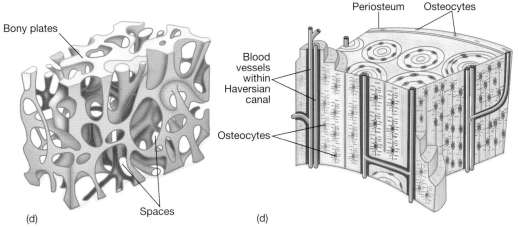

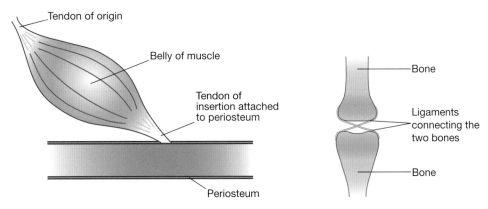

Figure 2.11   Tendons attach to muscle and bone.

Figure 2.12   Ligaments attach bone to bone.

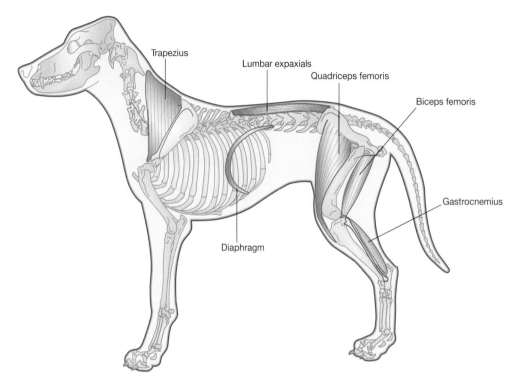

Figure 2.13 Some of the major muscles.

The trapezius is one of the muscles that help to move the forelimb.

The muscle of respiration is the diaphragm.

JOINTS

Where two or more bones meet, this is known as a joint. There are three classes of joint, all with differing amounts of movement.

1. **Fibrous** – no movement. As found in the suture joints of the skull.
2. **Cartilaginous** – slight movement. As found between vertebrae, between ribs and sternum, (known as the *amphiarthrosis*) at the mandibular symphysis (between the two halves of the lower jaw), at the pubic symphysis (between the two halves of the pelvis; the slight movement helps to widen the birth canal during labour), known as the *synarthrosis*.
3. **Synovial** – free moving. Found on the appendicular skeleton. The ends of bone in a synovial joint have a thin layer of cartilage, the articular cartilage, and a fluid lubricant within the joint capsule called synovial fluid (see Figure 2.14).

An example of a typical synovial joint is the knee joint or stifle joint (Figure 2.15). It includes the femur, tibia and fibia. The patella (a sesamoid bone) guides the quadriceps tendon over the stifle, and inside, cruciate ligaments keep the joint stable.

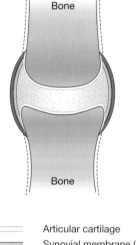

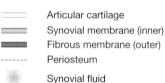

———	Articular cartilage
▬▬▬	Synovial membrane (inner)
▬▬▬	Fibrous membrane (outer)
- - - - -	Periosteum
⬤	Synovial fluid

Figure 2.14 A synovial joint.

Types of synovial joint

There are five types of synovial joint, classified according to the shape of the two surfaces that move against each other – the articular surfaces.

1. **Plane or gliding joints** – two flat surfaces that glide over each other, e.g. between vertebrae, carpals, tarsals.

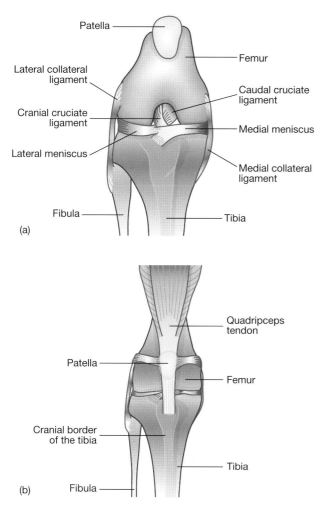

Figure 2.15   Stifle joint. (a) Cranial view; (b) caudal view.

2. **Pivot joint** – one bone slots into another, allowing rotation, e.g. between the first and second vertebrae (the atlas and axis) when shaking the head.
3. **Condyloid or ellipsoid joint** – football-shaped surface of one bone fits into the cupped surface of another, e.g. between the skull and the first cervical vertebra (atlas), allows nodding and tilting of the head.
4. **Hinge joint** – cylinder-shaped bone inserts into cupped surface of another. Similar to condyloid, but only allows one type of movement, e.g. elbow, stifle.
5. **Ball and socket joint** – consists of a ball (head) at the end of one bone fitting into a socket in an adjacent bone. Allows movement in all directions, e.g. hip joint, and between humerus and scapula.

Types of joint movement

Movement of a joint is always related to the structure of that joint. Some are limited to one type of movement, and others can move in several directions (Figure 2.16).

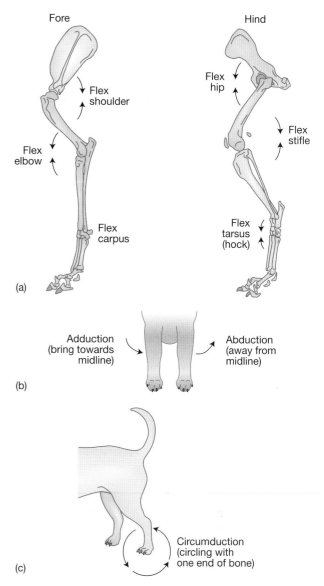

Figure 2.16   Joint movement. (a) Flexion; (b) adduction/ abduction; (c) circumduction.

- **Flexion** – bend, a closed joint (see Figure 2.16a)
- **Extension** – straighten, an opened joint
- **Abduction** – to take away from the midline
- **Adduction** – to bring together, move towards the midline (Figure 2.16b)
- **Pronation** – paw down in normal position
- **Supination** – rotation of paw inwards (as a cat eating meat from a tin)
- **Circumduction** – draw circles with one end of bone (see Figure 2.16c).

SKIN

The skin or integument forms the covering of the body. The outer layer, the epidermis, is made up of stratified epithelial tissue, with two other layers beneath, the

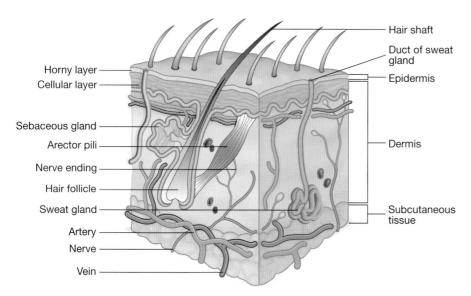

Horny layer
Cellular layer
Sebaceous gland
Arector pili
Nerve ending
Hair follicle
Sweat gland
Artery
Nerve
Vein

Hair shaft
Duct of sweat gland
Epidermis
Dermis
Subcutaneous tissue

Figure 2.17 Dermis and epidermis.

dermis and hypodermis (subcutaneous tissue) (see Figure 2.17).

Functions:

- **Protection** – prevents water loss from the body, and stops harmful substances (toxins, pathogens) from entering the body.
- **Production** – glands in the skin can produce: *Sebum* – an oily substance, helps 'waterproof' the coat. *Sweat* – produced to help cool an animal (mainly on the pads of the feet). *Pheromones* – animal perfume, for communication. *Milk* – from the mammary glands, produce food for the newborn. Skin can also produce *vitamin D*, with the help of sunlight.
- **Storage** – in lower layers, fat can be stored for energy and insulation.
- **Sensory** – sensitive to touch, pain, pressure, temperature.
- **Heat control** – thermoregulation. The blood supply to skin can be reduced to lower heat loss from the body. Erecting hair can trap a layer of air to insulate the body.
- **Communication** – pheromones, as mentioned before, e.g. from the anal glands, used for marking territory at defecation. Visually, animals can erect hairs – raising hackles – when threatened.

SPECIAL SENSES

Taste, smell, vision, hearing and balance, the special sensations detected by receptors in the head.

SIGHT

The organ of sight is, of course, the eye. The bony socket of the orbit houses the eye and gives a degree of

protection caudally. Externally, two eyelids – palpebrae – cover the front of the eye protecting and keeping the front surface (cornea) moist.

The lacrimal gland (under the medial dorsal lid) produces tears that are washed over the cornea by the eyelids. Most animals have an extra or third eyelid – the nictitating membrane – also for protection.

The eye itself has several layers (see Figure 2.18):

- **Cornea** – clear front surface of the eye. Allows light to enter and can change shape slightly to aid focusing. The cornea is continuous with the white of the eye or sclera.
- **Sclera** – supporting framework, helps keep the shape.
- **Choroid** – middle layer, contains blood vessels for nourishment.
- **Retina** – inner layer. Nervous coat, connected to the optic nerve. Contains photoreceptors that respond to light: rods providing night vision, and cones responding to bright, coloured light. Nerve fibres leave the retina at the optic disc to join the optic nerve.

Internally, the eye is split into two chambers (see Figure 2.18). The anterior chamber contains aqueous humour, a watery fluid. The posterior chamber contains vitreous humour, a gelatinous substance.

Where the eye divides into the two chambers, the choroid (middle layer) projects inwards (Figure 2.18).

Ciliary body – the inner projection of the choroid.
Suspensory ligaments – attached to the ciliary body. Hold the lens in place.
Lens – clear, solid, biconvex structure that changes shape to allow focusing. Light enters the eye

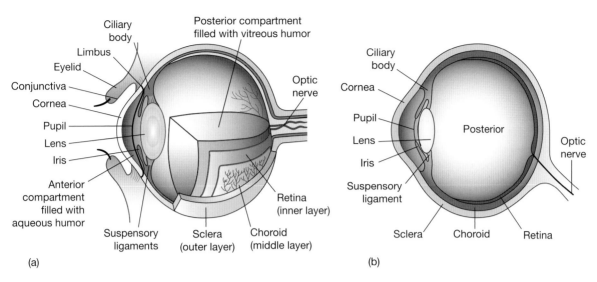

Figure 2.18   The eye.

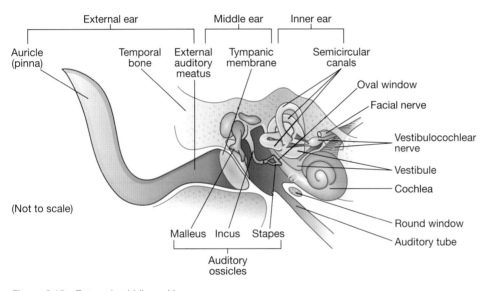

Figure 2.19   External, middle and inner ears.

through a hole in the iris that can change its size, called the pupil.

Iris – a further projection inwards of the ciliary body. Surrounds the pupil, the coloured part of the eye. Contraction and relaxation of muscles in the iris can alter pupil size, controlling the amount of light entering the eye. Think of a cat's eyes in bright and dim light, and how different they look.

HEARING AND BALANCE

The mammalian ear is concerned with both hearing and balance. There are three parts: external, middle and inner (Figure 2.19).

External ear

The outer ear flap or pinna made up of skin and cartilage, can be moved by voluntary muscles. The ear canal is the L-shaped canal entering the skull and ending at the tympanic membrane, the 'ear drum', which separates the external and middle ear.

Middle ear

The middle ear runs from the tympanic membrane to the oval window. The middle ear is filled with air and has three tiny bones that touch each other. These bones or auditory ossicles transmit sound vibrations from the tympanic membrane to the oval window. The small bones are called:

Malleus – hammer-shaped
Incus – anvil-shaped
Stapes – stirrup-shaped.

The tube that connects the middle ear to the pharynx is called the Eustachian tube and opens on swallowing. This allows air pressure to equalise on either side of the ear drum, e.g. the 'ear popping' experienced when in a lift or on an aeroplane.

Inner ear

This is really the 'business end' of the ear. The inner ear is filled with fluid and contains two main structures (Figure 2.19), one for hearing, the cochlea, and one for balance, the semi-circular canals.

The cochlea is shaped like a snail's shell and is filled with fluid. The middle portion of the cochlea contains a special structure called the organ of Corti, which has specialised hair cells that transmit the sound vibrations via the vestibulocochlear nerve to the brain.

The semi-circular canals are three loops filled with fluid. At the base of each loop, an area of specialised epithelium called crista ampullaris has hair cells embedded in a jelly-like mass. With body movement, the jelly moves, sending a message through the hairs to the brain via the vestibulocochlear nerve. When the animal stops moving, the fluid carries on and continues to displace the jelly (which gives us that dizzy feeling after spinning around).

Hearing

Sound waves enter the ear via the pinna and travel through the external canal to the tympanic membrane. This vibrates (like the skin of a drum), and in turn causes the malleus, incus and stapes to vibrate, transferring the waves to the oval window. The vibration from this causes waves in the fluid of the cochlea and moves the small hairs in the organ of Corti. The vibrations are then picked up by the vestibulocochlear nerve and sent direct to the brain, where the vibration is interpreted as sound.

TASTE AND SMELL

Taste, or gustation, comes from the taste buds that lie in the mucous membrane on the tongue, pharynx and larynx.

Smell, or olfaction, ties in closely with the sense of taste (try eating an apple whilst smelling an onion!). The mucous membrane of the nasal cavity contains the small receptors which send messages directly to the brain via the olfactory nerve.

Smell is a very important sense for both dogs and cats and is highly developed in both. Dogs especially use smell for a whole host of activities, including communication, territorial and sexual behaviour, tracking and, of course, sniffing out food.

In many vertebrate animals, an 'extra' organ has nerve endings found in the roof of the mouth. This extra organ is called the Jacobson's organ. Working with the nose, it helps the animal 'taste' the air. It is well developed in snakes, which explains why they continually flick out their tongues, tasting the air, always on the lookout for food.

Major body systems – Part 1

Victoria Aspinall

THE RESPIRATORY SYSTEM

Respiration is the exchange of gases between an animal and its environment.

The function of the respiratory system is to take oxygen from the air into the body (inspiration) and to excrete carbon dioxide from the body into the air (expiration).

The respiratory tract

The respiratory tract is the pathway along which the inspired and expired gases travel to and from the area of gaseous exchange within the lung tissue. The respiratory tract lies in the thoracic cavity or chest – Figure 3.1.

The parts of the respiratory tract are:

- The nose and nasal chambers
- The pharynx
- The larynx
- The trachea
- The bronchi and bronchioles
- The lungs.

Nose and nasal chambers (Figure 3.2)

The nose forms the entrance to the respiratory tract. It consists of a nosepad which is penetrated by a pair of C-shaped nostrils or nares. Each nostril leads into a nasal chamber. There is a pair of nasal chambers lying parallel to each other and dorsal to the oral cavity or mouth. The floor of the nasal chambers is extended into the pharynx at the back of the oral cavity by the soft palate.

Within the nasal chambers are delicate scrolled bones known as the ethmoturbinate bones. The nasal chambers and the ethmoturbinate bones are covered in ciliated mucous membrane which is well supplied with blood capillaries and fine nerve fibres. Leading from each nasal chamber is the frontal sinus and the maxillary sinus. These are air filled cavities lying within the bones of the skull (Figure 3.2).

As the inspired air passes through the nasal chambers it is warmed and moistened. Any smells in the air are detected and nerve fibres to the brain transmit the information. Particles such as dust, pollen or disease-causing organisms are trapped by the mucus in the nasal chambers and prevented from reaching the remainder of the respiratory tract.

Pharynx

The pharynx is a crossover between the respiratory and digestive systems. It consists of a wide muscular tube at the back of the nasal and oral cavities (Figure 3.2). It is lined with lymphoid tissue and mucous membrane. There are six openings into the pharynx:

- Oral cavity
- Nasal chambers
- Larynx leading to the trachea
- Oesophagus
- Two Eustachian tubes, each leading from the middle ear.

The function of the pharynx is to regulate the passage of air from the nasal chambers into the larynx and trachea and the passage of food from the oral cavity into the oesophagus.

Larynx

The larynx is a collection of interconnecting cartilages forming a box-like structure lined by mucous membrane. The epiglottis is the most cranial of the cartilages

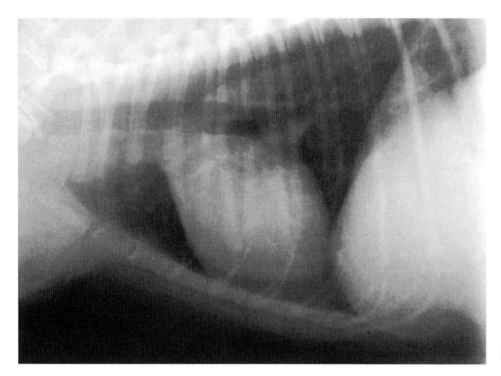

Figure 3.1   Radiograph showing lateral view of the thorax of the dog.

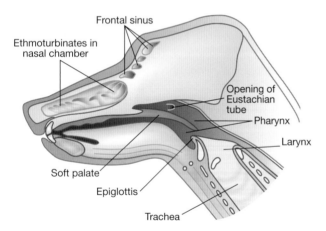

Figure 3.2   Left lateral view of head of dog to show nasal cavities and pharynx.

and is attached to the ventral border of the larynx. Its function is to regulate the passage of air down the larynx and prevent food entering the trachea during swallowing. Lying within the larynx are the vocal cords. Movement of the cords during inspiration and expiration produces sounds.

Trachea

The trachea is a tube made of C-shaped rings of hyaline cartilage linked by connective tissue and smooth muscle. It is lined by ciliated columnar epithelium which helps to trap particles in the inspired air and prevent them getting into the lungs. The cartilage rings keep the trachea open and allow an unimpeded passage of air into the lungs.

The trachea runs down the midline of the neck and enters the thoracic cavity.

Bronchi and bronchioles

In the thoracic cavity, at a point above the base of the heart, the trachea divides into a right and left bronchus, each of which supplies the lung on the corresponding side.

The bronchi have a similar structure to that of the trachea except that the cartilage rings are complete and the diameter of each tube is smaller.

Within the lungs, each bronchus divides into smaller and smaller tubules known as bronchioles. This arrangement of tubules transports the respiratory gases into and out of the lung tissue.

The lungs

When examined with the naked eye, the lungs are pale pink and feel spongy to the touch. They are divided into the right and left lung each consisting of several lobes which are dissimilar in size and shape (Table 3.1). In life the lungs almost completely fill the thoracic cavity (Figure 3.3).

Within the lung tissue, the smallest bronchioles continue to divide and lead into narrower respiratory bronchioles ending in minute air – filled sacs known as alveoli (Figure 3.4). These are lined by a membrane which is one cell thick and known as the pulmonary membrane.

Table 3.1 Comparison between the lobes of the right and left lungs	
Right lung	**Left lung**
Apical or cranial lobe	Apical or cranial lobe
Cardiac or middle lobe	Cardiac or middle lobe
Caudal or diaphragmatic lobe	Caudal or diaphragmatic lobe
Accessory lobe	–

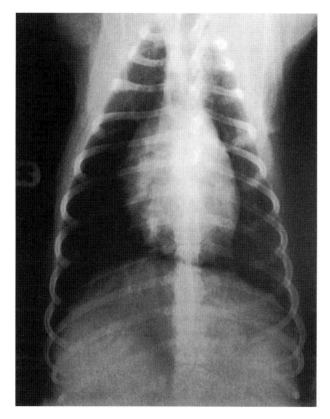

Figure 3.3 Radiograph showing dorsoventral view of the thorax of the dog.

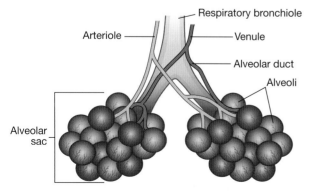

Figure 3.4 Terminal air passages.

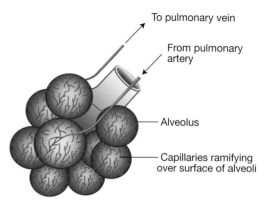

Figure 3.5 Capillary network surrounding the alveoli of the lungs.

Each alveolus is surrounded by a network of blood capillaries (Figure 3.5). These are branches of the pulmonary vein which carries oxygenated blood from the lungs to the heart. Deoxygenated blood is carried to the lungs from the heart by the pulmonary artery. These blood vessels form the pulmonary circulation.

The thoracic cavity

This is the most cranial of the three body cavities and is formed by the ribs, sternum, diaphragm and thoracic vertebrae (see Figure 3.3).

It contains the:

- lungs
- trachea
- heart, its associated blood and lymphatic vessels
- oesophagus.

The thoracic cavity and the lungs are covered in a double layer of pleural membrane. Between the two layers is the pleural cavity. This contains a little watery fluid which acts as a lubricant during respiration (Figure 3.6).

Lying between the ribs are the intercostal muscles. Dividing the thoracic cavity from the abdominal cavity is the diaphragm (Figure 3.7). This is a dome-shaped sheet of muscle stretched between the most caudal pairs of ribs. These two sets of muscles are responsible for inspiration (Figure 3.7).

Breathing

Breathing takes place as result of movements of the thorax (Figure 3.7). It occurs in two stages:

1. **Inspiration** – the intercostal muscles contract and pull the ribs outwards. The diaphragm contracts and flattens. This results in an increase in volume of the thorax and the lungs. Pressure in the lungs is lowered and air is drawn into the lungs.

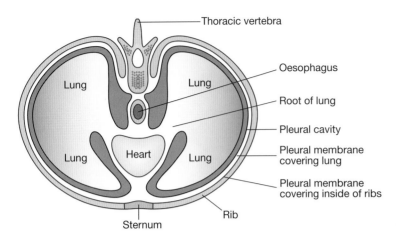

Figure 3.6 Transverse section through the thoracic cavity to show the position of the pleural cavity.

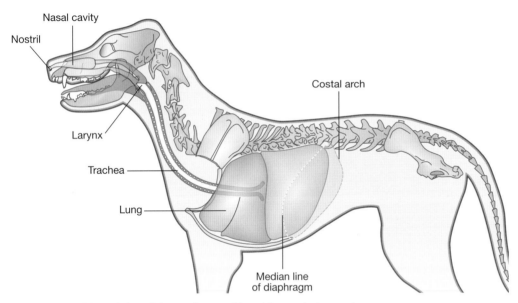

Figure 3.7 Left lateral view of dog to show position of the respiratory system.

2. **Expiration** – the intercostal muscles and the diaphragm relax and the ribs return to the resting position. The volume of the thorax and lungs reduces, pressure in the lungs rises and air is forced out of the lungs.

Gaseous exchange

This is the exchange of gases between the lung tissue and the blood and between the blood and the tissues of the body (Figure 3.8).

Oxygen is taken into the body in the inspired air and travels down into the alveoli of the lung tissue. Oxygen molecules diffuse across the thin pulmonary membrane into the blood capillaries surrounding the alveoli. Oxygen is then picked up by the haemoglobin in the red blood cells and is carried to the tissues of the body.

At the same time carbon dioxide produced by metabolic reactions in the tissues dissolves in the blood plasma and is carried to the alveoli of the lungs. Carbon dioxide molecules diffuse from the blood into the lungs and the gas passes out in the expired air.

Inspired atmospheric air contains a mixture of gases, including oxygen and carbon dioxide (Table 3.2). The relative proportions of oxygen and carbon dioxide change when the air is expired. Only about a quarter of the oxygen in the air diffuses into the blood, the remainder passes out unchanged. Carbon dioxide is produced by metabolism in the cells, so expired air contains a higher proportion of carbon dioxide than inspired air (Table 3.2).

Respiratory rate

The respiratory rate is the number of times an animal breathes in one minute (Table 3.3). The rhythm and

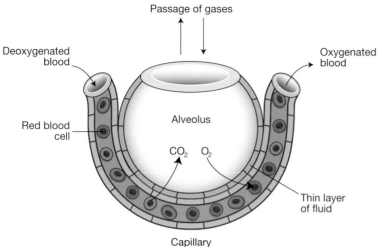

Passage of gases

Deoxygenated blood

Oxygenated blood

Red blood cell

Alveolus

CO_2 O_2

Thin layer of fluid

Capillary

Figure 3.8 Diagram to show diffusion between an alveolus and a blood capillary.

Table 3.2 Comparison between the gases in inspired and expired air

Gas	Inspired air	Expired air
Nitrogen	79%	79%
Oxygen	21%	16%
Carbon dioxide	0.04%	4–5%
Water vapour	Trace	Levels rise
Inert gases	Trace	No change

Table 3.3 Normal range of respiratory and pulse rates of the dog and cat

	Dog	Cat
Respiratory rate	10–30 breaths/min	20–30 breaths/min
Pulse rate	60–120 beats/min	110–180 beats/min

depth of respiration can also be measured. All three factors are linked to the metabolic rate of the animal and can be affected by:

- **Sleep** – the rate slows to a basic rate.
- **Exercise and excitement** – rate will rise but will depend on the fitness of the animal.
- **Pain** – rate may rise but the depth may become shallower.
- **Environmental temperature** – rate will rise as the temperature rises. A dog will pant to reduce its body temperature by the evaporation of saliva on its tongue.
- **Raised body temperature due to systemic infection** – rate will rise.
- **Anaesthesia and sedation** – rate and depth may fall due to depression of respiratory centres in the brain.

THE CARDIOVASCULAR SYSTEM

This consists of four parts:

- The heart
- The circulatory system
- The blood
- The lymphatic system.

The heart

Structure of the heart
The heart is a muscular four-chambered organ, whose function is to pump blood around the body (Figures 3.1 and 3.3).

The heart wall (Figure 3.9)
From the outside inwards, this consists of:

- **Pericardium** – fibrous tissue sac enclosing the heart.
- **Myocardium** – made of cardiac muscle which is capable of continuous rhythmic contraction for the whole of an animal's life.
- **Endocardium** – layer of simple epithelial cells that also covers the heart valves.

Chambers of the heart (Figure 3.9)
The heart is divided into a right and left side by the interventricular septum. Each side consists of two chambers:

- An atrium
- A ventricle.

The wall of the left ventricle is thicker than that of the right ventricle.

Heart valves (Figure 3.9)
The opening between the atrium and ventricle on each side is guarded by an atrioventricular valve:

- The right valve has three cusps or flaps and is called the tricuspid valve.

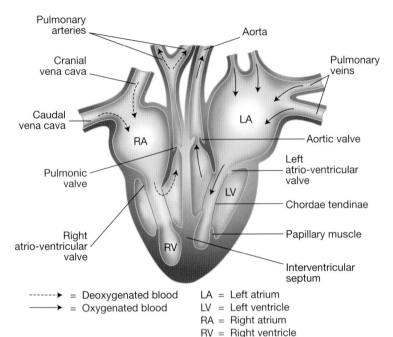

Figure 3.9 Cross-section through the heart to show structure.

- The left valve has two cusps and is called the bicuspid or mitral valve.

The function of the atrioventricular valves is to prevent backflow of blood as it is forced from the atrium into the ventricle. The edge of each valve is attached by fibrous strands known as chordae tendinae, to the heart wall. These prevent the valves from everting during contraction of the heart.

At the exit from each ventricle into the major blood vessels are the semilunar valves. These are:

- **Pulmonic valve** – at the base of the pulmonary artery as it leaves the right ventricle.
- **Aortic valve** – at the base of the dorsal aorta as it leaves the left ventricle.

The function of the semilunar valves is to prevent blood flowing back into the ventricles as the heart relaxes.

Blood flow through the heart (Figure 3.10)

Blood flows through the heart as a result of alternate contraction and relaxation of the heart muscle. The sequence is:

1. Blood enters the right atrium from the major veins of the body, the caudal and cranial venae cavae.
2. The right atrium contracts and forces blood into the right ventricle.
3. The atrium relaxes and the ventricle contracts forcing blood out of the pulmonary artery and into the pulmonary circulation of the lungs. The tricuspid valve closes preventing blood re-entering the right atrium.

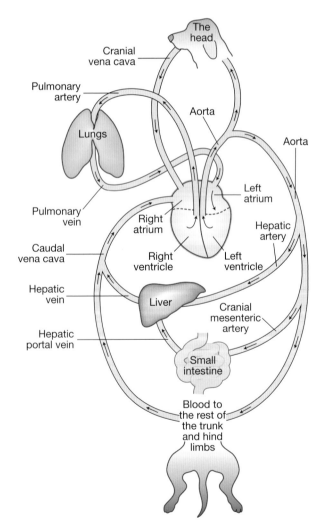

Figure 3.10 The flow of blood through the heart.

4. Blood returns from the lungs and enters the left atrium via the pulmonary vein.
5. The left atrium contracts and forces blood into the left ventricle.
6. The atrium relaxes and the left ventricle contracts forcing blood out of the dorsal aorta and round the systemic circulation of the body. The bicuspid valve closes preventing blood re-entering the left atrium.

The circulatory system

The circulatory system is a network of blood vessels whose function is to transport blood around the body.

Blood vessels (Figure 3.11)
There are three types:

1. **Arteries** – these carry blood away from the heart. Further away from the heart, the diameter of the vessels gets smaller and the walls become thinner – they are known as arterioles.
2. **Capillaries** – these are thin-walled vessels found within the tissues. Oxygen and nutrients are able to diffuse through the thin walls and reach the cells. Carbon dioxide diffuses into the blood. Capillaries form networks of vessels.
3. **Veins** – these carry blood towards the heart. As they leave the tissues, the capillaries combine to form small veins or venules and these become veins (Figure 3.12). Some veins in the legs have valves in their walls to prevent blood flowing back to the feet (Figure 3.11).

The circulation can be divided into two systems:

▪ **Systemic circulation** – the blood vessels supplying most of the body.
▪ **Pulmonary circulation** – the blood vessels carrying blood between the lungs and the heart.

These two systems are connected and work as a continuous series of vessels through which blood is pumped by the heart.

Systemic circulation
Arterial network (Figure 3.13)
Oxygenated blood leaves the left ventricle of the heart in the largest artery of the body, the dorsal aorta. As it passes through the body it gives off pairs of arteries to all the organs of the body. Some arteries supplying the digestive tract are unpaired. Examples of these arteries can be seen in Table 3.4.

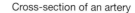
Cross-section of an artery

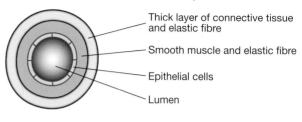
Thick layer of connective tissue and elastic fibre
Smooth muscle and elastic fibre
Epithelial cells
Lumen

Cross-section of a vein
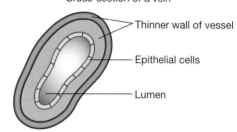
Thinner wall of vessel
Epithelial cells
Lumen

Longitudinal section through a vein
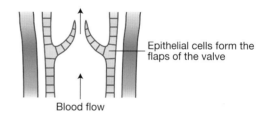
Epithelial cells form the flaps of the valve
Blood flow

Cross-section through a capillary
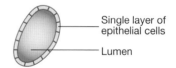
Single layer of epithelial cells
Lumen

Figure 3.11   The structure of blood vessels.

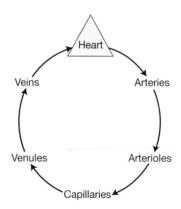

Figure 3.12   The network of blood vessels in the body.

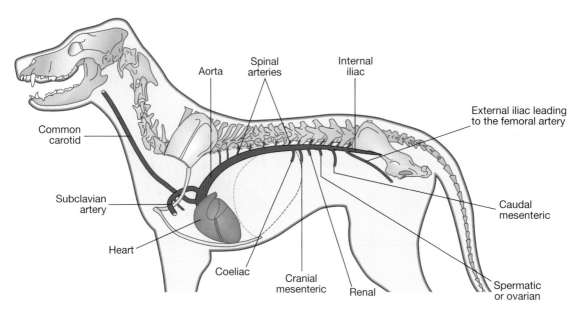

Figure 3.13 The major arteries of the dog.

Venous network (Figure 3.14)

In the tissues, the blood gives up its oxygen and nutrients and collects carbon dioxide and waste products. This deoxygenated blood returns to the heart by the veins which follow a similar pattern to the arteries and drain into the largest vein in the body, the caudal vena cava. This empties into the right atrium of the heart and from there to the lungs in the pulmonary circulation (Table 3.4).

Hepatic portal system (Figure 3.15)

This is part of the systemic circulation and drains the small intestine. The breakdown products of digestion such as amino acids and glucose, pass into the hepatic portal vein and are carried to the liver. Here they are metabolised and converted to materials needed by the body. Waste products produced by the liver travel in the hepatic vein to the caudal vena cava.

Pulmonary circulation

Deoxygenated blood from the systemic circulation leaves the right ventricle of the heart in the pulmonary artery and is carried to the lungs. In the lungs the artery breaks up into capillary networks around every alveolus. Blood in the capillaries picks up oxygen from the inspired air.

The capillary networks combine and eventually form the pulmonary vein which pours oxygenated blood into the left atrium of the heart. This is pumped into the left ventricle and around the body in the systemic circulation.

Table 3.4 Examples of the arteries and veins supplying the major organs of the body

Artery	Organ	Vein
Common carotid artery	Head and neck	Jugular vein
Right and left subclavian arteries lead to axillary and brachial arteries in each forelimb	Right and left forelimbs	Brachial and cephalic veins
Spinal arteries	Areas around vertebral column	Spinal veins
Coronary arteries	Heart muscle	Coronary veins
Renal artery	Kidney	Renal vein
Coeliac artery (unpaired)	Stomach, spleen and liver	Gastric, splenic and hepatic veins
Cranial mesenteric (unpaired)	Small intestine	Cranial mesenteric
Caudal mesenteric (unpaired)	Large intestine	Caudal mesenteric
External and internal iliac lead to femoral artery in each hindlimb	Right and left hindlimbs	Femoral and saphenous veins
Coccygeal artery	Tail	Coccygeal vein

Pulse rates

The pulse rate of an animal is the number of times the heart beats every minute. It can be measured at any point where an artery runs close to the surface. Suitable sites are shown in Table 3.5. The pulse rate reflects the metabolic rate of the animal and shows similar changes to that seen in the respiratory rate (Table 3.3).

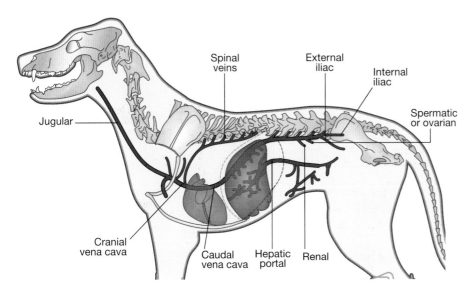

Figure 3.14   The major veins of the dog.

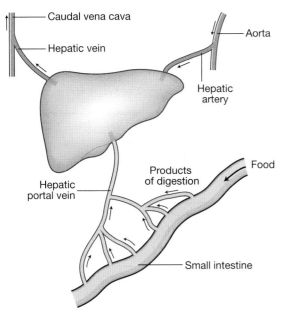

Figure 3.15   Hepatic portal system.

Table 3.5 Blood vessels of clinical importance		
Name of blood vessel	Site in the body	Veterinary use
Cephalic vein	Cranial surface of the lower forelimb	Intravenous injection (venepuncture)
Femoral vein	Medial aspect of inner thigh	Intravenous injection
Saphenous vein	Lateral aspect of the hock	Intravenous injection
Lingual vein	Underside of the tongue	Intravenous injection (used only under GA)
Coccygeal vein	Underside of tail	Intravenous injection (not commonly used in the dog and cat)
Brachial artery	In the axilla, on medial side of forelimb	Pulse rate; pressure point in first aid
Femoral artery	Medial aspect of inner thigh	Pulse rate; pressure point in first aid
Coccygeal artery	Underside of tail	Pulse rate; pressure point in first aid
Lingual artery	Underside of tongue	Pulse rate

THE BLOOD

Composition of blood

Blood consists of a collection of different cells suspended in a liquid matrix known as plasma (Figure 3.16).

Blood cells (Figure 3.17)
- **Red blood cells** or **erythrocytes** – contain haemoglobin and carry oxygen around the body
- **White blood cells** or **leucocytes**
  1. Granulocytes
     Neutrophils – most common white cell – defence against pathogens and other foreign material.
     Eosinophils – seen in cases of allergies and parasitism
     Basophils – seen in cases of allergies and parasitism
  2. Agranulocytes
     Monocytes – defence against pathogens and other foreign materials

Blood
Plasma (55%–70%)
Blood cells
Serum
Fibrinogen
Leucocytes (white blood cells)
Erythrocytes (red blood cells)
Platelets
Granulocytes
Agranulocytes
Neutrophils
Esoinophils
Basophils
Monocytes
Lymphocytes

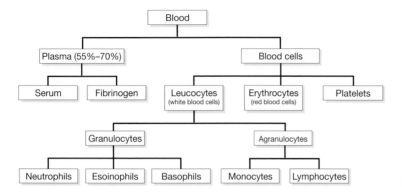

Figure 3.16 The constituents of blood.

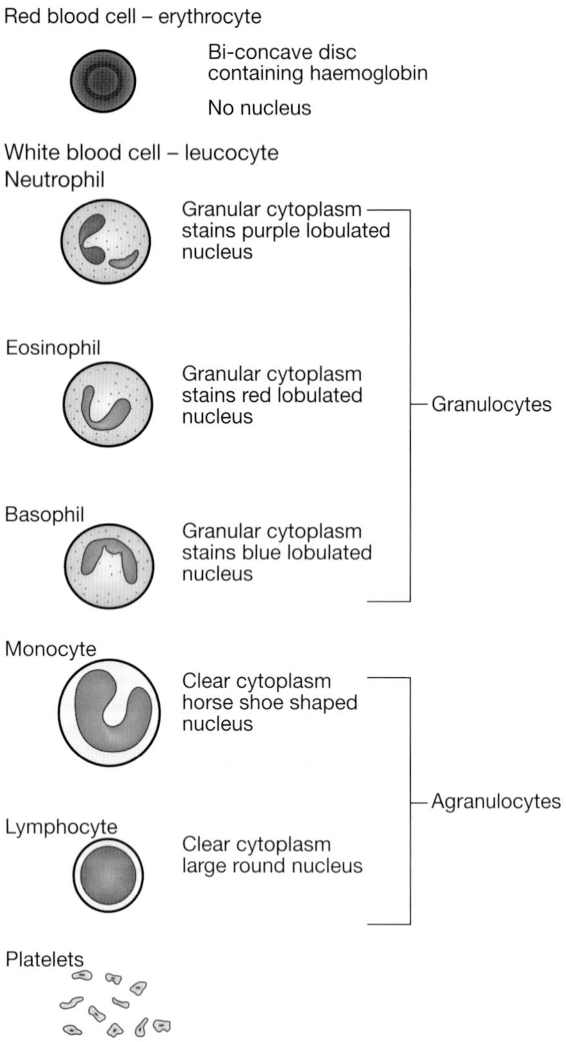

Red blood cell – erythrocyte
Bi-concave disc containing haemoglobin
No nucleus
White blood cell – leucocyte
Neutrophil
Granular cytoplasm stains purple lobulated nucleus
Eosinophil
Granular cytoplasm stains red lobulated nucleus
Granulocytes
Basophil
Granular cytoplasm stains blue lobulated nucleus
Monocyte
Clear cytoplasm horse shoe shaped nucleus
Agranulocytes
Lymphocyte
Clear cytoplasm large round nucleus
Platelets

Figure 3.17 Blood cells.

Lymphocytes – main cell involved in the formation of antibodies against specific diseases. Part of the defence of the body.

- **Platelets** – cell fragments needed in the clotting of blood.
- **Plasma** – makes up 55–70% of blood and is the part of the blood that remains when a blood sample is spun in a centrifuge. It contains all the materials that are transported in the blood e.g. hormones, proteins, waste products and mineral salts.

Serum is a yellow-coloured liquid that is left when blood clots naturally.

Functions of blood

These are to:

1. Carry oxygen from the lungs to the cells of the body
2. Collect carbon dioxide from the cells and take it to the lungs
3. Carry nutrients around the body
4. Carry hormones produced by the endocrine glands to their target organs
5. Collect waste products produced by the cells and take them to the liver and kidneys for excretion
6. Play a part in the control of body temperature
7. Maintain the balance of the body fluids
8. Play a part in the balance of the pH of the cells and tissues
9. Be responsible for the defence system of the body
10. Stop haemorrhage by the clotting mechanism.

The lymphatic system

The lymphatic system consists of a network of vessels and lymph nodes which collect and filter lymph and return it to the circulation via the heart.

The function of the lymphatic system is to:

- return tissue fluid to the circulation
- filter potentially damaging material from the lymph
- produce antibodies and lymphocytes for the defence of the body
- transport digested fat from the intestine to storage sites around the body.

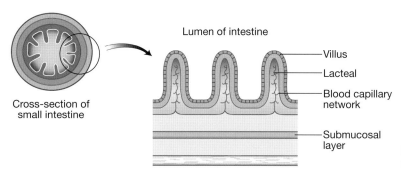

Figure 3.18 Villus structure in the walls of the small intestine.

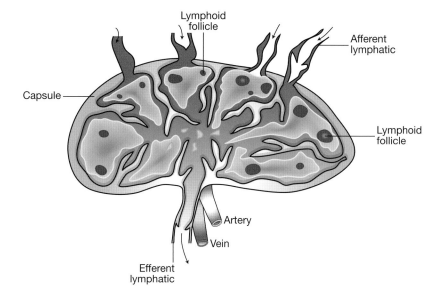

Figure 3.19 Cross-section of a lymph node.

Lymph is tissue fluid. It is of a similar composition to plasma but contains less protein and more lymphocytes.

Lymphatic circulation

Within the tissues and organs, lymph leaks out of the networks of blood capillaries and bathes the cells. It diffuses into thin walled lymphatic capillaries which drain into larger vessels, some of which have valves in their walls to prevent the pooling of lymph in the legs and feet. The large vessels empty into the right atrium of the heart. In this way the tissue fluid rejoins the circulation of the blood.

The major lymphatic vessels are:

- **Thoracic duct** – drains the hind limbs, the caudal parts of the body and the left forelimb and runs through the thoracic cavity towards the heart.
- **Right lymphatic duct** – drains the right forelimb.
- **Tracheal ducts** – drain the head and neck.

Within the finger-like villi of the mucous membrane lining the small intestine are specialised lymphatic capillaries known as lacteals (Figure 3.18). Digested fat, in a milky fluid known as chyle, diffuses into the lacteals and then passes into the cisterna chyli. This lies at the distal end of the thoracic duct in the cranial abdomen. Here chyle is added to the rest of the lymph and is carried by the thoracic duct to the heart.

Lymph nodes (Figure 3.19)

As lymph is carried in the lymphatic vessels it passes through areas of lymphoid tissue known as lymph nodes. Each node is surrounded by a connective tissue capsule.

Lymph enters the node through several narrow afferent vessels and leaves by a single wider efferent vessel. Inside each node are 'islands' of lymphoid tissue which filter the incoming lymph and remove any foreign material. Cells within the lymphoid tissue are able to form antibodies against specific pathogens picked up by the lymph.

Each area of the body and every organ is associated with one or more lymph nodes which monitor the levels of inflammation in that area. Many of these nodes are too deep to feel but some are more superficial and can be palpated as indicators of the health of the area they drain. The palpable lymph nodes of the dog are shown in Figure 3.20.

In other parts of the body there are also areas of lymphoid tissue which are important in the defence against disease. These are:

- **Spleen** – attached to the greater curvature of the stomach. It is not essential for life but is important in the production of lymphocytes and the storage of red blood cells.
- **Tonsils** – lie in the walls of the pharynx and monitor materials entering the digestive and respiratory systems. Inflammation is known as tonsilitis.
- **Thymus gland** – lies in the entrance to the thoracic cavity. It is relatively large at birth but disappears as the animal reaches adulthood. It is an important site for the formation of lymphocytes.
- **Lymph follicles** – smaller masses of lymphoid tissue are found around the body in areas such as in the walls of the small intestine.

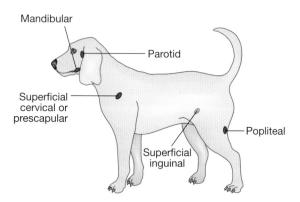

Figure 3.20   Palpable lymph nodes of the dog.

THE DIGESTIVE SYSTEM

The digestive system is adapted to ingest or take food into the body, digest it or break it down into small molecules ready for absorption and finally excrete the indigestible remains as faeces. Each organ within the digestive system is designed to perform a particular part of the digestive process.

The parts of the system are (Figure 3.21):

- **Mouth** – including teeth, tongue, lips and cheeks
- **Pharynx**
- **Oesophagus**
- **Stomach**
- **Small intestine** – duodenum, jejunum, ileum
- **Large intestine** – caecum, colon, rectum, anus.

There are several accessory glands whose secretions are vital for effective digestion. These are:

- **Salivary glands** – lie around the area of the mouth. Produce saliva
- **Pancreas** – secretes digestive enzymes into the duodenum. Also secretes the hormone insulin which regulates levels of glucose in the blood
- **Liver** – variety of functions linked to body metabolism
- **Gall bladder** – stores bile which contains bile salts produced by the liver.

Teeth

The teeth are hard structures embedded in the gums of the upper and lower jaws.

- Tooth structure (see Figure 3.22)
- Tooth shape and function (see Table 3.6).

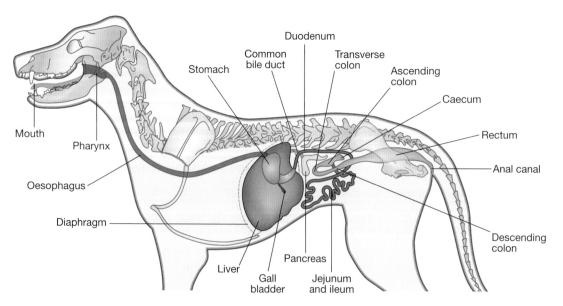

Figure 3.21   Left lateral view of dog to show position of the digestive system.

Permanent and deciduous teeth

Dogs and cats have two sets of teeth during their lives. These are:

- **Deciduous teeth** – also called the 'milk' teeth. These are present in the jaw at birth and push through the gum or erupt during the first weeks of life. They are generally smaller and whiter than the permanent teeth.
- **Permanent teeth** – these replace the deciduous teeth after they fall out. They remain in the jaw for the rest of the animal's life.

Examination of the teeth of the puppy or kitten is not an accurate method of telling the age of an animal but knowledge of the times at which each type of tooth should be present in the jaw can be used to gauge the approximate age. This may be important when deciding whether a young animal is old enough to be weaned. Using Table 3.7 you can see that you should start to wean a puppy as the deciduous incisors start to erupt, i.e. at 3–4 weeks, and weaning should be complete by the time all the deciduous premolars are present in the jaw, i.e. by 8 weeks.

Dental formulae

Each individual animal of a particular species has the same number of teeth in its jaw. These are written down as a dental formula which allows the vet to monitor how many teeth have been lost as a result of disease and old age (Figure 3.23).

Each tooth is referred to by its initial letter – I is for incisors, C is for canines and so on.

Numbers are used to show how many of each tooth type there are in the upper and lower jaws. The total number is then multiplied by 2 to give the total number of teeth in the mouth.

These are the dental formulae for both the permanent and deciduous dentitions:

Dog: $I\frac{3}{3} C\frac{1}{1} PM\frac{4}{4} M\frac{2}{3} \times 2 = 42$

Puppy: $I\frac{3}{3} C\frac{1}{1} PM\frac{3}{3} \times 2 = 28$

Cat: $I\frac{3}{3} C\frac{1}{1} PM\frac{3}{2} M\frac{1}{1} \times 2 = 30$

Kitten: $I\frac{3}{3} C\frac{1}{1} PM\frac{3}{2} \times 2 = 26$

NB. There are no molars in the deciduous dentition.

Table 3.6 Tooth shape and function

Tooth type	Shape	Function
Incisor	Small, pointed with a single root. Found at front of jaw	Fine nibbling and cutting meat off the bone
Canine (eye) teeth	Curved with large single root. One on each side of the upper and lower jaws. Deeply embedded in the jaw bone	Holding meat firmly in the mouth
Premolar (cheek teeth)	Flatter surface with several cusps or tubercles. Two or three roots	Shearing and grinding in association with teeth in the opposing jaw.
Carnassial – last upper premolar and first lower molar on each side of mouth	Largest teeth in the jaw. Several cusps and at least three roots	Very powerful teeth. Cutting and shearing meat. Unique to carnivores
Molar (cheek teeth)	Similar to premolars but larger with three roots	Shearing and grinding

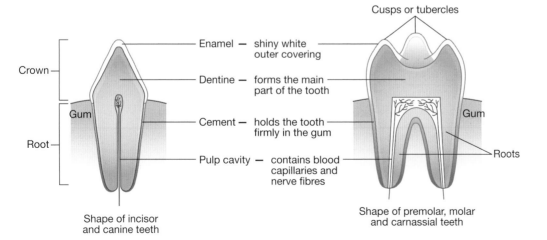

Figure 3.22 Tooth structure.

Structure of the digestive tract

This is a tubular system responsible for digestion and absorption of the food taken into the body. The majority of the system is found within the abdominal cavity (Figure 3.21).

Food is taken into the mouth where it is chewed, mixed with saliva from the salivary glands and formed into small pieces or boluses. This process involves the use of the lips, tongue, teeth and cheeks (Figure 3.24).

Table 3.7	Eruption times of teeth in the dog and cat	
Tooth type	**Deciduous dentition**	**Permanent dentition**
1. Dog		
Incisors	3–4 weeks	3.5–4 months
Canines	5 weeks	5–6 months
Premolars	4–8 weeks	4–5 months – first premolars
		5–7 months – remainder
Molars	Absent	5–7 months
2. Cat		
All teeth	Starts at 2 weeks and is complete by 4 weeks	Very variable. Starts at 12 weeks and is complete by 6 months

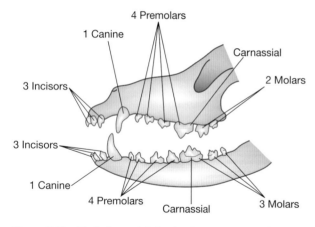

Figure 3.23 Skull of an adult dog to show permanent dentition.

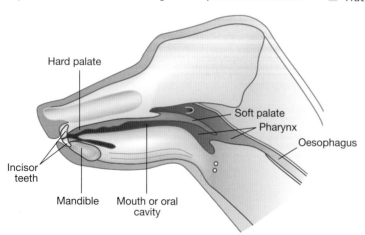

Figure 3.24 Left lateral view of head of dog to show digestive system.

Each bolus passes through the pharynx and travels down the digestive tract by means of muscular contractions known as peristaltic waves.

Food passes into the:

1. **Oesophagus** – this runs down the neck, passes through the thoracic cavity (Figure 3.25) and diaphragm and enters the stomach through the cardiac sphincter.
2. **Stomach** – a sac-like organ lying on the left side of the anterior abdominal cavity (Figure 3.26). Food mixes with acid gastric juices secreted by the stomach lining and the digestion of protein begins.
3. **Small intestine** – partially digested food now known as chyme, leaves the stomach by the pyloric sphincter and enters the duodenum. It passes along the jejunum and ileum (Figure 3.27). The lining of the small intestine is covered in minute finger-like villi (singular: villus) and digestive glands which secrete intestinal juices containing enzymes. Within the small intestine the process of digestion is completed and absorption of the products of digestion begins.
4. **Large intestine** – the remaining food material passes along the caecum, colon and rectum and out of the body via the anus (Figure 3.28). The large intestine is shorter and wider than the small intestine. Water is absorbed from the food and solid faeces are excreted.

The process of digestion

A balanced diet consists of:

- Protein
- Carbohydrate
- Fat
- Vitamins
- Minerals
- Water.

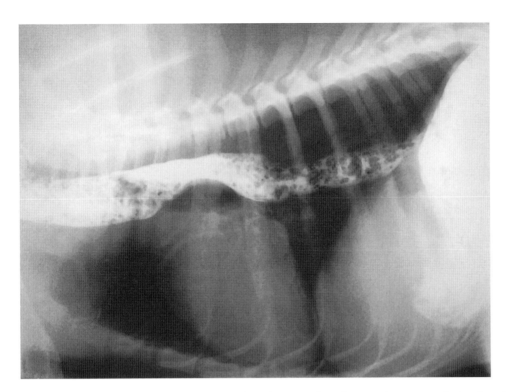

Figure 3.25 Radiograph showing lateral view of the thorax to show the oesophagus one minute after a barium meal. This dog has a mega-oesophagus.

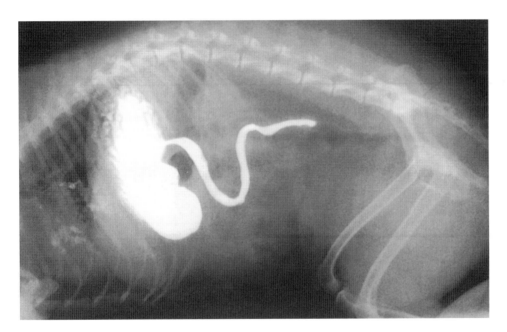

Figure 3.26 Radiograph showing lateral view of the abdomen of a dog to show stomach and duodenum 30 minutes after a barium meal.

Food eaten by the animal is broken down into small chemical units by the digestive tract in several stages:

■ **Mouth** – food is mixed with saliva which softens the food and makes it easier to swallow.

■ **Stomach** – gastric juices are added. These include hydrochloric acid and the enzyme pepsin which begins to digest protein. Acid chyme is produced.
■ **Small intestine** – intestinal juices secreted by glands lining the walls, by the pancreas and by the gall

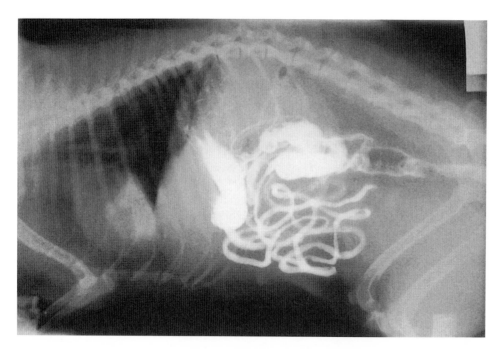

Figure 3.27 Radiograph showing lateral view of the abdomen of a dog to show the small intestine 1 hour after a barium meal.

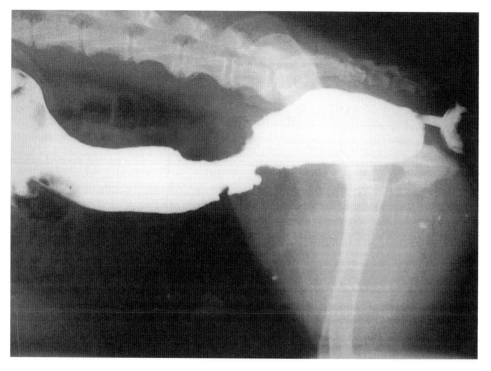

Figure 3.28 Radiograph showing lateral view of caudal abdomen to show descending colon and rectum – barium enema. This dog has a colonic tumour.

bladder are added to the chyme. These contain many different enzymes each of which digest a specific constituent of food, e.g.
- proteins are broken down by trypsin to produce amino acids.

- carbohydrates and sugars are broken down by amylase, maltase, sucrase and fructase to produce simple sugars such as glucose.
- fats are broken down by bile salts and lipase to produce fatty acids and glycerol.

In this way the constituents of food are broken down into small molecules – amino acids, glucose, fatty acids and glycerol – which are absorbed into the bloodstream of the animal.

The process of absorption

Absorption of the small molecules produced as result of digestion occurs through the villi lining the walls of the small intestine.

Each villus contains (Figure 3.18):

- a loop of blood capillaries which lead via the hepatic portal vein to the liver (Figure 3.15)
- a lymphatic capillary called a lacteal which leads via the cisterna chyli into the lymphatic system.

Amino acids and sugars pass through the walls of the villi into the blood capillaries. They are carried to the liver, by the hepatic portal vein, where they are metabolised and used by the cells of the body.

Fatty acids and glycerol pass into the lacteals as a milky solution known as chyle. This enters the lymphatic system and is then poured back into the bloodstream in the heart.

The indigestible remains of the food pass down the large intestine and out of the body as faeces.

Further reading
Aspinall, V., O'Reilly, M. (2004) Introduction to Veterinary Anatomy and Physiology. Elsevier, Oxford.

Lane, D.R. (ed) Jones Animal Nursing, 5th edn. Pergamon, Oxford.

Lane, D.R., Cooper, B. (eds) (1999) Veterinary Nursing, 3rd edn. Butterworth Heinemann, Oxford.

Phillips, W.D., Chilton, T.J. (1991) A-Level Biology. Oxford University Press, Oxford.

Roberts, M.B.V. (1986) Biology for Life, 2nd edn. Nelson, Walton on Thames.

Major body systems – Part 2

Selena Burroughs

REPRODUCTIVE SYSTEM OF THE CAT AND DOG

Basic structure and function

The following sections will describe the structure and function of both male and female reproductive systems of the cat and dog. The basic structure of the cat and dog are very similar and unless stated, the text will apply to both species of animal.

The female reproductive system (Figs 4.1 and 4.2)

The function of this system will be to produce ova (eggs), which are then fertilised if the animal has been successfully mated in the fallopian tube. The fertilised egg will travel to the uterus where it implants and grows.

The basic system consists of:

- Ovaries
- Fallopian tubes
- Uterus
- Vagina
- Vulva

Ovaries

The cat and dog each have two ovaries that lie within the abdominal cavity just behind the kidney. They receive oxygenated blood from the ovarian artery, which stems from the aorta. The function of the ovary is to produce the eggs and the hormones oestrogen and progesterone; both of which will be mentioned later in the oestrus cycle.

Fallopian tube

These two tubes may also be called **uterine tubes** or **oviducts**.

They are found between the ovary and the horn of the uterus. They do not actually join to the ovary but have a layer of mesentery surrounding them to help form a sac called the ovarian bursa. On the end of the fallopian tubes are finger-like projections called **fimbrae**. The function of these is to attract the egg released from the ovary into the fallopian tube.

Fertilisation of the egg and sperm will occur in the fallopian tubes.

The uterus

This structure can be subdivided into the two horns where the fertilised egg implants and grows throughout pregnancy and the main body where the fully grown foetuses pass through during parturition.

The walls of the uterus are made up of smooth muscle called the myometrium. The mucus epithelial lining is called the endometrium.

The cervix

This can be found at the base of the body of the uterus. It acts as a sphincter muscle controlling the opening into the uterus.

The cervix will relax and open:

- during oestrus to allow sperm to be fertilised in the fallopian tube
- during parturition to allow the fetus through.

At all other times the cervix should stay closed to stop any pathogens getting into the uterine area which could lead to the medical condition called a pyometra (which translated means 'infection in the uterus').

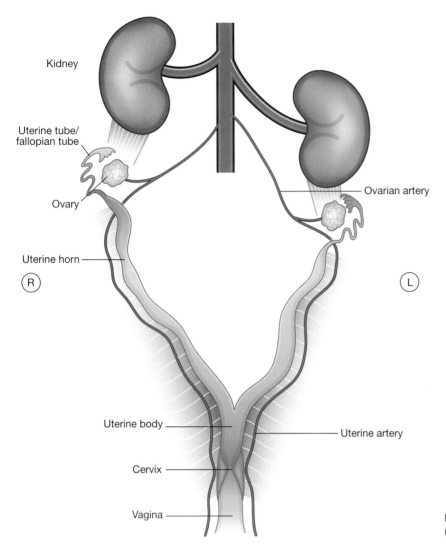

Figure 4.1 Female reproductive system (ventrodorsal).

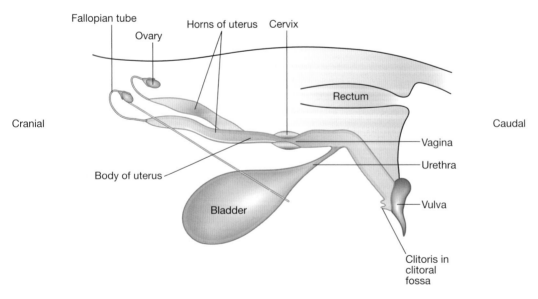

Figure 4.2 Female reproductive system.

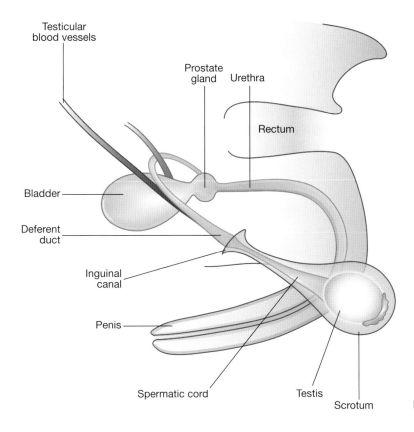

Figure 4.3   Male reproductive system (canine).

The vagina

Lying within the vagina is the opening of the urethra, which would then lead to the bladder. The vagina has various functions.

- It allows a passageway for the foetuses during parturition
- The muscular lining aids with the 'tie' in mating
- Allows urine to flow through via the urethra.

The vulva

The vulva consists of two folds of muscular tissue that keeps the area sealed. This will help protect against any potential pathogens entering the system. This area is normally soft but can become turgid and swollen when the animal is in season.

External genitalia

The vulva can be seen externally in the bitch and queen. This lies ventral to the anus in the standing animal.

The male reproductive system (Figs 4.3–4.5)

The function of this system is to produce, nourish, store and transport the male gamete, which is the sperm.

The basic structure consists of:

- The testes
- Epididymes
- Vas deferens
- Testicular blood vessels
- Prostate gland
- Bulbo urethral gland (cat only)
- Urethra
- Penis
- Prepuce.

The testicle

In the normal healthy male dog and cat there should be two testicles present lying within the hairless sac called the scrotum. Up until approximately 12 weeks of age the testicles will be inside the abdominal cavity. As the animal matures they start to descend via the inguinal canal into the scrotal sac. The testicles lie outside of the body cavity to keep them at a lower temperature than the internal organs. High temperatures will inhibit sperm production.

The two areas of the testicle responsible for sperm being formed are the seminiferous tubules and interstitial space.

Sperm formation sequence

The hormone testosterone is produced from the interstitial space in the cells of Leydig

↓

This stimulates production of sperm from the spermatogenic cells in the seminiferous tubules

↓

The secretion from the Sertoli cells in the seminiferous tubules nourishes sperm

↓

The sperm will continue to grow and when they are mature they will detach themselves and travel to the epididymis.

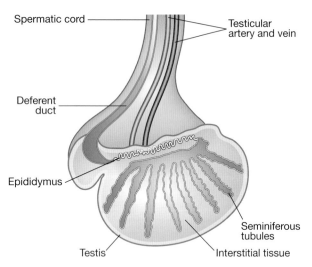

Figure 4.4 The testicle.

The epididymis

This coiled structure stores the sperm when they are mature. The structure lies on the side of the testicle.

The spermatic cord

The spermatic cord extends from the testicle. The cord houses the following structures:

- Vas deferens, also called the deferent duct
- Testicular blood vessels
- Nerves
- Muscles responsible for lowering and raising the testicle
- Lymph vessels.

Vas deferens

This tube-like structure, which can also be called the deferent duct, is responsible for transporting the sperm from the testicle towards the urethra to then be carried out of the penis. It runs from the epididymis to the urethra. It is made up of fibromuscular tissue and is one of the structures that make up the spermatic cord.

Testicular blood vessels

The testicle is supplied with oxygenated blood via the testicular artery, which stems from the aorta. Deoxygenated blood is carried away via the testicular vein. This will join the vena cava. Testicular blood vessels are contained within the spermatic cord.

Prostate gland

This gland secretes a watery fluid called seminal fluid. It is secreted into the urethra and has three main functions:

- It helps to neutralise acidic urine

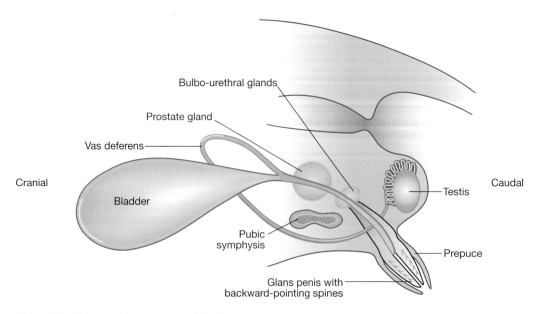

Figure 4.5 Male reproductive system (feline).

- It provides nutrients for sperm
- It helps to uncoagulate the sperm and make them more mobile.

This gland is developed and influenced by the hormone testosterone. Enlargement of this gland can be common in the uncastrated dog with excess testosterone levels.

The bulbo-urethral glands in the cat are further down the length of the urethra and have similar properties to that of the prostate gland. These are not found in the dog.

The urethra
The urethra runs from the neck of the bladder, through the penis and opens at the external urinary meatus. It is layered with epithelium tissue and transports both semen and urine.

The penis
Differences in the cat and dog penis include the direction of the glans of the penis. In the cat the penis points caudally and has sharp spines on the end of the glans, which will help with stimulation of the queen to cause ovulation in mating. In the dog the penis points cranially and does not have these spines.

The prepuce
The prepuce located at the end is a tubular fold of skin and is lined with mucus epithelium. This helps protect the end of the penis.

External genitalia
The external genitalia in a dog can easily be identified. With the male cat the penis lies ventral to the anus in the standing animal. Determination of the sex of cats can be made by comparing the distance between the genitalia and anus. The gap between the two will be larger in the male and less in the female.

OESTRUS CYCLE
The bitch

Bitches are classed as seasonally monoestrus, which means that they will have a single fertile period or 'season' within a period of time. Most bitches will come into season in the spring and autumn. This however is not necessarily normal in all breeds.

Puberty in the bitch will depend on the individual. Generally smaller breeds will reach puberty and have their first season from the age of 9–12 months. Larger breeds may not have their first season until 24 months of age.

There are four stages that make up the cycle:

1. Pro-oestrus
2. Oestrus
3. Metoestrus (sometimes called dioestrus)
4. Anoestrus.

The term 'heat' or 'season' describes two stages of the cycle, pro-oestrus and oestrus.

When describing each stage, the following things should be considered:

- length of the stage
- behavioural signs displayed
- clinical signs displayed
- hormonal action.

Table 4.1 describes the stages individually.

Table 4.1	Stages of the bitch's oestrus cycle			
Stage	Duration	Clinical signs	Behavioural signs	Hormonal action
Pro-oestrus	Average 9 days	Swelling of vulva Bloody discharge	Urination more often to spread their pheromones. Bitch attracted to male but no mating occurs	High level of oestrogen, which will cause the external signs of the season. FSH is causing the egg in the ovary to ripen
Oestrus	Average 9 days	Straw coloured discharge	Bitch will allow coitus (mating)	A surge of LH will cause the egg to be released from the ovary. This is known as ovulation
Metoestrus	30–64 days	Vulva less swollen	If successful mating has occurred, pregnancy will occur. Pseudopregnancy (false pregnancy) may occur here	Progesterone is released from the walls of the ruptured follicle to help maintain a pregnancy. In pregnant animals prolactin is released to develop mammary tissue for milk production
Anoestrus	4 months	Period of inactivity	Bitch should show no abnormal signs of behaviour. This would be the ideal time to spay a bitch	No hormonal activity for the majority of this stage; towards the end FSH levels start to rise to develop the egg

Figure 4.6 shows the relative time durations of each part of the oestrus cycle.

Ovulation in the bitch

Eggs develop within the ovary. The hormone follicle stimulating hormone (FSH) will stimulate their growth. They each develop in a fluid filled follicle called the Graafian follicle. The follicle wall will secrete the hormone oestrogen. This will cause the bitch to show signs of being in season and prepare the genital tract formating.

When the egg is mature, a surge of luteinising hormone (LH) will cause the follicle to rupture and cause the egg to be released from the ovary towards the fallopian tube.

After ovulation the empty follicle develops into a solid structure called the corpus luteum. This produces the hormone progesterone that is responsible for maintaining pregnancy (Figure 4.7).

The queen

The queen is known as seasonally polyoestrus which means that they will have many fertile periods or 'seasons' within a period of time. Queens usually cycle every 2–3 weeks in the Spring, Summer and Autumn. This is due to the longer and warmer daylight hours.

Puberty can vary in the queen but usually their first breeding season is between 5 and 9 months.

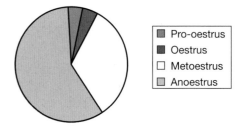

Figure 4.6 The oestrus cycle.

- ■ Pro-oestrus
- ■ Oestrus
- □ Metoestrus
- ▨ Anoestrus

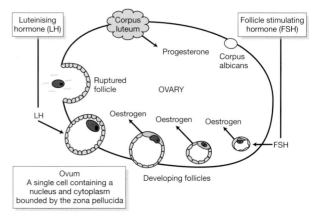

Figure 4.7 Development of the egg.

Table 4.2	Stages of the queen's oestrus cycle			
Stage	**Duration**	**Clinical signs**	**Behavioural signs**	**Hormonal action**
Pro-oestrus	1–4 days	Swelling of vulva Bloody discharge if seen. Cats are usually very keen to clean themselves	Vocalisation Rubbing and rolling on the floor	High level of oestrogen, which will cause the external signs of the season. FSH is causing the egg in the ovary to ripen.
Oestrus	5–8 days	The queen will accept the male for mating	Loud 'calling' sounds from the queen and signs of lordosis	Mating will stimulate the releases of LH, which will cause ovulation
Interoestrus This stage follows oestrus when mating has not occurred or a mating has not resulted in pregnancy. In the breeding season, the queen would return to pro-oestrus after this period of rest	10–14 days	No visible signs	No signs displayed	
Anoestrus	5 months	Period of inactivity through the winter months	Queen should show no abnormal signs of behaviour. This would be the ideal time to spay a queen	No hormonal activity for the majority of this stage; towards the end FSH levels start to rise to develop the egg

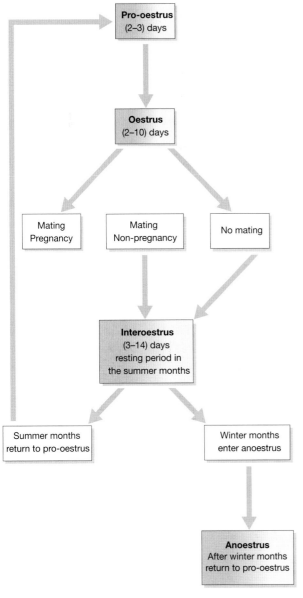

Figure 4.8   The queen's oestrus cycle.

There are four stages that make up the cycle:

- Pro-oestrus
- Oestrus
- Interoestrus
- Anoestrus.

The same points should be considered when describing each stage as in the bitch's cycle. Table 4.2 highlights the key aspects of this cycle with the cycle being explained in diagrammatic form in Figure 4.8 and Figure 4.9.

Ovulation in the queen

Queens are known as induced ovulators. They have to be induced via the mating procedure to cause ovulation. Stimulation whilst mating from the spines of the male's penis causes a surge of LH. This surge will cause ovulation to occur.

Following ovulation and successful fertilisation, progesterone will be released from the corpus luteum to maintain the pregnancy.

THE URINARY SYSTEM

Basic function and structure

The main function of the urinary system is to remove waste products from the body in the form of urine. Other functions include:

- helps regulate water and sodium levels in the blood
- converts the fat soluble form of vitamin D to water soluble
- the kidneys secrete the hormone erythropoietin that stimulates the production of red blood cells.

The structure both in the male and female, cat and dog includes (see Figure 4.10):

- two kidneys
- two ureters
- one bladder
- one urethra.

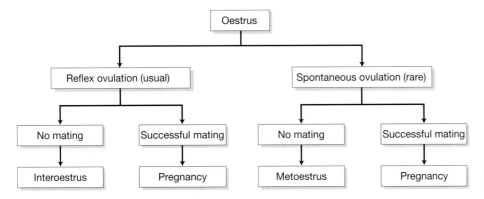

Figure 4.9   Oestrus cycle table of signs.

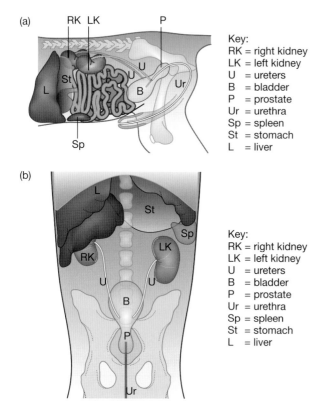

Figure 4.10   (a) Lateral and (b) ventrodorsal view of urinary system.

The kidney

Location

As can be seen from the lateral view diagram (Figure 4.10) the kidneys are closely attached to the dorsal body wall, with the right kidney being more cranial than the left.

Structure

The depressed area of the kidney where blood vessels enter and leave and also the ureters leave is called the hilus. The renal artery that brings oxygen stems from aorta, with the renal vein going straight from the kidney into the vena cava.

When looking at the kidney the darker red outer section is called the cortex, with the paler red inner section called the medulla.

The kidney is made up of several million cells called nephrons or sometimes called renal tubules. It is their function to help produce the fluid we know as urine. The renal pelvis is the structure within the kidney where the fluid collects after it has been through the nephrons before going into the ureters. These structures can be seen in Figure 4.11.

The kidney nephron (Figure 4.12)

Within these cells urine is formed to then be passed to the bladder via the ureters and then discharged through the urethra.

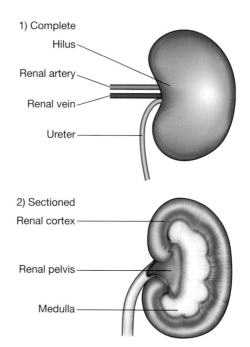

Figure 4.11   The kidney.

To aid understanding you can break the kidney nephron down into stages to describe the flow of fluid and eventual formation of urine (Table 4.3).

The ureters

These are paired structures that run from the hilus of the kidney to the bladder. They transport urine from the kidney to be stored in the bladder (Figure 4.13).

The bladder

This is the large organ that stores urine. The outer wall consists of smooth muscle and elastic tissue to aid in the act of urination. The act of passing urine can also be called micturition. The bladder is lined with transitional epithelium, which allows the walls of the bladder to stretch as it fills. As the bladder fills it extends cranially along the floor of the abdomen.

Where the ureters enter the bladder there is a flap valve (Figure 4.14). This stops any backflow of urine. Once the urine has entered the bladder, it should not retrace up the ureters. The urine is stored in the bladder until the animal wishes to urinate. There is a sphincter muscle at the neck of the bladder and when urination occurs, this muscle will relax and allow the urine to flow into the urethra.

The urethra

This is a single tube that allows urine to flow from the bladder to the outside. In the male it will travel to the

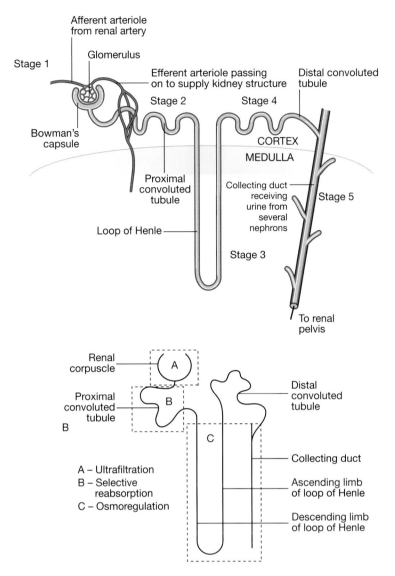

Figure 4.12   The kidney nephron.

Table 4.3	Function of the kidney nephron
Stage	**Description**
1	Blood enters the glomerulus from the renal artery under high pressure. The glomerulus is a network of capillaries, which will filter small molecules into the Bowman's capsule, e.g. urea, glucose, amino acids, water, salts.
2	Selective reabsorption of nutrients such as glucose, amino acids and water occurs through the walls of the proximal convoluted tubule. Hormones control this.
3	The loop of Henle is where the urine is beginning to concentrate even further. Water and salts are being reabsorbed back into the blood stream if the body requires them. This is called osmoregulation. Hormones control this.
4	The fluid now enters the distal convoluted tubule, which then joins a collecting duct.
5	The urine from this nephron and several others will all collect in the same collecting duct. It will then travel to the renal pelvis where it is taken to the bladder via the ureters.

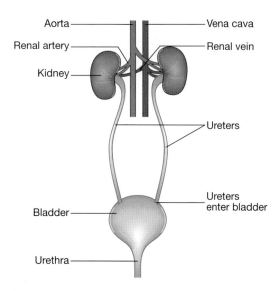

Figure 4.13 The urinary system (ventrodorsal).

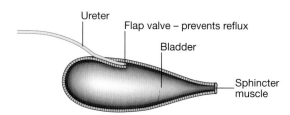

Figure 4.14 Flap valve and sphincter muscle.

end of the penis and in the female it will join the reproductive system at the opening of the vagina to then be discharged through the vulva.

THE ENDOCRINE SYSTEM

The endocrine system is a collection of ductless glands throughout the body that secrete hormones. Hormones are released into the bloodstream and travel to a target organ or tissue, where they exert a specific effect.

Example: FSH
Follicle stimulating hormone (FSH) is released from the pituitary gland

↓

FSH travels through the bloodstream to the target organ of the ovary

↓

When it reaches the ovary it causes an egg to develop and mature.

Figure 4.15 shows the major endocrine glands in a dog. Each gland produces at least one hormone or chemical messenger.

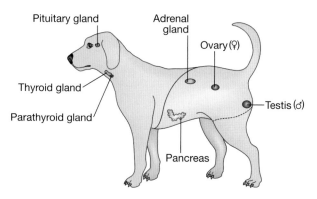

Figure 4.15 Major endocrine glands.

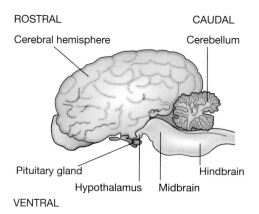

Figure 4.16 Position of the pituitary gland.

Sites of the glands

Pituitary (Figure 4.16)
This gland is situated in the base of the brain. It can be divided into two sections: the anterior pituitary, which secretes six hormones and the posterior pituitary, which secretes two hormones.

Thyroid
Situated either side of the upper part of the trachea, close to the jugular vein. The thyroid gland secretes two hormones.

Parathyroid
There are a total of four parathyroid glands in the body. They are situated either end of the thyroid gland as can be seen in Figure 4.17. They secrete one hormone.

Pancreas (Figure 4.18)
This is situated in the 'U' of the duodenum of the small intestine. It is a lobular, pink organ which secretes both digestive enzymes, for the breakdown of food, as well as hormones.

Adrenal glands (Figure 4.19)
These paired glands are situated close to the kidney but are not connected. The gland can be divided into

CRANIAL

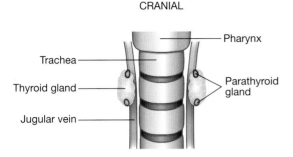

Figure 4.17   The thyroid and parathyroid glands.

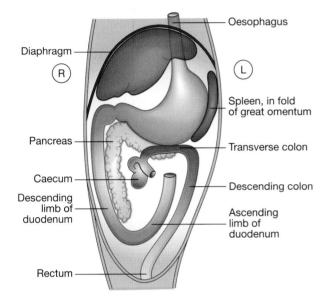

Figure 4.18   Position of the pancreas.

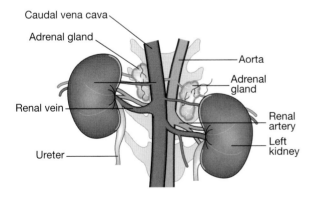

Figure 4.19   Position of the adrenal glands.

the cortex and medulla sections. They secret three hormones.

Ovaries

The two ovaries in the un-neutered female secrete a total of three hormones.

Testicles

The two testicles in the un-neutered male secrete two hormones.

Table 4.4 gives the names of the hormones released from each gland, their target organ or tissue and their effect.

THE NERVOUS SYSTEM

Basic structure and function

The main functions of the system are:

- to receive information from external stimuli
- to receive information from the body tissues
- to interpret information received
- to send impulses throughout the body to stimulate movement and activity.

The nervous system is composed of two parts:

1. **Central nervous system (CNS)** – made up of the brain and spinal cord.
2. **Peripheral nervous system** – consisting of all the other nerves throughout the body.

Nerves can be classed as either:

- **Sensory nerves:** these afferent nerves lead towards the CNS. They receive information from the external environment. (Afferent meaning towards a structure.)
- **Motor nerves:** these efferent nerves lead away from the CNS. They send impulses to stimulate a reaction for the information originally received. (Efferent meaning leading away from a structure.)

These can be further classed as visceral or somatic:

1. **Visceral nerves:** A *visceral motor nerve* will take instructions to the involuntary muscle of the body, e.g. smooth or cardiac muscle and a *visceral sensory nerve* will bring back information on their action.
2. **Somatic nerves:** A *somatic motor nerve* will take instructions to the voluntary muscles of the body, e.g. skeletal muscles. *Somatic sensory nerves* will bring back information on their action.

Structure of a nerve cell

The basic cell of nervous tissue is called a **neuron**. When these cells are joined together they form what

Table 4.4 Hormone secretion and function in the dog and cat

Gland	Hormone secreted	Target organ/tissue	Effect
Anterior pituitary	Thyroid-stimulating hormone	Thyroid gland	Stimulates the thyroid gland to produce the hormone thyroxine
	Adrenocorticotrophic hormone	Adrenal gland	Stimulates growth of gland and the production of cortisol
	Growth hormone	Body tissue	Stimulates the growth of bones and tissues in the body
	Follicle-stimulating hormone	Ovary and testicle	Causes the egg and sperm to grow and mature
	Luteinising hormone	Ovary and testicle	Causes the egg to ripen and be released from the ovary; in the male it stimulates the production of testosterone in the cells of the testicle
	Prolactin	Mammary tissue	Develops growth of the mammary gland and stimulates milk production
Posterior pituitary	Antidiuretic hormone	Kidney nephrons	Stimulates water re-absorption within the nephron into the bloodstream
	Oxytocin	Uterus and mammary gland	Causes contraction of uterus during parturition and also causes the release of milk from the mammary gland
Thyroid gland	Thyroxine	Body tissues	Helps control the body's metabolic rate
	Thyrocalcitonin	Blood	Helps to regulate the blood calcium levels
Parathyroid	Parathormone	Body and blood tissues	Helps with the regulation of blood calcium levels
Pancreas	Insulin	Blood, liver	Lowers blood glucose levels
	Glucagon		Raises the blood glucose level by converting the storage form of glucose (glycogen) in the liver to a useable form
Adrenal glands – cortex	Glucocorticoids	Various body systems	Acts as an anti-inflammatory, stimulates appetite, increases blood glucose levels and also increases water loss in the kidney nephron
	Mineralocorticoids – aldosterone	Body and blood tissues	Helps to maintain the correct balance of sodium and potassium in the body
	Sex hormones	Gonads and body tissue	Not thought to be of much significance as main sex hormones are released elsewhere in the body
Adrenal glands – medulla	Adrenaline Noradrenaline	Body	Both hormones have a similar effect in preparing the body for emergencies; they cause the heart rate, respiration rate and blood pressure to rise
Ovaries	Oestrogen (from the walls of the developing follicle)	Female reproductive	Prepares the reproductive tract and genitalia for oestrus; this hormone will promote the external signs of the female being in season
	Progesterone (from the corpus luteum)	Uterus, placenta	Maintains pregnancy
	Relaxin	Pelvic ligaments	Relaxes the ligaments around the pelvis to allow an easier birth
Testicles	Testosterone (from the cells of Leydig in the interstitial space)	Male reproductive	Promotes the production of sperm; also develops the male sexual characteristics such as heavier muscular make up
	Oestrogens	Sperm developing in the seminiferous tubules	Oestrogen will nourish the sperm developing in the testicle

we know as nerves. They allow impulses to travel their length to transmit a message (Figure 4.20).

In every neuron, the structure will consist of the elements shown in Table 4.5.

The nerve impulse

Impulses start at the dendrites of a neuron and pass along the axon to the nerve endings. From there the

Table 4.5	Structure of the nerve cell
Name	**Function and structure**
Cell body	Contains the nucleus.
Cell processes	These lead to and from the cell body. There are two types of process, axons and dendrites.
Axons	These carry impulses away from the cell body. They are long and only one comes from each nerve cell. A sheath of connective tissue called the neurilemma surrounds the whole axon. The axon may be also be insulated by a sheath of fatty substance called myelin. Impulses will travel faster in myelinated nerves. Nutrients and oxygen are taken in to the neuron by gaps along the axon called the nodes of Ranvier. There are branching nerve endings at the end of the axon which transmits the impulses to the next dendrite of the next neuron.
Dendrites	These carry impulses towards the cell body. They are short and one or more can lead towards the cell body.
Synapse	This is the junction between each neuron. Communication between the neuron relies on chemicals transmitting the impulse. This chemical is called acetylcholine.

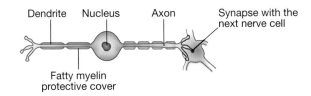

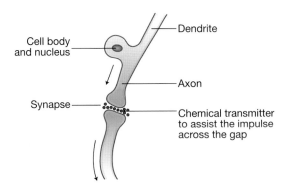

Figure 4.20   The neuron and synapse.

nerve impulse will travel onto another neuron via the **synapse**. The area of nerve-synapse-muscle is called a **neuromuscular junction**.

Reflex action

This is a simple, rapid, automatic response to a stimulus. The action is not under conscious control and does not involve the brain, only the spinal cord.

The pathway between the stimulus and the effect can be called a **reflex arc**.

Structures involved in a reflex action are:

- the receptor, e.g. sensory cells in the skin
- a sensory neuron

- a connector neuron which transmits impulses from the sensory and motor neuron
- a motor neuron
- an effector, e.g. a muscle.

A simple example of a reflex arc can be seen when an animal stands on something sharp. The response is quick and will hopefully cause limited damage (Figure 4.21).

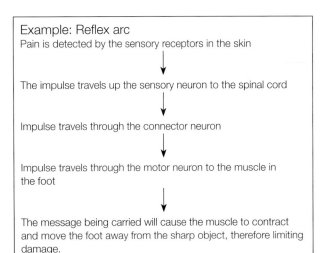

Autonomic nervous system

This system consists of the visceral nerves of the body. These nerves run to all the internal organs of the body, blood vessels, smooth and cardiac muscle. The body has no control of these nerves.

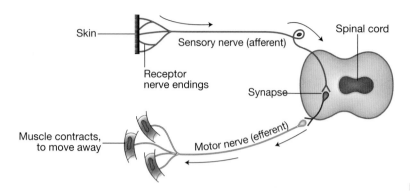

Figure 4.21   Reflex arc.

Table 4.6 Actions of the sympathetic and parasympathetic system	
Sympathetic	**Parasympathetic**
Prepares body for action	Prepares body for relaxation
Increases heart rate	Slows heart rate
Dilates arteries in skeletal muscles	Dilates arteries in gut
Slows gut movement	Speeds gut movement
Dilates bronchioles of lungs	Constricts bronchioles of lungs
Causes hair to stand erect	Hair not erect

Table 4.7 The brain	
Forebrain	Consists of two areas called the cerebral hemispheres. Receives and processes information from all over the body. Contains the hypothalamus gland which helps regulate the function of the pituitary gland.
Midbrain	Receives impulses from the eyes, ears and helps with muscle control.
Hindbrain	Helps control the heartbeat and respiration. Also helps co-ordinate muscular activity in the body.

The system can be divided into two sections:

- sympathetic nervous system
- parasympathetic nervous system.

Although the actions of these systems are totally opposite to each other, most organs would have both types within them. Working together they balance and control the function of the organ.

Table 4.6 summarises the actions of both systems.

To summarise, the sympathetic nervous system produces actions to prepare the body to meet a situation of stress or excitement. The parasympathetic produces actions when the animal is relaxed and not anxious.

The central nervous system

This consists of the brain and the spinal cord. Both are composed of nerve fibres and cell bodies.

The brain (Table 4.7 & Figure 4.22)

The role of the brain is to co-ordinate the body's functions. It receives messages from the sensory nerves, processes it and causes either an immediate reaction, or stores information for later use.

(a) Lateral view

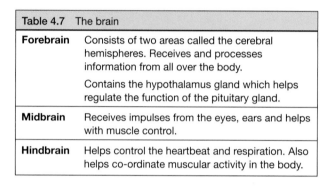

(b) Longitudinal section

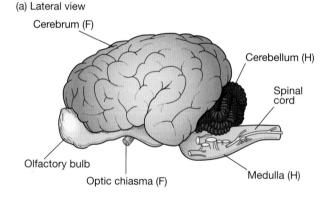

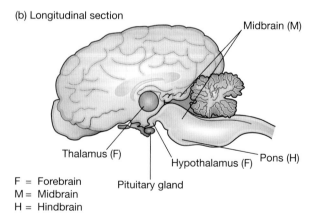

F = Forebrain
M = Midbrain
H = Hindbrain

Figure 4.22   (a) Lateral view and (b) longitudinal section of the brain.

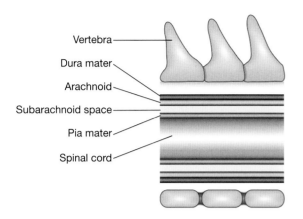

Figure 4.23   Longitudinal view of the meninges.

The brain can be divided into three parts – the fore-brain, midbrain and hindbrain – although they are not easily distinguishable.

The spinal cord

The spinal cord extends from the hindbrain, through the base of the skull and on to the pelvis. It is housed within the vertebral column and has many branching spinal nerves running from the main cord.

The cord is covered by the **meninges**. Three layers of membrane make up the meninges:

- dura mater
- arachnoid layer
- pia mater.

The meninges cover and help protect both the brain and the spinal cord. Inflammation of these is called meningitis, which can be a life-threatening condition (Figure 4.23).

Cerebrospinal fluid

Cerebrospinal fluid (CSF) is found surrounding the brain and in the spinal cord. It can also be found in the subarachnoid space which is the area lying between the arachnoid layer and pia mater of the meninges.

Its function is to help protect the brain against sudden movement or trauma. CSF is a clear fluid and is similar in properties to plasma.

Further reading

Aspinall, V., O'Reilly, M. (2004) Introduction to Veterinary Anatomy and Physiology. Butterworth Heinemann, Oxford.

Dallas, S. (2001) Animal Biology and Care. Blackwell Science, Oxford.

Lane, D.R., Cooper, B. (eds) (2003) Veterinary Nursing, 3rd edn. Butterworth Heinemann, Oxford.

Tartaglia, L., Waugh, A. (2002) Veterinary Physiology and Applied Anatomy. Butterworth Heinemann, Oxford.

Villee, C.A., Solomon, E.P., Martin, C.E. et al. (1989) Biology, 2nd edn. Saunders College Publishing, Orlando, USA.

Veterinary animal management

Canine and feline husbandry

Sally Bowden and Elizabeth Easter

HOUSING

This section describes housing for dogs and cats kept as household pets. Commercial premises such as boarding kennels and catteries are not included. These are subject to specific guidelines and legislation.

Siting

Today, the majority of pets live with their owners inside the home. However, with careful thought to the animals' needs, it is possible to house a dog or cat outside.

Whilst keeping a pet in the home increases contact between pet and owner, allows close monitoring of health and behaviour and provides more constant environmental conditions, there may be advantages in keeping a pet outside. For example, well constructed kennels are easy to keep clean and may be more practical if a large number of animals are kept.

Construction materials

There are many types of material available. Serious consideration should be given before selection of construction materials. Table 5.1 outlines some advantages and disadvantages of commonly used materials.

Design and layout

Whether outside or inside, it is equally important to consider where the housing is sited.

If the animal is to be housed outside, the following points should be taken into account:

- A position which allows some sun and protection from North/North-East weather is ideal.
- The ground should have a slight slope tilting away from the sleeping quarters to avoid pooling of water and urine. Drainage should be considered.
- The housing should be sited avoiding disturbance or annoyance to neighbours.

If the animal is to be housed inside, the following points should be taken into account:

- Most animals feel more secure when a permanent area is selected as their sleeping quarters – avoid constantly moving their bedding.
- Try not to select an excessively busy area – even animals need their own space!
- Areas where the temperature can fluctuate greatly should be avoided, e.g. conservatories.

Common designs and layouts for outside kennelling

- **Sleeping quarters** – This area should be protected from wind and rain, will require some form of heating and should have a raised bedding area. For smaller dogs and cats, 'chalet-style' kennelling is available, which provides a raised indoor area.

■ **Exercise area** – This should be secure to prevent escape or theft. It should have a solid floor for hygiene reasons and should still provide some protection from the weather, e.g. a roof or screen.

■ **Dimensions** – The sleeping quarters should be large enough to allow ample room for the animal to lie down and stretch out without difficulty. In addition, there should be space for bowls and litter trays as appropriate. Ideally, the headroom should allow for a person to enter. The exercise area should be at least three times the size of the sleeping quarters, although it must be appreciated that all dogs require additional exercise.

■ **Security and ventilation** – Sadly, theft of valuable animals is on the increase and this should be taken into account. Additionally, the housing should be escape-proof – remember both cats and dogs can climb to considerable heights. Ventilation should ensure adequate provision of oxygen and remove carbon dioxide, excessive water vapour (humidity) and odours efficiently without causing a draught.

■ **Resources** – Services such as electricity and water should be considered at the planning stage if they are to be easily installed. Remember that if artificial lighting is installed, it should mimic the natural daylight pattern as much as possible – disturbances in photoperiod may cause stress.

Kennel contents

Heating

In most cases, pets kept inside the house do not need supplementary heating. However, an additional heat source may be required in the following situations:

■ if there is no central heating
■ geriatric/juvenile animals
■ pregnant or lactating animals
■ postoperatively
■ during illness.

Supplementary heating is most commonly used for animals that are housed outside. Below are some examples of other heating methods:

■ **Heat lamps** – Usually infra-red bulb emitting heat. Not intended for use as a light source. Suspended above bedding area at a safe height.
■ **Heat mats** – Waterproof mat placed underneath bedding area. Several types have been developed. Heat is provided by electric cable. More recently cordless microwaveable pads have become popular.
■ **Fan heaters** – May be wall-mounted or free-standing. Warm air is blown from the front of the heat source by a fan.
■ **Hot water bottles** – Useful but short-lived source of heat.
■ **Oil radiators** – Oil-filled radiator heated by electricity. Slow to heat up and cool down.

Table 5.1 Construction materials – advantages and disadvantages		
Material	**Advantages**	**Disadvantages**
Wood	Relatively inexpensive Easy to work with Attractive	Easily chewed Splinters Porous – difficult to clean and may harbour micro-organisms
Concrete blocks/bricks	Strong Secure Draught proof Long lasting	Expensive Porous and not easy to clean unless sealed
Melamine	Relatively inexpensive Easy to clean Draught proof and insulating	Chewable Difficult to work with Can harbour micro-organisms if cracked
Wire mesh	Very durable Strong if good quality Allows ventilation	Difficult to clean Not attractive May be draughty
Glass	Allows natural light Easy to clean	Breakable Expensive, especially toughened glass

> - All local heat sources are potentially dangerous. Animals MUST be able to move away if they need to cool down.
> - Cables should be placed out of the animal's reach to avoid electrocution by chewing. Care must be taken to ensure that the appliance is kept away from water. Circuit breakers should always be used as an additional safety measure.
> - There have been reports of microwaveable pads bursting and leaking their contents causing burns, so they should always be discarded if damage is evident.

Beds

There are many forms of bed available. Table 5.2 outlines some of the common types.

Bedding

The choice of bedding must be carefully considered. Good bedding must be insulative, absorptive and easily cleaned (Figure 5.1). Table 5.3 shows the advantages and disadvantages of commonly used bedding materials.

Other kennel contents

- Litter trays
  Conventional plastic are the most widely used.
  Hooded trays provide privacy and can be more visually acceptable if used in the home. They are also less accessible to young children.
  Odour-eating trays are available which have charcoal filters.
- Cat litter

Table 5.4 outlines commonly used types of litter.

Environmental enrichments

Environmental enrichment is altering the living environment of an animal to provide opportunity for them to express their natural behaviour. In this country it is common practice to provide environmental enrichment for captive wild animals but it is equally important to enrich the environment of domestic pets. It does not have to be an expensive exercise – some of the best enrichments have been made from common household items, e.g. scrunched-up newspaper! Examples of enrichments:

- Scratching posts for claw maintenance.
- Toys such as chews, balls for chasing and pulling toys on string for cats to 'hunt'.
- Commercially available toys, such as 'Kong'® toys, which can be stuffed with food.
- Kennelled animals may also benefit from larger enrichments such as climbing frames, constructing surfaces of different heights and textures, paddling pools and tunnels.

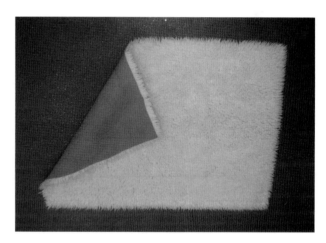

Figure 5.1 Photograph of 'Vetbed'®.

Table 5.2 Beds – advantages and disadvantages		
Name	Advantages	Disadvantages
Plastic moulded	Strong Easy to clean Durable Draught-proof	Visually unattractive Chewable
Wicker basket	Warm Visually attractive	Difficult to clean – many crevices to harbour parasites May snap and leave sharp edges
Bean-bag	Very warm Mould to animals shape – supportive	Difficult to clean Polystyrene balls are poisonous Easily damaged Difficult for arthritic animals to use
Fabric-covered foam	Warm Draught-proof, especially igloo-style Washable	Chewable Become thin and unsupportive after prolonged use

Table 5.3 Bedding – advantages and disadvantages

Name	Advantages	Disadvantages
Dry-top absorbent (Vetbed®)	Easy to clean Dries quickly Surface remains dry, with liquids being absorbed to the underside Can be sterilised	Expensive Require brushing to keep in good order
Blankets and towels	Can be obtained cheaply Warm and comfortable when dry	Cold when wet Take a long time to dry
Newspaper	Cheap Warm Easily available Useful as kennel liner	Does not provide padding Ink may stain pale coated animals Soggy and cold when wet
Foam	Provides excellent cushioning Warm Can be covered with waterproof material	Large pieces are difficult to clean and are expensive Becomes thin and unsupportive after prolonged use
Shredded paper	Cheap and easy to obtain Warm	Soggy and cold when wet Bulky to store and dispose of Messy

Table 5.4 Cat litter – advantages and disadvantages

Name	Advantages	Disadvantages
Mineral-based, e.g. Fuller's Earth (clay-like substances)	Available in clumping and non-clumping varieties (Clumping enables easy removal of soiled litter)	A lot of litter is needed to allow the clumps to form Non-clumping varieties need be totally replaced after soiling, although less litter is needed
Wood-based	Lightweight Biodegradable Highly absorbent Pleasant smelling	Messy Bulky
Vegetable-based	Clumping Biodegradable	Can be more difficult to obtain and more costly than other types
Paper-based	Recycled Biodegradable	Messy Newspaper-based product can stain

Pheromones

The use of pheromones, or 'pheromonatherapy', is becoming popular. F3 facial fraction ('Feliway'®) for cats and 'Dog Appeasing Pheromone' ('DAP'®) via a spray or plug-in air diffuser has been found to reduce stress and anxiety in a range of situations and could be used to alleviate anxiety in animals unused to the kennel or cattery environment.

FEEDING

Due to the advances in science and technology, we now know more about the impact of good and bad nutrition on both humans and animals than in the past. Therefore, awareness of nutritional requirements is of fundamental importance to all those caring for animals.

Nutritional requirements

A nutrient is defined as 'any food constituent that helps support life' (Lewis *et al.* 1994). There are six main groups of nutrients, some of which also provide the body with energy.

All energy comes from the sun. It is never destroyed, but changes form as it passes from one living thing to another (Figure 5.2). Energy is needed by the body for metabolic processes to take place, e.g. digestion, respiration.

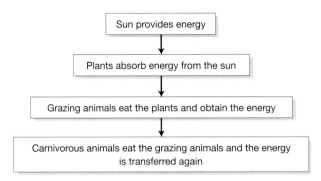

Figure 5.2 Diagram of energy transfer.

Energy producing nutrients:

- fat
- carbohydrate
- protein.

Non-energy producing nutrients:

- vitamins
- minerals
- water.

Protein

Protein is required by dogs and cats for the growth and repair of body tissues. All basic food materials contain protein but the amounts and quality vary. All proteins can be broken down into **amino acids**, their most simple form. Some amino acids are absolutely essential in a dog and cat food to maintain health. This is because they cannot be made by the body from other substances. There are 11 essential amino acids required in canine food and 12 needed in feline food, the additional one being taurine.

The essential amino acid taurine is only available from meat sources, hence the cat is an obligate carnivore. A vegetarian diet would result in taurine deficiency, causing degeneration of the retina which leads to blindness.

The more essential amino acids there are in a protein source, the higher its biological value.

Fat

Fat is a highly digestible nutrient which acts as a concentrated and palatable source of energy. It is twice as efficient as an energy provider than protein or carbohydrate. Most fat in dog and cat food is of animal origin. Fat is also necessary to supply the three **essential fatty acids** (EFAs) which are needed for many metabolic functions within the body.

Dogs can convert any of the EFAs into another within the body tissues. Therefore, if only one EFA was present in the food in a sufficient amount, then the other two could be manufactured and there would be no deficiency. However, cats cannot do this and have a dietary requirement for all three EFAs.

If no EFAs were present in the food then signs of deficiency would be seen, e.g. scurfy skin and poor growth.

Fat is also vital to act as a carrier for the fat soluble vitamins which are A, D, E and K.

Carbohydrate

There are two types:

1. **Digestible** – 'starch' such as cereals and rice which are broken down into simple sugars and used as an easily available energy source.
2. **Non-digestible** – 'fibre'. This makes the food bulky which helps to control the rate at which food moves through the digestive tract (transit time) and the rate of absorption of other nutrients. It does not produce energy as it cannot be digested.

There is no absolute requirement for carbohydrate in canine or feline food, although it is often added as it is a cheap energy source.

Vitamins

These are needed in minute quantities for vital metabolic processes. With the advent of modern pet foods, vitamin deficiency (hypovitaminosis) is extremely uncommon and it is far more common to find problems when animals have been given too much of a specific vitamin (hypervitaminosis).

Vitamins can be described in two ways – fat soluble (A, D, E and K) and water soluble (B complex and C).

Table 5.5 shows the functions of vitamins and common signs of excesses and deficiencies.

Minerals

Minerals are inorganic substances. Sometimes, on a pet food can, these are referred to as 'ash'. Macrominerals are those which are needed in larger quantities than microminerals (trace minerals). Minerals are found in the body in the form of ions.

Table 5.6 shows the functions of minerals and common signs of excesses and deficiencies.

Water

By far the largest component of the body, water makes up approximately 60–70% of fat-free bodyweight, although this varies with age. Water is used by the body to maintain electrolyte balance, maintain body temperature, remove wastes and is a major component of blood and lymph, among other functions.

'Balanced diet' and life stage feeding

A balanced diet is one which provides all necessary nutrients at optimal levels. Optimal level of nutrients

Table 5.5   Vitamins

	Functions	Hypervitaminosis	Hypovitaminosis	Note
Fat soluble vitamins				
A	Skin and bone health. Maintains sight and hearing	Skeletal disease, anorexia and weakness	Failing vision and other diseases of the eye. Weakness and increased susceptibility to infection	Unlike dogs, cats cannot convert the precursor carotene into vitamin A. It must be provided preformed in the diet and is only available from animal sources
D	Closely related to calcium and phosphorus metabolism – related to bone structure	Soft tissue mineralisation and organ dysfunction	'Rickets' – malformed bones and teeth	Formed in the skin in the presence of UV light
E	Reproductive function and has antioxidant effect	Anorexia	Reproductive failure, 'yellow fat disease' – pansteatitis	
K	Blood clotting	Not recorded	Clotting problems	Manufactured in large intestine by gut flora
Water soluble vitamins				
Thiamin (B1)	Various metabolic functions	Not recorded	Weight loss. Weakness. Neurological signs	Some raw fish contains thiaminase, an enzyme which destroys thiamin so animals fed this type of diet are predisposed to thiamin deficiency
Riboflavin (B2)		Not recorded	Skin disease, weakness and fertility problems	
Niacin		Sore, itchy skin	'Blacktongue' – ulceration of tongue and mucosa	
Pyridoxine (B6)		Not recorded	Anaemia and convulsions	
Biotin		Not recorded	Skin disease and weakness	Avidin in raw egg whites prevents biotin absorption
C	Skin and blood vessel health	Not recorded	Does not occur as dogs and cats manufacture their own	

Table 5.6 Minerals

	Major functions	Hypermineralosis	Hypomineralosis	Notes
Macrominerals				
Calcium (Ca)	Bone development and maintenance. Muscle contraction	Slow growth and thyroid problems. Causes phosphorus deficiency	Can occur due to high phosphorus content of food, e.g. muscle meat. Causes skeletal disease. Acute calcium deficiency can occur in whelping bitch (eclampsia)	The calcium:phosphorus ratio is vital. It must not exceed 1.4:1 (ideal = 1.1:1)
Phosphorus (P)		Renal damage Calcium deficiency	Often caused by calcium supplementation	
Potassium (K)	Osmoregulation and muscle function	Uncommon but often fatal if occurs	Muscle weakness, drooping of head and stiff limbs	Hypokalaemia may be seen in renal cases
Sodium (Na)	Osmoregulation and blood pressure control	If acute: thirst, pruritus and anorexia If chronic: increased blood pressure, heart and renal disease	Polyuria, weight loss and agalactia	There is a high sodium content in many commercial pet foods
Magnesium (Mg)	Necessary for the function of many enzymes	Diarrhoea and urolithiasis	Skeletal disease and convulsions	High magnesium levels in pet foods have been linked with urolithiasis
Microminerals				
Iron (Fe)	Haemoglobin manufacture	Very rare	Anaemia	
Zinc (Zn)	Component of several enzymes	Causes calcium or copper deficiency	Skin disease and poor healing	Recognised disease in Huskies
Copper (Cu)	Bone and blood formation	Liver disease	Skin problems and increased susceptibility to disease	Toxicity is a recognised problem in Bedlington Terriers

Table 5.7 Nutritional requirements for normal, healthy adult dogs and cats

	Protein	Fat	Carbohydrate	Energy
Dog	15–25%	>8%	No absolute requirement but often present as it is a cheap, easily available source of energy	(62.2 × bwt/kg) + 144.4 = metabolisable kilocalories per day
Cat	>25%	>10%		65–70 metabolisable kilocalories per kilogram per day

These figures are expressed as a percentage on a dry matter basis (with all water removed from the food).
Source: Lewis et al., 1994.

differs between species and also changes depending on activity level and age. Feeding an animal a balanced diet throughout its life is known as 'life stage feeding'

Table 5.7 details nutritional requirements for normal, healthy adult dogs and cats.

Nutritional requirements of a puppy or kitten
Young animals require more protein and energy in their food for growth of tissues. An increase in some minerals is required, e.g. calcium and phosphorus but it is important that these are fed at the correct ratios to each other.

Nutritional requirements of a pregnant or lactating animal (Figure 5.3)
Provided the pregnant animal is already on a suitable diet it is not necessary to alter the food intake until the last third of gestation. At this time an increase in protein and energy is required for foetal growth. This may involve an increase in the volume fed, but it is important to remember that a pregnant animal has a smaller stomach capacity due to the enlarged uterus and should be fed little and often.

Nutritional requirements of an active or working animal (Figure 5.3)
These animals will use more energy and will therefore require a higher level in the diet. Extra protein will be needed to mend 'wear and tear' of body tissues.

Nutritional requirements of an elderly animal
Generally, geriatric animals require lower energy levels in their food as they lead less active lives. Constipation may occur and high fibre food can be fed to regulate transit time. Absorption of nutrients may be less efficient and it could be necessary to increase vitamin and mineral intake at the correct ratio.

Geriatric animals often have renal disease. As the waste product of protein breakdown – urea – is excreted from the body via the kidneys, it is not advisable to feed excesses of protein to such animals. However, feeding too little protein can result in the body breaking down its own tissues, so it is important to feed protein of a high biological value at optimal levels.

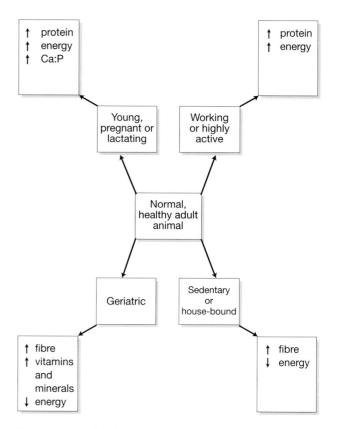

Figure 5.3 Model of changing nutritional requirements.

Types of food

Although dogs are omnivorous (eat both animal and plant matter) and cats are carnivorous (see section on protein), foods are available for both species in the following forms:

Commercial diets
■ **Canned food** – Moist processed food usually containing a combination of meat and cereal. It is traditional in this country to feed a mixer biscuit with moist food although there is no nutritional advantage to doing this in most cases (unless the food is complementary – see below).

Table 5.8   Advantages and disadvantages of various pet foods

Food type	Advantages	Disadvantages
Home-made	Food is 'fresh' so owner can see raw ingredients and knows exactly what is being fed	Changing ingredients, therefore, nutrient levels very difficult to measure Can be expensive, especially for medium/large dogs Encourages 'picky' eating habits Time consuming for owners
Canned	Balanced Some owners prefer the look of the food – 'more natural' Palatable	Bulky to store Can be expensive Once opened, food will go stale (although it is possible to freeze some foods for later use)
Tins and mixers	Balanced Some owners prefer the look of the food – traditional	Bulky to store Mixers add to expense for no nutritional reason (unless complementary tins are fed)
Dry	Balanced Tends to be more economical Perhaps some advantage of cleaning teeth (but do not over-estimate its effectiveness)	Generally less palatable Many owners do not like its appearance
Semi-moist	Individual sachets Owners like look of food Palatable	Expensive

- **Dried** – Usually made up of individual biscuits or kibbles. Although dried food looks like cereal, good quality products are, in fact, meat-based.
- **Semi-moist** – Sealed packets containing soft processed food. Less common than other forms of food.

Tinned vs dry

REMEMBER, it is the ingredients and nutrient content that is more important than the form in which the food comes.

Home-made food

This is less common with the advent of modern commercial pet foods. Should this method be selected, it is important to bear in mind that a detailed knowledge of specific nutrients is necessary to ensure a balanced diet. Malnutrition is much more likely to occur in an animal fed on home-made food.

Raw food

In recent years, certain groups have begun advocating feeding a raw diet, including bones, to dogs. Although this is a rather controversial method, if it is selected it should be thoroughly researched and food should be correctly sourced.

It should be borne in mind that feeding large quantities of one type of raw food could cause nutritional problems, e.g. some types of raw fish flesh contains the enzyme thiaminase, which breaks down thiamine and can lead to a deficiency of this vitamin if fed in large quantities.

Complete and complementary

Most commercial foods are complete, i.e. they contain all nutrients necessary for a balanced diet. However, some foods are complementary which means they are not balanced if fed alone. It is a legal requirement to state whether a food is complete or complementary on the label.

Table 5.8 shows the advantages and disadvantages of various pet foods.

Quantity of food

The amount of food needed will vary depending upon how calorie-dense the food is. In other words, the more calories per gram, the less quantity of food is needed to meet the animal's daily energy requirements. Feeding charts are usually provided on the label and should be used initially as a rough guide.

All animals should be weighed regularly. If there is a change in bodyweight then food quantity can be adjusted accordingly. It is common in pets to see weight gain rather than weight loss.

Frequency of feeding and watering

Generally speaking the feeding patterns between dogs and cats are different. Dogs are pack animals and as such, have evolved 'frenzy feeding' behaviour. This means that dogs tend to eat all food offered to them due to the threat of competition. Cats, as solitary hunters, are more inclined to partially complete a meal and return to it later.

The suggested feeding pattern for dogs and cats is at least twice daily. It is thought that once daily feeding can cause gastric overload and this may encourage regurgitation of all or part of a meal.

Food should be withheld prior to anaesthesia as passive vomiting may occur. This is when the cardiac sphincter opens to allow food to move back up the oesophagus and into the mouth. Food could then obstruct the airway, or be inhaled by the anaesthetised animal causing asphyxiation or aspiration pneumonia.

Fresh water in a regularly cleaned bowl must be available to dogs and cats at all times. In some veterinary practices it is common practice to withhold water for a period of time prior to anaesthesia. However, this is becoming increasingly uncommon as schools of thought change – dehydration is considered by many to be more of a risk to a patient than inhaling vomited fluid.

Dogs tend to visit their water bowls more frequently than cats, which are more inclined to drink from puddles and other alternative sources. Cats often prefer running water to still water – drinking fountains for pets are available. Bear in mind that animals may drink more during lactation and after exercise.

Alert Box!

- It is important to replenish water more frequently on hot days.
- Also, food is more likely to go stale or attract flies and should not be left uncovered for long periods of time.

Bowls/containers and utensils (Figure 5.4)

The animal's requirements and physical characteristics should be taken into account when selecting a suitable feeding bowl. Commonly used materials include ceramic, stainless steel and plastic. Ceramic bowls are heavy and durable but are difficult to clean and may break. Stainless steel bowls are easy to clean, durable and can be sterilised in an autoclave. However they can be chewed, are noisy and are quite lightweight. Plastic is cheap and available in many shapes but is light and can be scratched or chewed. Table 5.9 gives a description of different bowls and their use.

All equipment for food preparation should only be used for animals. It should also be kept separately during washing and storage. This is because there are

Table 5.9	Bowl types
Type of bowl	**Description and use**
Standard bowl	Straight sided bowl for general use.
Inward-sloping bowl	Bowl with inward-sloping sides, suitable for long-eared breeds.
Outward-sloping bowl	Bowl with outward-sloping sides, suitable for brachycephalic breeds.
Raised bowl	Bowl slots into a raised platform. Used for breeds susceptible to gastric dilation/torsion.
Timer bowl	Bowl with timer and lids which allows controlled feeding over a period of time. Useful for cats. It is important to check it is functioning correctly prior to each use.
Inflatable bowl	Flat-packed portable bowl. Used to offer water when away from the home.
Disposable bowl	Made from cardboard. These are useful when feeding animals with contagious diseases.
Travel bowls	Bowl with removable rim which prevents spillage during movement.
Water fountains	Constantly running water source. Useful for pets who need to be encouraged to drink, e.g. chronic cystitis sufferers.

some zoonoses which could be transmitted, such as the feline oral bacterium *Pasteurella multocida* or the protozoan *Toxoplasma gondii*.

The feeding process

Food storage

Food should be stored according to the manufacturer's recommendations. Generally, it should be kept in a dry environment away from fluctuations in temperature. Food kept in warm damp conditions tends to go stale rapidly. This does not just affect the taste, but also the nutritional content – vitamins will easily denature and fats can become rancid if food is stored incorrectly. Where possible, food should be kept in its original packaging, as this will protect it from the light. Plastic storage bins will help prevent infestation or damage from pests such as mice or weevils.

Careful stock control is important. If food is not correctly stored and rotated, it can easily become damaged or pass its expiry date.

New stock should be placed behind older items to ensure that there is no need to discard unused food.

Food preparation

It is good practice to follow basic hygiene measures such as washing your hands and cleaning surfaces prior to food preparation – animal food is as susceptible to contamination as human food!

It is also important to ensure frozen food has been thoroughly defrosted prior to feeding. Never re-freeze food that has defrosted.

Food kept in the fridge may need to be brought to room temperature prior to feeding – animals, particularly cats, do not always find cold food palatable.

Food should always be measured using an accurate method rather than estimating the amount 'by eye'. Otherwise, over a period of time it is easy to become lax and allow feed volumes to change.

Animal behaviour during feeding

Dogs (and sometimes cats) can behave differently at mealtimes due to excitement. Feeding more than one dog in the same area can lead to fighting or bullying over meals, particularly as one dog is likely to be dominant over the others. Try to feed in separate areas to avoid aggression and ensure each animal receives the correct amount of food. If it is not possible to do this dogs must be supervised throughout.

Never remove the feed bowl from an unfamiliar dog whilst it is eating. Many animals become protective over their food leading to aggression towards their handlers – not acceptable behaviour but it does occur nevertheless.

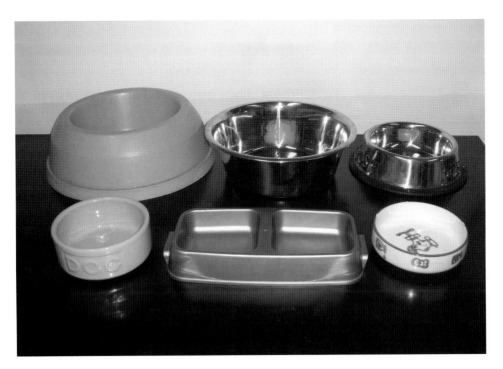

Figure 5.4 Photograph of different bowls.

Deviation in feeding and drinking habits

Deviation from normal eating or drinking habits could indicate disease. Any changes should be reported and recorded as soon as possible and closely monitored.

Refusal to eat (anorexia) often causes concern for pet owners. Once the possibility of disease is ruled out, it may be necessary to examine other causes. Commonly, this is a learnt behaviour, i.e. the owner offers attention or a treat when the animal refuses food so the behaviour is reinforced. Sometimes, ignoring the animal is the best approach! Healthy animals rarely go without food voluntarily for more than a few days.

Other methods of tempting an animal to eat include:

- Warming the food to blood temperature
- Offering smaller portions
- Mixing in a strong-smelling or favourite treat such as pilchard or Bovril®
- Feeding in a different bowl or area, e.g. somewhere quiet
- Hand feeding.

Nutritional problems

Before commercial pet food was widely available, nutritional disease was fairly common in dogs and cats. Today, however, it is quite unusual to see such problems but if they occur they are much more likely to be due to nutritional excesses than deficiencies.

Definitions

- **Undernutrition** – Insufficient quantities of one or more nutrients.
- **Overnutrition** – Excessive quantities of one or more nutrients.
- **Malnutrition** – 'wrong' nutrition; includes undernutrition or overnutrition.

Obesity

Obesity is now the most common nutritional disorder amongst dogs and cats in this country. It is most often seen in middle-aged, neutered, female animals.

Problems obesity causes include joint and locomotor problems, exercise intolerance and skin disease. Additionally, there is an increased likelihood of neoplasia and complications during surgery (Crane, 1991).

Vegetarian food

Meat-free food is becoming increasingly popular, for either moral or medical reasons. Dogs can tolerate vegetarian food as they can synthesise any unavailable nutrients in their own body tissues. As discussed previously, cats are unable to live solely on vegetarian food

and must have some food of animal origin (see section on nutritional requirements).

Feeding muscle meat

There remains a misconception that feeding large quantities of muscle meat, particularly to young animals, is healthier than feeding commercial pet food. This is not the case – muscle meat contains high amounts of phosphorus which causes an incorrect calcium:phosphorus ratio (see Table 5.6). Animals fed on high amounts of muscle meat may display signs of skeletal deformity.

'People food'

As our society has become more affluent people are spending more money and time on their pets which has increased their status. This sometimes leads to well-meaning owners trying to 'humanise' or spoil their animals by feeding food similar to theirs or giving too many treats. This kind of inbalanced diet may lead to nutritional disease, notably obesity.

Supplements

These are often given by well-intentioned owners who believe it is beneficial for their pet. Nutritional supplements should not be given unless they are needed for managing a specific condition and have been prescribed by a veterinary surgeon.

No supplements are needed for routine feeding if a good quality commercial food is fed. In fact, supplementing a good quality diet may lead to nutrient excesses or imbalance of ratios.

Common supplements used include cod liver oil and bone meal, which can cause skeletal abnormalities.

Clinical diets and electrolyte solutions

Altering the type of fluid and/or food given can aid recovery from, or in some cases control, disease.

Oral electrolyte solutions

When fluid is lost from the body various ions are also lost. If these are not replaced, acid–base balance may be disturbed. A common disorder resulting in fluid and ion loss is gastroenteritis (due to vomiting and/or diarrhoea).

A method of both fluid and ion replacement is an oral electrolyte solution (e.g. 'Lectade', Pfizer).

Clinical diets

A clinical diet is one which has been formulated to control or treat a specific condition. There are now many different ranges, e.g. Hill's Prescription Diet, Royal Canin/Waltham Veterinary Diet and Eukanuba Veterinary Diets.

Examples of common situations where a clinical diet may be used are:

- Feeding during recovery – a calorie dense, easily digestible, high protein formula is needed, e.g. Hill's a/d or Royal Canin/Waltham Concentration Diet.
- Treating obesity – a reduced calorie diet can be fed, e.g. Eukanuba Restricted-Calorie Formula or Hill's r/d.
- Chronic renal failure – moderated protein, low phosphorus levels, e.g. Royal Canin/Waltham Renal Diet or Hill's k/d.

GROOMING

Routine grooming is an important part of pet healthcare. This is particularly true of long-haired animals which may become matted. Animals with injury or disease may be reluctant or unable to groom themselves and may require special attention. Geriatric animals have slower hair re-growth and less sebaceous discharge leading to a drier skin and coat. Older animals are also more likely to be arthritic and may be unable to turn to groom.

Some breeds of dog may require specialist cosmetic attention carried out by professional dog groomers. Examples of such breeds include poodles and cocker spaniels. There are a variety of styles within each breed ranging from a 'pet trim' to various show cuts.

Equipment identification and use

To groom effectively a variety of equipment has been developed (Figure 5.5). Commonly used equipment is listed below:

- **Bristle brush** – Usually made of plastic with a wooden base. Most useful in short-haired breeds. May be used in long-haired breeds but often cannot reach through to the undercoat.
- **Pin brush** – Metal pins mounted on a rubber backed cushion. Care must be taken as pins may scratch the skin. Used for general grooming of silky and long coats with undercoat.

- **Slicker brush** – Rectangular board with short, bent wire teeth. Used in one direction to remove dead undercoat.
- **Rubber brush** – has long, thick rubber projections. Massages skin and removes dead undercoat.
- **Metal comb** – Can be wide, medium or fine-toothed. Used to break up knots and snags.
- **De-matting comb** – Comb with sharp edges. Used to break up or cut out large mats. Must only be used after careful instruction.
- **Straight-edged scissors** – General hair cutting, often used to trim feet and feathers. Great care must be taken when carrying out this procedure.
- **Thinning scissors** – Scissors designed to thin coat by only partially cutting hair sections. Often used on hind-quarters.
- **Hound glove** – Fits over hand. Small plastic projections or velvet surface. Used to polish smooth coated breeds.
- **Nail clippers** – Different types available. Most commonly used are plier, guillotine and volute spring cutters.
- **Electric clippers** – Usually used in cosmetic grooming or to remove large mats. Occasionally severely matted animals are completely clipped. A range of blades are available which will clip hair different lengths – the most common size used in veterinary practice is 40 which clips very short and is useful for the preparation of a surgical site.
- **Dryers** – There are various types including hand held and free-standing dryers. A drying cabinet provides a heated, enclosed space but must be used with care to prevent hyperthermia. Blasters are used before drying to force excess water from the coat.

Alert Box!

- Avoid the use of scissors on cats and rabbits – their skin is delicate and can be cut easily. Electric clippers or careful use of a de-matting comb is preferable.

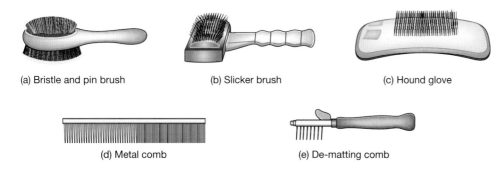

(a) Bristle and pin brush   (b) Slicker brush   (c) Hound glove

(d) Metal comb   (e) De-matting comb

Figure 5.5 Grooming equipment.

Care of grooming equipment

Good quality grooming equipment is expensive and should be maintained carefully. Bear in mind that it can potentially transmit infectious organisms from one animal to another (a fomite) and must be thoroughly disinfected after each use.

Cleaning and disinfecting equipment

The cleaning process is similar to that of surgical instruments.

- Remove any organic matter (e.g. hair) from equipment as this may inhibit the action of the disinfectant.
- Depending upon the disinfectant selected it may be necessary to use a separate detergent to remove sebaceous deposits.
- Disinfect equipment making sure that you adhere to the manufacturer's guidelines regarding dilution rates, contact time etc.
- Rinse equipment thoroughly in clean water.
- It is essential to dry equipment well and lubricate scissors and other moving parts to prevent rusting and stiffness.
- Careful thought should be given to the storage area. It should be kept clean, dry and tidy to prevent contamination or damage of equipment.

Disinfection and sterilisation of grooming equipment

All equipment should be thoroughly cleaned and disinfected after each use. Some grooming establishments use a specially manufactured UV light to disinfect equipment.

It is vital to sterilise any grooming equipment that has been used on an animal suspected of having a contagious disease. Equipment composed entirely of metal can be autoclaved, although this method can blunt sharp edges. Cold sterilising fluids can be used on most pieces of equipment.

Care of electric clippers and blades

Equipment needed:

- Nailbrush and toothbrush
- Non-abrasive cloth
- Appropriate disinfectant
- Clipper oil – used to lubricate moving surfaces after cleaning. Available in a tube or as a wash
- Clipper spray – used to cool blades and lubricate moving surfaces during use.

Daily care – check the plug, flex and casing before use. After use clipper blades should be removed and disinfected (see cleaning and disinfection routine above). The blades should also be oiled wherever moving surfaces meet before the next use. The clippers may accumulate hair which must be brushed away before wiping with an appropriate disinfectant. Any cloth used must be thoroughly wrung out to prevent drips of water entering the clipper casing.

Servicing – blades should be regularly sharpened. The clippers must be serviced as often as necessary which will vary depending on level of use.

Do:
- use a circuit breaker
- check the flex and casing before each use
- wear gloves when using disinfectants and clipper oil or spray. Some of these chemicals may irritate the skin. Some types of clipper oil are carcinogenic.

Do not:
- use dryers or clippers near wet surfaces or sinks
- use electrical equipment which has been dropped or damaged
- forget to sharpen clipper blades and service clippers regularly.

Bathing, drying and grooming an animal

When bathing, drying or grooming an animal it is important to ensure that they are secure and are not going to escape or injure themselves or their handler. Animals unused to being groomed may become stressed during the procedure. Reduce this as far as possible by:

- reassuring the animal verbally where appropriate
- keeping the surrounding area as quiet as possible
- having adequate assistance to facilitate the procedure.

Don't rush! Make calm and deliberate movements.

Preparation
- Check animal identification and record card
- Put on protective clothing, e.g. apron and gloves
- If necessary clip the nails (see box below)
- Gather correct equipment, such as towels, chamois leather, jug, cleaning agent and muzzle if necessary
- Place a non-slip mat in the bathing area.

<table>
<tr><td>

Clipping nails

- Restrain the animal correctly.
- Systematically inspect each nail.
- Clip at an angle below the 'quick' (the blood and nerve supply).
- If the nail is pigmented, be cautious and clip a little at a time.
- If you are unsure where to clip ask for assistance but if bleeding does occur apply pressure or a silver nitrate pencil.
- Don't forget to look for dew claws as these nails are not naturally worn down.

</td></tr>
</table>

Types of cleaning agent

- **Shampoo** – different types. Should always use a product designed for cats or dogs.
- **Medicated shampoo** – these are specifically formulated to treat particular conditions of the skin and coat, e.g. seborrhoea.
- **Topical medication** – conditions such as mange are sometimes treated with a topical wash which may not need rinsing. Care must be taken when using such products as they often have health and safety implications for the operator.
- **Conditioners** – for use after cleansing, conditioners can soften the coat, add shine and reduce tangling.

Bathing

1. Brush out knots using appropriate grooming equipment (see equipment identification and use).
2. Make sure water is at a constant acceptable temperature.
3. Wet animal thoroughly all over, protecting eyes with hand.
4. Shampoo starting with back. Avoid sensitive areas such as eyes, vulva and prepuce.
5. Massage shampoo into body and leave for recommended time.
6. Rinse thoroughly (if necessary). Check thick areas of the coat and areas that are difficult to reach to ensure all product is removed.
7. Repeat if necessary.
8. Remove excess water using towel or chamois leather.
9. Towel dry by rubbing coat vigorously taking care not to tangle the coat of long or silky breeds.

Drying

It is important to ensure the animal does not get cold and the environmental temperature should be checked and monitored.

<table>
<tr><td>

Tip

When applying shampoo, squeeze a small amount onto your hands and rub them together to spread the shampoo evenly across your palms. Then rub the shampoo onto the coat – this will allow a more even distribution of shampoo.

</td></tr>
</table>

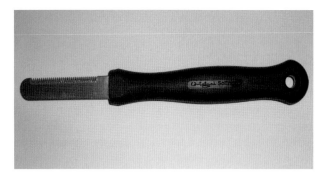

Figure 5.6 A stripping knife.

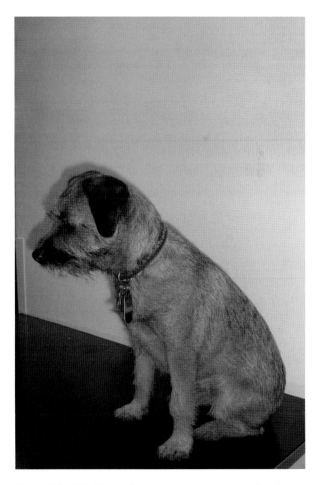

Figure 5.7 This Border Terrier has been stripped rather than clipped to maintain the coarse coat texture.

Remove as much water as possible by towel drying and squeezing excess water from legs and body. Comb through gently to ensure no tangles are present.

A number of appliances may be used to finish the drying process, including blasters and hand-held dryers. Care must be taken with the use of dryers as they can get very hot and may even burn the skin. It is a good idea to keep your hand in the path of the hot air in order to monitor the temperature and lift the hair as it is drying. This is known as 'fluff drying' and can also be carried out using a brush.

Grooming

Dry coats should be brushed through. Finishing off may involve clipping in some breeds. Wire-haired breeds, e.g. border terrier, may need stripping (Figures 5.6 and 5.7). This is the removal of hair by plucking with fingers or use of a 'stripping knife'. Clipping wire-haired coats tends to change their texture so it becomes much softer. This is commonly seen in West Highland white terriers.

References

- Crane, S. (1991) Journal of Small Animal Practice 32:275–282.
- Lewis L. et al. (1994) Small Animal Clinical Nutrition, 3rd edn. Mark Morris Institute, Kansas, USA.

Further reading

- Henderson, A. (ed) (1996) The Henston Small Animal Veterinary Vade Mecum, 15th edn. Henston Veterinary Publications, Peterborough.
- Lane, D., Cooper, B. (eds) (2003) Veterinary Nursing, 3rd edn. Butterworth Heinemann, Oxford.
- Lewis, L. et al. (2000) Small Animal Clinical Nutrition, 4th edn. Mark Morris Institute, Kansas, USA.
- Wills, J., Simpson, W. (1994) The Waltham Book of Clinical Nutrition. Pergamon, Oxford.

Management of the cat and dog

Joy Venturi Rose

Chapter objectives

This chapter describes:

- Identification of dog and cat breed groups
- House training
- Handling and restraint – general points
- Selection and fitting of collar and lead
- Exercising a healthy dog
- Obedience training
- Breeding dogs and cats

IDENTIFICATION OF DOGS AND CATS

A pedigree animal is one where the parentage for several generations is known. Generally the term will refer to selected breeds of animals with a known parentage where its 'breed type' has been especially selected for over many generations.

A cross-bred animal results from the reproduction of parents each of which were different breeds. Where the parents of an animal were of mixed or nondescript breeds the offspring are called mongrels.

DOGS

The governing body for pedigree dogs in the UK is the Kennel Club (1 Clarges Street, London). They register puppies from pedigree parents registered with them, issue registration documents and copies of pedigrees. The registration document will also record other details such as whether the parents have been X-rayed for hip or elbow dysplasia and had their eyes examined for any signs of hereditary disease before being bred from.

The breeds are sub-divided into seven Kennel Club groups. The importance of this is that dogs were all originally bred for certain jobs of work and their temperament and appearance relate to the instincts and conformation originally selectively bred for in order to best carry out their work. Nurses need to be able to advise clients regarding the normal attributes of a breed they own or are considering. Sometimes their preferred choice may not be suitable for their lifestyle. For example, an elderly couple living in a small flat should probably avoid a young Irish setter as they can be boisterous and require a lot of exercise.

Toy group (Table 6.1)

These are all small dogs but represent a big variety in coat types and temperaments. Most tend to have quite sparky temperaments despite their small frame. Often bought purely as companion dogs, their intelligence is not always recognised and they can become rather dominant unless their owners ensure they are trained and not just treated as a cuddly toy. Note the toy poodle has now been moved to the utility group.

Table 6.1 Toy group	
Affenpinscher	Italian Greyhound
Australian Silky Terrier	Japanese Chin
Bichon Frise	King Charles Spaniel
Bolognese	Lowchen (Little Lion Dog)
Cavalier King Charles Spaniel	Maltese
Chihuahua	Miniature Pinscher
Chinese Crested	Papillon
Coton De Tulear	Pekingese
English Toy Terrier	Pomeranian
Griffon Bruxellois	Pug
Havanese	Yorkshire Terrier

Utility group (Table 6.2)

Most of these dogs represent breeds whose specialist jobs often no longer exist in the modern world, e.g. the Bulldog (fighting bulls) and the Dalmatian (running under the axles of horse drawn carriages to look both attractive and guard the occupants). Another example is the spitz breed, recognised by their compact square bodies, prick ears and thick coat with the tail curved over the back. Note the similar looking Alaskan malamute is in the working group.

Gundog group (Table 6.3)

All these breeds were bred to work with the hunting man and his gun. All the breeds have flop-over ears for protection, but coat types and recommended tail lengths vary depending on the terrain normally worked. Some breeds include varieties with either long, short or wire coats, e.g. Hungarian vizsla.

There are four sub-groups each representing a distinct task required in the field. Temperaments reflect this role with the retrievers generally being the most stoical within the group.

The spaniels are bred to hunt through thick undergrowth all day, find the game, flush it and then retrieve if required. The setter breeds and (English) pointers are required to hunt or quarter in wide open spaces such as moors, point or set the game when found, flush it on command, so that it can be shot, but not retrieve. This is left to the retrievers who wait patiently with the handler or gun, only being sent to retrieve the game, tenderly to hand, undamaged for the pot, after it has been found by a spaniel, pointer or setter.

The hunt, point and retrievers (HPRs) all originate from Europe and are multi-purpose, being bred to carry out all three roles but in different types of terrain. They are active, fairly high strung, breeds.

Working group (Table 6.4)

This group includes dogs bred for specialist roles. The guarders (Rottweiler, Dobermann and Mastiffs), the search and rescue dogs (St Bernard and Newfoundland) and the sled and guard dogs (Siberian husky). Most guard dogs first warn their victims with noise but the mastiffs work silently and then knock their victims to the ground with force and weight. Trained correctly and given plenty of appropriate mental stimulation these dogs are intelligent and devoted companions although they might be rather protective of their owner. The

Table 6.3 Gundog group	
Chesapeake Bay Retriever	Pointer
Curly Coated Retriever	Gordon Setter
Flat Coated Retriever	English Setter
Golden Retriever	Irish Setter
Labrador Retriever	Irish Red and White Setter
Nova Scotia Duck Tolling Retriever	**HPRs**
Kooikerhondje	Bracco Italiano
American Cocker Spaniel	Brittany
Cocker Spaniel	German Shorthaired Pointer
Clumber Spaniel	German Wirehaired Pointer
English Springer Spaniel	Hungarian Vizsla
Field Spaniel	Hungarian Wirehaired Vizsla
Irish Water Spaniel	Italian Spinoni
Sussex Spaniel	Large Munsterlander
Welsh Springer Spaniel	Weimaraner

Table 6.2 Utility group	
Boston Terrier	Tibetan Spaniel
Bulldog	Tibetan Terrier
Dalmatian	Chow Chow
French Bulldog	Canaan Dog
Lhasa Apso	Japanese Akita
Poodles Toy, Miniature	Japanese Shiba Inu
Standard	Japanese Spitz
Miniature Schnauzer	Keeshund
Schnauzer	German Spitz Mittel
Shar-Pei	German Spitz Klein
Shih Tzu	Schipperke

Table 6.4 Working group	
Bullmastiff	Alaskan Malamute
Mastiff	Newfoundland
Neopolitan Mastiff	Bouvier Des Flandres
Tibetan Mastiff	St Bernard
Boxer	Siberian Husky
Dobermann	Giant Schnauzer
Rottweiler	Great Dane
Bernese Mountain Dog	

rescue breeds are gentle giants but with dense coats for protection and often have to work independently, more on instinct rather than by obedience.

Pastoral group (Table 6.5)

These dogs were all bred to either herd livestock or assist in driving (droving) them to market or to guard livestock. The herders are often very intelligent and can achieve high levels of skill and obedience. They need to be quick and fearless to move a stubborn herd so can be protective and snappy if provoked or not controlled. Bred to replace or support the shepherd the livestock, guarders often live alone with just the flock. Aloof and with the courage to attack a wolf or thieves they often have profuse coats and are not for the novice owner with little time to spare.

Terrier group (Table 6.6)

The sizes of dog in this group can range from large (Airedale and Kerry Blue terriers) to small (Glen of Imaal terrier and Dandie Dinmont terrier). Coat types are either short or wiry. All were originally bred for catching and flushing (by incessant barking) or killing 'pest' animals such as rats and foxes. Many will have needed to work inside burrows or earths out of sight of the owner. Therefore this group contains breeds which tend to be plucky and independent. If not controlled, they can be excessively yappy and display a more than healthy interest in other domestic pets if not socialised with them early.

Hound group (Table 6.7)

Originally bred as hunters. These dogs are divided into two sub-groups depending on the method they employ to pursue their prey. The sight hounds (e.g. greyhound, deerhound) and the scent hounds such as beagles and bloodhounds. Usually the dogs are kept in packs and aggression to humans is not tolerated. Therefore, they are usually very sociable animals with both other dogs and people. However, the sight hounds need careful control if they are not to get into the habit of chasing any cat or small animal they set eyes on. The scent hounds love to hunt so find it difficult to listen to words of command whilst exploring an interesting smell. Training is possible with both groups but from

Table 6.6 Terrier group

Airedale	Kerry Blue
Australian	Lakeland
Bedlington	Manchester
Border	Norfolk
Bull Terrier	Norwich
Bull Terrier (Miniature)	Parson Russell
Staffordshire Bull Terrier	Scottish
Cairn Terrier	Sealyham
Dandie Dinmont	Skye
Fox (Wire and Smooth)	Soft Coated Wheaten
Gen of Imaal	Welsh
Irish	West Highland White

Table 6.5 Pastoral group

Herders and drovers	Livestock guarders
Bearded Collie	Briard
Belgian Shepherd Dog	Estrela Mountain Dog
Border Collie	Hungarian Puli
Rough Collie	Komondor
Smooth Collie	Maremma Sheepdog
German Shepherd Dog	Pyrenean Mountain Dog
Lancashire Heeler	Samoyed
Old English Sheepdog	Hungarian Kuvasz
Shetland Sheepdog	
Swedish Vallhund	
Welsh Corgi (Cardigan)	
Welsh Corgi (Pembroke)	

Table 6.7 Hound group

Sight	Scent
Afghan	Basset Hound
Basenji	Basset Griffon Vendeen (Grand and Petit)
Borzoi	Beagle
Greyhound	Bloodhound
Ibizan Hound	Dachshund
Irish Wolfhound	Elkhound
Deerhound	Finnish Spitz
Pharaoh Hound	Foxhound
Saluki	Hamiltonstovare
Sloughi	Otterhound
Whippet	Rhodesian Ridgeback

an early age requires patience and controlled practice in 'risk' situations.

CATS

The governing body for pedigree cats in the UK is the Governing Council of the Cat Fancy (GCCF) (4–6 Penel Orlieu, Bridgwater, Somerset). They perform similar regulatory and registration roles for cats as does the Kennel Club for dogs.

Cats are divided into breeds and are allocated a breed number. The breeds are subdivided into sections according to type and hair length and then in most cases, further subdivided by colour into separate breeds.

Longhaired section

- *Persians*: solid cobby body, sturdy legs, short tail, round head and short nose. Wide variety of coat and eye colours. Usually good tempered but need grooming from 7 weeks of age in order to become accustomed to what will be a daily task all their lives.
- *Exotic*: a short-haired version of the Persian produced by crossing the Persian and British shorthair.

Semi-longhair section

- *Birman*: similar shaped body to the Persian but its legs and tail are a little longer and the nose is of medium length. It is a good tempered breed and the coat is easier to keep groomed than the Persian. The coat colours are the same as for the Siamese but uniquely it has white feet caused by a gene called 'white gloving'.
- *Turkish van*: The body shape is moving away from the Persian being longer with a wedge-shaped head, long nose and large upright ears. The coat is long and silky but quite easy to groom and they lose a lot of their coat in the summer, looking almost shorthaired. They are pure white with auburn or cream patches on the face and a tail of the same colour. Eyes are light amber or blue or one of each.
- *Maine coon*: originating in the USA it is one of the largest of pedigree cats with a glossy waterproof coat. It is a medium foreign type (a type starting to take on the characteristics of a longer rather than shorter body) and comes in a variety of colours.
- *Ragdoll*: moderately foreign type head, long muscular body, fairly long legs and long tail. They come in the same colours as the Siamese as well as varieties with white feet and undersides (mitted) and bi-colours (two colours, one being white).
- *Norwegian forest cat*: medium foreign type similar to the Maine coon but with a triangular head and rather high-set ears leading to a different expression. Siamese coat pattern and lilac and chocolate not accepted.

British section

- *British*: shorthaired, powerful compact cats with sturdy bodies and legs, short tails, round heads with small ears set wide apart as are its large, round eyes. It has a short, straight nose. The dense coat requires more grooming than a Siamese but not as much as a Persian. A wide variety of coat and eye colours.
- *Manx*: Although in the British shorthair section it does have some differences apart from the absence of a tail. It is short backed with hind legs longer than the front ones. It has a longer nose and taller ears. The hairs of the outer (top) coat are longer than the thick undercoat. Colour as other British shorthairs but not Siamese pattern. There is a rare long haired variety called the Cymric.

Foreign section

Very sociable cats which are rather vocal, like the Siamese, and tend to seek attention.

- *Russian blue*: vivid green eyes also occasionally seen with black or white coats.
- *Abyssinian*: distinguished by the coat pattern which is usually described as 'ticked tabby' with the base colour of each hair having two or three bands of a different (usually darker) colour on it.
- *Somali*: longhaired version of the Abyssinian.
- *Cornish rex*: has a short fairly fine coat with a curl or wave to it caused by a recessive gene which prevents the cat having a normal top coat.
- *Devon rex*: similar type of coat to the Cornish Rex but with a different body type having a wider face, very large ears and a strongly marked stop to the nose.
- *Selkirk rex*: a rare longhaired rex.
- *Korat*: blue coat with silvery tipping which is slightly longer than most of the foreign shorthairs.
- *Asians*: originally developed from a cross between a Burmese and a chinchilla-coloured Persian but have the same type, coat and character as Burmese.
- *Tonkinese*: a cross between Burmese and Siamese, not really a true breed.
- *Singapura*: derived from Singapore, a stocky cat with large eyes and ears, short close coat ticked with brown on a lighter coloured background.
- *Ocicat*: a recently developed, quite large, spotted cat.

■ *Bengal*: a result of cross-breeding with the wild Asian leopard cat. Selective breeding has produced a good-tempered cat with a spotted tabby type coat.

Burmese section

Short fine, glossy coats requiring little grooming. They are mid-way in type between the British and the Siamese. Lively cats, they can be demanding but are usually very affectionate and talkative to their owners. They do not always like being left alone.

Oriental section

The Oriental shorthair is a self-coloured cat similar to the Siamese in type. They come in many colours and usually take their name from this, e.g. oriental blue or oriental caramel ticked tabby but the brown colour is called Havana and the white is called foreign white.

Siamese section

This breed is well known and the seal point is perhaps the most common. However, they also come in a wide range of other colours including tabby and tortoiseshell patterns. An affectionate and vocal breed they can be demanding but their extrovert characters make them popular pets. The Balinese is a longhaired Siamese.

Rare breeds of cat include a hairless cat – the sphynx – and the Scottish fold, which has folded-over ears.

TRAINING THE DOG

Training is usually made much easier if starting with a young puppy. Young means between 7 and 16 weeks. This is a major socialisation stage which enables habituation of the puppy and moulding of its character and behaviour to suit the human social environment. After this age many of the puppy's character and behaviour traits will have been formed and, although it is still quite possible to teach an 'old' dog new tricks, it may require a more patient and thoughtful handler to do so.

Disposal of faeces and cat litter in the surgery

Pet excrement in the surgery is treated as clinical waste and staff should wear gloves and follow good hygiene

---

House training puppies and kittens

Puppies

1. Puppies normally want to urinate or defecate as soon as they wake up, have been fed or have been playing. So straight away they should be put outside and given a chance to perform.
2. As the pup urinates or defecates a cue word spoken in a soothing voice should be used at the same time, e.g. 'toilet'.
3. Accidents should be ignored, where an incident is witnessed the pup should be calmly put outside (it may not have finished) and the cue word used as above. In future owners should be careful to observe pre-toileting behaviour such as agitation or circling and try to be quicker in moving the pup to a suitable place. Punishment is to be avoided as it can frighten the pup into only soiling when it thinks the owner is not looking and making future training difficult.
4. Pups do not usually like to soil their own bed and the use of a puppy cage, which is not too large, is useful overnight or when the pup is unsupervised. Between four and eight hours is the maximum period for young puppies between excretions dependent on breed and individual. Meals and exercise should be planned to help the pup to last the night, gradually increasing time as it matures.

Kittens

1. Kittens normally want to urinate or defecate as soon as they wake up, have been fed or have been playing. So straight away they should be put outside or into the litter tray and given a chance to perform.
2. A variety of substrates/cat litter can be tried and one similar to that used by the kitten in its previous environment is the best one to use to start with.
3. Gradually, the preferred substrate can be added using more of the new and less of the old over time.
4. As the kitten gets used to the litter tray it can gradually be moved, over a few days or weeks, and short distances at a time to outside or a preferred area of the house. Kittens and cats do not like performing toilet behaviour close to where they are fed or sleep so the litter tray should not be put in these areas
5. The litter tray should be cleaned regularly or the cat will stop using it. It should also be in a relatively quiet area so the cat is not easily disturbed.

Owners should always clean up their dog's faeces in public places using a plastic bag. This is placed in local authority disposal points where possible.

procedures. Pregnant women should not clean out cat litter trays without using face masks and gloves.

Owners often do not realise how actions, which they see as humorous or harmless in a young puppy, can become established and cause problems later on. If an 8- to 12-week-old puppy is taken for a gentle walk, in a spacious but strange area it could run off, but its reactions are likely to be the opposite because it is worried about its new surroundings and is without the company of its litter mates or any other dogs. The owner is the only thing with which it is really familiar and confident. Therefore it will rely on the owner being the leader and will eagerly follow not wishing to get itself lost. If it wanders then the owner, who is bigger and faster, is instantly able to fetch it back, further compounding their superiority and pack leader status. This behaviour pattern, when repeated several times, is imprinted on the puppy's brain and problems with not coming when called will largely be avoided.

Contrast this with the new owner who has only ever allowed the new puppy to exercise in its own garden, usually because its vaccination programme is not complete. The puppy will feel confident in these familiar surroundings. If it happens to be making its own entertainment, perhaps chewing an old flower pot whilst being called by its owner, it will, most probably, not feel obliged to come. Often the owner, thinking the puppy is at least keeping out of mischief, does not enforce the command and misses an ideal opportunity to practise the recall when the puppy's attention is distracted. The owner must ideally either work harder to make themselves more interesting than the puppy's distraction, such as by clapping their hands, offering a food titbit or starting to play with a more interesting toy, or go and get the puppy whilst repeating the recall command, and then making a fuss of it.

Puppy parties or other events can be very useful; it is recognised that the very slight risk of infection is the lesser evil when compared to the behavioural problems that are created by incorrect socialisation of young puppies. This period is also very important for a puppy's training development. Yes, things should be kept light-hearted but the educational purpose of everything done with the puppy should be appreciated. If the puppy carries out an action which is displeasing a suitable course of action is for the owner to say a sharp 'NO' and quickly give a counter command to perform a more suitable alternative action, such as 'SIT', and then praise it for carrying out this act.

After 14 weeks of age, puppies which have not experienced a wide variety of situations, different people and dogs are inclined to find new situations either too exciting or too worrying. This distracts them from concentrating on what the owner wants. Ignored commands result in the speedy acquisition of bad habits. The pup is also larger and faster and more difficult for the owner to restrain or go and get.

Training is also about daily management and the prevention of problems. For example, if a puppy runs off with shoes or other objects and is reprimanded every time, it will eventually refuse to bring items to its owner. The correct action would be for the owner to encourage it to bring the object to hand, give it a lot of praise and then make sure important things are kept out of reach in future.

Punishment

Appropriate punishment is more difficult to enforce than owners realise. It must be within half a second of the action to be punished and at an intensity which worries the puppy but cannot damage it mentally or physically. This is not the easiest judgement for owners to make and can result, if carried out wrongly, in the puppy developing fear aggression, insecurities or phobias. In addition, punishment, to be effective, usually also needs to be repeated whenever the puppy commits the misdemeanour and in a variety of different circumstances. If not the puppy may just wait until the owner's back is turned before attempting the misdemeanour and not be cured. Therefore, reward-based training is preferable using titbits, toys, games or praise which includes verbal or physical (tactile) reinforcers. They need to be given within half a second of the action to be rewarded for effective association to take place.

If punishment is absolutely necessary, it should be after careful consideration and in the form of a withdrawal of human attention or rewards until the puppy complies. If this is not possible a remote punishment, not directly attributable to the owners, is preferable. Some trainers shake the pup by the scruff combined with a growling noise made in the throat, in the same way its mother would – whilst this can work with some dogs it can provoke an attack from others, especially in older dogs.

All puppies develop at different rates but by 6 months of age most, with appropriate training, should be able to come when called, sit and stay, down and stay, and walk to heel on, and ideally off, the lead.

Basic obedience

- **Start on day 1:** The longer training is delayed, the harder it will become. Training can take the form of games but always ones which the owner wins.
- **Single word cue words (commands) are best:** Owners should write down their cue words and the action they refer to. Different single-syllable words should be used to avoid confusing the puppy.

Keep life simple. Giving the appropriate cue word (command) as a puppy voluntarily carries out an action and then rewarding with a titbit, toy or praise is an easy and surprisingly effective way to start.

- **Speak clearly at normal level:** Dogs hear more acutely than humans but associate words by the sounds they produce. Mumbled sounds become altered. Shouting is counterproductive as the puppy becomes habituated with nothing left in reserve for genuine emergencies.

- **Always reward response to a cue word:** Social animals, like dogs, seek to please their leaders. Owners can show this with the voice or actions such as 'good dog', stroking, a game or titbits. Where puppies are timid then proportionally more praise to increase their confidence is required. If the pup is more excitable then a toned down gentle stroke or quiet 'good dog' may be enough. More praise is generally required when a puppy learns new things and to consolidate learning as compared to once it is proficient at responding to a cue word. Rewards must be given within 0.5 seconds of the pup responding to form an positive reinforcement association.

- **Give cue word as the pup carries out the desired action:**
  Teaching the sit: The titbit is held above the pup's head and moved slightly backwards as the head comes up the bottom starts going down (a little gentle assistance on the bottom is OK if absolutely necessary) and a sit is obtained, give cue word ('SIT') and then give the titbit or praise. Over time gradually increase the time spent in the sit before the reward is given and cue in the word 'STAY'.
  Teaching the down: The puppy should be in front or beside the handler, preferably in the sit position. The titbit is enclosed in the hand which is wiggled slightly on the floor and moved gently forward as the dog goes down to investigate. Cue in the 'DOWN' and reward. Over time gradually increase the time spent in the down before the reward is given. Putting the dog on the lead and using a chair which the dog starts to crawl under for the titbit can help with some dogs.
  Teaching the recall: Start in a secure area if necessary. A second person should hold the dog on the lead or by the collar and the owner should move a few yards away, stand still for a few seconds and then say the dog's name and 'COME'. Use additional encouragement such as clapping hands, a whistle, funny voice, showing a toy or titbit as required. As the dog reaches the owner they

should take hold of the collar and instantly give a meaningful reward. This can be followed by a sit and reward. Repeat as necessary and over time the second person can provide progressively more difficult 'managed distractions' by stroking or playing with the dog so that the owner has to work harder with their encouragement to get the dog to come.
Teaching heel work: Select appropriate equipment. Encourage the pup to walk by left side using titbits and praise. Plenty of direction changes interspersed with 'SIT' should be given to keep the pup's attention on the owner.

- **Commands should never be given which owners cannot enforce:** If owners are too tired or cannot be bothered, then commands are better not given. Puppies should never think there are some occasions when they can disobey. Instead future 'dummy' situations should be stage-managed so that a puppy is given every opportunity to get it right and is praised for his efforts. Eventually habits are formed which can be repeated in all environments. For example, if there is difficulty with recalls they should be practised in 'alley way' situations – these limit the possibility of running off sideways and help form a habit of coming straight into the handler. The owner can run backwards clapping their hands so the pup can chase up this exciting creature. Progressively wider areas can be used before graduating to a larger parks or fields where the temptation to run off is greater.

- **Training should be short, sweet and varied:** Ten minutes' formative training a day is enough coupled with ensuring daily management commands are obeyed. Training with dogs, like children, is an ongoing activity and the best training sessions are often the impromptu ones, which result from having to cope with real-life situations. Feeding time is excellent for teaching the sit, down and stay – with the reward, of course, being dinner.

- **Being in the right frame of mind and always ending sessions on a positive note:** Owners should not attempt training if in a bad mood or short of time as things will go wrong. Dogs, like us, have off days. If the lesson is not going well it should be ended by getting the dog to do something simple, praising it and putting the pup somewhere quiet, preferably by itself, to think about it. A later attempt at the session will often see surprising improvement.

- **Training requires lots of repetition over time:** Even simple procedures may need repeating many times to form habits in the dog's mind. This will take several weeks or months because the dog would be bored if forced to carry out the necessary repeats over a short time period. Owners need to learn to anticipate their dog's reactions in a variety of situations as preventative training rather than cure is best. Dogs need 'saving' from some of their natural instincts which if not moulded and channelled correctly, can result in accidents or anti-social behaviour.

■ **When things go wrong:** Mistakes will be made but are best acknowledged, thought about and avoided in the future. Once trained dogs, like athletes, need regular practice to keep up to standard and owners should always be prepared to return to basics if necessary.

Even after dogs have been taught a given behaviour sometimes they will fail to respond. Repeating commands which are disobeyed is useless. Instead, where possible, the owner should remain silent, evaluate the situation and think about how the puppy can be induced to comply on a later occasion. Owners need to ensure that the puppy is motivated, or tricked, into pleasing them and then making it worth their while.

Ignoring or behaving in a cool off-hand manner with the pup for a period by refusing to give into attention demands, such as jumping up or giving a paw, will render it mentally more likely to obey as it becomes hungry for human attention. Mostly, dogs should earn rewards from humans and not be given them for free.

RESPONSIBLE PET OWNERSHIP

Owners should not take on pets unless they can afford to feed them and give them veterinary attention when required. They also need time to exercise adult dogs at least twice a day for 20 minutes. Most pet cats and pet bitches that will not be required for breeding are best neutered. This is usually carried out around six months for cats and after the first season for bitches.

BREEDING
Definitions

■ *Puberty*: The age at which sexual maturity is reached. Normally between 6 and 12 months in the dog, with small breeds reaching it earlier. In cats it is reached between 6 and 15 months, with foreign breeds and kittens born early in the year tending to be earlier than British breeds. In the male animal it is signalled by the ability to produce sperm and mate and in the female by the onset of the first heat or season.

■ *Seasonally monoestrus*: An animal, for example the bitch (female dog), which has one reproductive cycle (heat) in a breeding season.

■ *Seasonally polyoestrus*: An animal, for example the queen (female cat), which has more than one reproductive cycle within a breeding season.

■ *Pro-oestrus*: The first part of a reproductive cycle where the female starts to become attractive to males, although she does not yet mate.

■ *Oestrus*: The second part of a reproductive cycle during which the female produces eggs from her ovaries (ovulation) and will accept the male for mating.

■ *Metoestrus*: The period after ovulation where areas on the surface of the ovaries called corpus lutea (corpus luteum = singular) are formed after the ova (eggs) have ovulated (ruptured). These areas are important because they produce the hormone progesterone, which is responsible for maintaining pregnancy.

■ *Inter-oestrus*: The short period between each reproductive cycle of one breeding season such as occurs in the queen. During this time the reproductive organs are 'repriming' ready to enter another proestrus.

■ *Anoestrus*: The longer period of time after the last or only reproductive cycle in a breeding season and before the next breeding season begins. During this period there is no reproductive activity going on.

■ *Gestation*: The period of time between the fertilisation of the egg by the sperm and the birth of the young.

■ *Graafian follicles*: Found in the ovaries and are where the ova are produced.

■ *Pituitary gland*: Endocrine (hormone-producing) gland at the base of the brain.

■ *Parturition*: The time of birth, also called labour.

■ *Post parturient*: The time after the birth.

■ *Lactation*: The time the female is feeding the young with milk from the mammary glands.

■ *Neonate*: A new-born puppy or kitten before the eyes are open.

■ *Colostrum*: The first milk produced by the mother which contains antibodies to give the young immunity to certain diseases. It also contains red blood cells to help boost the neonate's blood circulation.

The bitch's reproductive cycle

The bitch is seasonally monoestrus and has one reproductive cycle approximately every 6 months. When this happens owners will say their bitch is in season or in heat (see Table 6.8). It lasts for approximately 3 weeks. Wild

Table 6.8	Stages of the bitch's reproductive cycle		
Stage and average length	Behavioural signs	Physical signs	Physiology
Pro-oestrus, 8–13 days	Increased urination; possible irritability with other bitches; attractive to the male but will not allow mating	Bloody vaginal discharge; swollen vulva	Graafian follicles in ovary start to mature under the influence of follicle stimulating hormone (FSH) secreted by the pituitary gland; they also produce increasing amounts of oestrogen
Oestrus, 4–7 days	The bitch stands for the dog; the tail is held to one side and the vulva is presented more dorsally to assist penetration (so-called winking)	Bloody discharge reduces, becoming clearer; vulva softens	The higher levels of oestrogen and progesterone which the follicles also start to produce switch off the secretion of FSH (negative feedback) and the pituitary gland produces luteinising hormone (LH) instead; ovulation now occurs
Metoestrus, 30–64 days	The bitch will no longer accept the dog and starts to return to normal by about 21 days after the first signs of pro-oestrus; metoestrus includes the stage of pregnancy or, in the non-mated bitch, false pregnancy, when milk can be produced	The discharge dries up completely and the vulva returns to normal adult size	Where each ova is produced on the surface of the ovary a corpus luteum is formed and this produces more progesterone which maintains pregnancy if the bitch is mated. If not mated the corpus lutea eventually regress and prolactin is produced which is responsible for the formation of milk in the mammary glands
Anoestrus, approx 4 months	No reproductive activity	None	

dogs such as the wolf have one season a year and this pattern is mirrored in comparatively recently domesticated breeds of dog such as the Basenji. Bitches are best bred at their second or third season. And stud dogs first used at about 18 months.

The queen's reproductive cycle

The queen is seasonally polyoestrus and the breeding season starts around February and runs through to September (depending on daylight length), with the peak of sexual activity being early in the year (see Table 6.9). It is best to plan breeding for when the cat is at least a year old. Puberty is 6 months to a year with Siamese and short-haired cats tending to reach it earlier than longhaired Persian cats.

Mating

All animals should be routinely wormed and have an up to date vaccination booster prior to mating.

The bitch

It is usual to take the bitch to the dog and best for at least one of the pair to be experienced. The couple should be introduced on leads as the bitch may be quite ferocious with the dog if she is not in standing oestrus or is somewhat shy. Once the behaviour of the bitch has settled, which will only happen if she is in standing oestrus,

and if they are in a secure area, the dog can be let off the lead. The pair may wish to court each other by playing which can last up to 20 minutes. The bitch can also be let off at this point providing the attendant/s are able to restrain her again, once the dog has mounted her successfully, achieved penetration and the 'tie' or 'lock' is established. The dog will turn once he has tied with the bitch (Figure 6.1) and they will stand back to back for between 10 and 40 minutes. Sometimes the bitch may vocalise during the mating and the dog may yelp when he turns but this is usually short-lived. Gently but firmly holding the bitch's mouth closed if she continues can help to reduce the sound and her anxiety. It is important that the pair are not allowed to drag themselves around or alter from the standing position too much therefore some restraint is necessary (see Figure 6.2). Eventually the bitch's constrictor vestibularis (cingulum), a sphincter muscle at the junction between the vagina and vestibule, which has held the dog behind the swollen bulbus glandis of his penis, will relax and the tie will finish. The dog will usually lick himself back into place although sometimes he may need assistance to roll back the prepuce and slide it over the still swollen bulbus glandis (see Figure 6.3) For pedigree breeding there will usually be a repeat mating 48 hours later although in the wild the bitch may be mated several times over a few days. The bitch must be kept away from other dogs for at least a week after she has been mated as it is still possible for

Table 6.9 Stages of the queen's reproductive cycle

Stage and average length	Behavioural signs	Physical signs	Physiology
Pro-oestrus, 1–4 days	Not clearly defined; merges with oestrus; increased vocal behaviour (calling) but will not accept male	Few, there is no bloody discharge	Follicle stimulating hormone produced by pituitary gland matures Graafian follicles which produce increasing amounts of oestrogen
Oestrus, 5–8 days	Arching of the back (lordosis); tail to one side; rolling; wanting to go out for long frequent periods; accepts males	Mating (usually repeatedly); artificial vaginal stimulation can be performed; spontaneous ovulation possible but rare	Reflex release of luteinising hormone from pituitary gland causing final maturation of ovarian follicles and induced ovulation of ova; progesterone levels then start to increase
Interoestrus, 10–14 days	If not mated, there is a short period of sexual inactivity before the next pro-oestrus	No mating	No ovulation
Or metoestrus	Occurs if the queen has been mated or if infertile mating or the queen has been artificially stimulated using a vaginal probe such as a thermometer	Pregnancy; false pregnancy	Formation of corpus luteum; production of progesterone and later prolactin
Anoestrus	Normal period of sexual inactivity, usually between September and March	None	

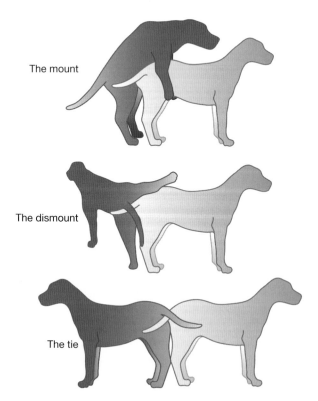

The mount

The dismount

The tie

Figure 6.1 Canine mating procedure.

another dog to fertilise some/more eggs resulting in a litter with more than one father.

The gestation period is 63 days from fertilisation of the eggs. However, they take 2 days to mature after ovulation and as the sperm can last up to a week in the bitch's reproductive tract, the time of mating may not exactly correlate to the time of fertilisation, which means parturition can occur up to a week early or late. The extremes of the range are likely to produce much smaller litters.

The queen

The queen is taken to the stud cat as he needs to be very confident of his territory in order to mate her. He will have sprayed his living area with urine and normally the queen will be moved in alongside for a period of socialisation and then be let into his area. The stud will mate her by grasping her by the scruff with his teeth. He will mount her first with his front legs and then his hindlegs, he will begin pelvic thrusting which is followed by penetration and ejaculation. The time from neck bite to penetration may be very short or last up to 5 minutes. Penetration usually lasts a few seconds. The queen will then let out a piercing scream, the post-coital yell, during or immediately after withdrawal

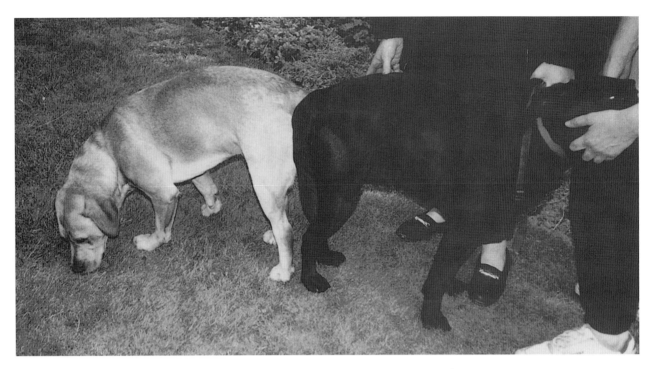

Figure 6.2 The tie – some restraint is necessary to avoid the pair dragging each other around.

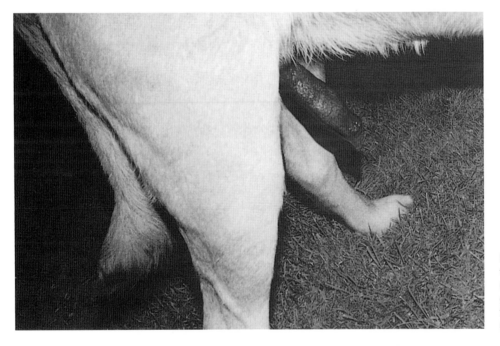

Figure 6.3 Engorgement of the canine penis post coitus (mating) showing the bulbus glandis proximal (nearest to body) and glans distally (furthest away from body).

of the male. She will try to free herself, strike out at him with her claws and lie on her side rolling, rubbing and licking her vulva. The tom will retreat and lick his penis. After a variable amount of time she will gradually become more receptive and another mating will occur. This pattern is repeated several times over 24 hours. They will normally be kept together for 1–3 days. Gestation is on average 65 days, range 61–70 days.

Parturition (Table 6.10)

The bitch should be introduced to her whelping box, so that she can be completely used to it and not anxious, at least 3 weeks before the puppies are due. If this is not done it can cause problems at the time of parturition and if the puppies arrive early the bitch may be reluctant to use this 'new' area (Figure 6.4).

Table 6.10   Signs and stages of parturition

Stage of labour	Bitch	Queen
First stage: Progressive relaxation and dilatation (opening) of the cervix	Variable time span of 6–20 hours Temperature will have gradually dropped over several days to a low of around 36°C (98–99°F) 12 hours prior to start of labour Panting and restlessness Bed making (scratching, tearing and chewing up) Possible light green mucoid discharge from the vagina. May vomit	Variable timespan 2–24 hours Temperature drop to 37–38°C (99–100°F) Nesting behaviour Restlessness (pacing) Vocalisation Rapid breathing Licking of the vulva
Second stage: Delivery of the fetuses once the cervix is fully dilated (open) and the fetal head is engaged in the birth canal	Contractions of the uterine and abdominal muscles which get progressively stronger Green-black fluid loss from rupture of the placenta (allantochorion) Licking at the vulva Eventual birth of the puppy. Average time between births is approx. 20 minutes but variable especially with large litters where two-hour gaps for the last puppies are common	Clear or blood tinged (brown) fluid loss Regular uterine and abdominal contractions Licking at the vulva Eventual birth of the kitten. Average time between births is approx. 20 minutes but can be variable. Queen usually finishes parturition 2–10 hours after birth of first kitten
Third stage: Expulsion of the fetal membranes (afterbirths). In animals which have multiple young this is repeated in a variable fashion between births	The puppy may be born enclosed in the intact membranes which the bitch should break, or the membrane may rupture and the puppy is not born in the membrane but is still attached by the umbilical cord. The bitch may break the cord and the membrane may remain in the vagina or retract into the uterus to be expelled later. Most bitches will eat the membranes which normally cause a black diarrhoea for a few days but this is quite normal	As for the bitch

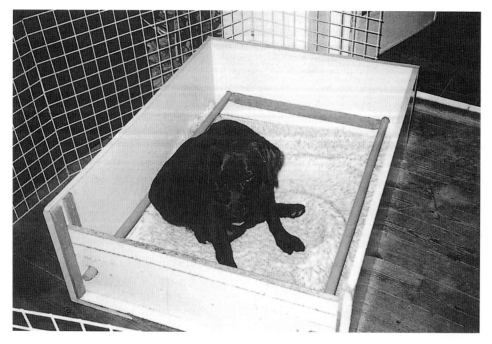

Figure 6.4   The whelping box. Note creep rails around the edge to avoid the dam crushing the new-born puppies. Some of the front side slats are removable to allow easier entry and exit for dam and puppies. Queens will require a similar arrangement but smaller and usually with a lid and a hole in the front for access.

The queen may need to be introduced even earlier as it will probably be necessary first to get her used to the whelping bed and then gradually moving it to the preferred birth area. Queens are well known for deciding to give birth in airing cupboards or on beds because they have not been given sufficient time to be gradually introduced to the owner's preferred area. The queen is not so malleable as the bitch in this respect and some compromises may need to be made.

The birth should be supervised if possible but the attendant should take an observing role and not interfere unless absolutely necessary. Most animals will cope instinctively with the birth by licking away the amnion (outer sac which the neonate is born in) and tearing through the umbilical cord. This licking stimulates the neonate's respiration and circulation and it will quite quickly find a nipple and start to suck. Sometimes the new mother is unsure what to do with the first born or may ignore or show fear during the first delivery because it has been painful. In this case the attendant may need to give assistance by ensuring the amnion is broken and the newborn's airways are clear. The umbilical cord should be severed ideally by placing a sterile artery forceps about two inches from the puppy and cutting the cord on the side away from the puppy with scissors. If forceps are not available, tearing the cord rather than cutting is necessary.

Signs and stages of parturition

The owner or attendant should record the progress of the parturition (see Table 6.11 and Figs 6.5–6.10). If the bitch or queen has been straining strongly for two hours without anything being born it is possible they will need veterinary attention. Therefore the veterinary surgeon needs to be informed after one hour of purposeful straining without delivery so that appropriate advice can be given to the owner.

Colostrum

It is important for the new-born to receive the first milk or colostrum from its mother within 48 hours. After this time the gut of the neonate becomes closed to the larger components of colostrum such as antibodies and they are unable to be absorbed.

Warmth and care

The young puppy or kitten is unable to regulate its body temperature by shivering during the first 6–8 days of life and will require an ambient temperature of around 80°F (26.6°C) for the first 10 days. This is the

Table 6.11	Record of parturition progress			
Time	Straining	Sex	Colour	Weight
1.02 am	Fluid passed			
1.05 am	+ (Just visible)			
1.12 am	+			
1.20 am	+			
1.23 am	+			
1.25 am	++ (More purposeful)			
1.31 am	++			
1.40 am	++			
1.46 am	+++ (Strongly)			
1.50 am	+++			
1.52 am	+++			
1.54 am	+++			
1.55 am	Birth. Afterbirth delivered	M	Black	308 grams
2.30 am	+			
2.35 am	+			
2.40 am	++			
2.44 am	+++			
2.47 am	+++			
2.50 am etc.	Birth. Afterbirth not seen	F	Black	280 grams

temperature in the nest made up of the body heat from both the mother and the puppies or kittens. Therefore unless the litter consists of only one or two puppies or kittens the environmental temperature will be much lower, about 65–70°F (18.3–21°C). Care should be taken that heat lamps are not placed too near the puppies or heat pads are not turned up too high. If neonates are too hot or cold they will be very noisy and not settle even after feeding. Cold neonates may huddle in mounds on top of one another and the weaker ones can quickly die. Hot puppies may spread out too far away from each other and their mother and spend excessive amounts of time on their backs exposing their underparts in an attempt to keep cool and this can lead to dehydration.

The mother stimulates urination and defecation by licking the perineal region. This is something the nurse must simulate, if required to rear orphaned puppies or kittens, by rubbing the area with a small swab or cotton wool after each meal until urination and defecation has occurred.

Vetbed with a layer of newspaper underneath for absorbency is probably the best bedding (see

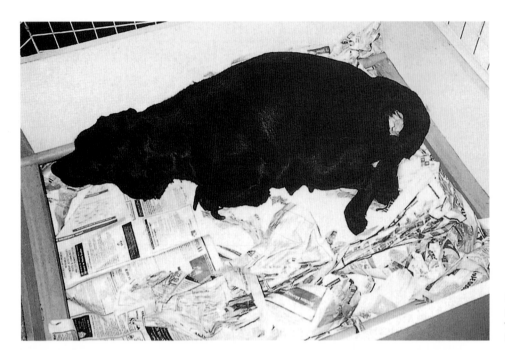

Figure 6.5 Second stage parturition. Positive straining with extended neck, arched back and raised tail.

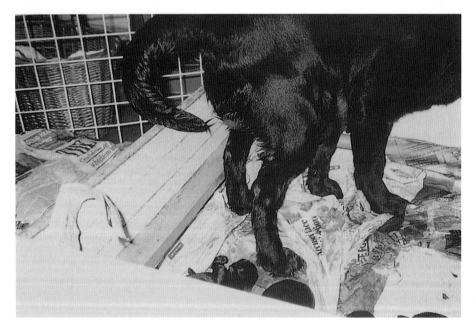

Figure 6.6 The puppy within the amnion is just visible at the vulva.

Figure 6.10). Until the young are on solid food the mother will clean up their urine and faeces by licking it up. As this mainly consists of milk it is not as distasteful as it sounds. As the young move onto solid food, which coincides with them becoming much more active, mum will become less keen to clean up after her offspring meaning more work for the owner. The mother will require two or three times her normal amount of balanced diet at this time, which must be fed in several small meals each day and access to plenty of fluids. Supplements are not necessary if a balanced diet, such as a preparatory growth diet, is fed.

The eyes of the young open from about 10 days of age, although focusing is not fully developed.

Weaning

Weaning starts at approximately 3 weeks in the dog and about 4–5 weeks in the cat. It should not be a sudden or dramatic occasion but a gradual interest by the offspring in solid food. The simplest measure is to offer some sloppy food in a low sided dish. The youngsters will get into the food dish and either start licking or, having got food on themselves, lick it off each other.

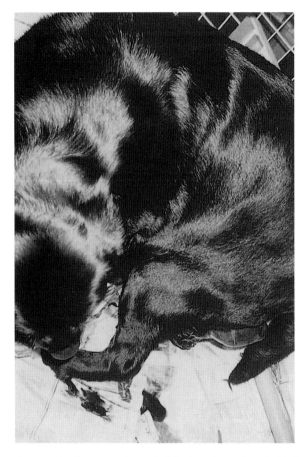

Figure 6.7 The puppy is nearly fully born. Note that the bitch has shredded lots of paper and that birth is a wet and bloody process so layers of newspaper which can be renewed as necessary are usually more useful than other bedding during the three stages of labour.

Once these tentative attempts to eat solid food have been mastered there will be a few weeks of the youngsters being fed two or three times a day with sloppy solid foods such as a preparatory puppy or kitten food, whilst still being fed by the mother. Gradually the mother will spend less and less time with her offspring and allow shorter time for them at the 'milk bar'. Her milk naturally starts to dry up as demand becomes less because the young start to get more nourishment out of their solid food.

An updated Breeding of Dogs Act came into force in January 2000 and requires anyone breeding puppies for a business or breeding five litters a year to obtain a local authority licence. Prior to this, the Act required anyone with more than two breeding bitches to obtain a licence.

HANDLING AND RESTRAINT

Many animals which attend the veterinary practice may be frightened, in pain or overexcited. All of these problems can be made worse by inexperienced or incompetent handling, inappropriate restraint methods, the use of unsuitable, or poorly fitting equipment or the incorrect use of such equipment.

Prevention

Thoughtful handling can often prevent an animal panicking and causing avoidable handling or restraint problems. Always ensure that collars are tight enough not to slip over the animal's head. If an animal thinks it can

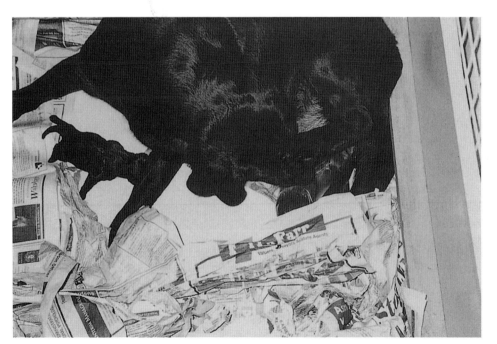

Figure 6.8 The puppy is born in the amnion which the mother is starting to lick away. Note a previously born puppy in the box. If the mother is very agitated prior to or during the birth of other puppies they can be temporarily moved to a separate box providing they are kept warm. They can be returned to suckle between births and moved again as necessary.

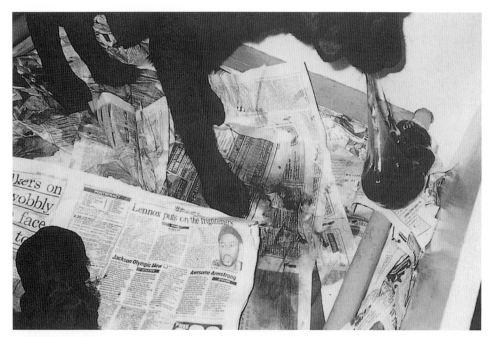

Figure 6.9 The bitch removing the puppy from the amnion and tearing the umbilical cord. Naturally this can be quite a violent process but probably also helps to stimulate the puppy's vital processes. This mother was quite rough with the cord and pups during this stage but none acquired umbilical hernias which are normally an inherited not acquired condition.

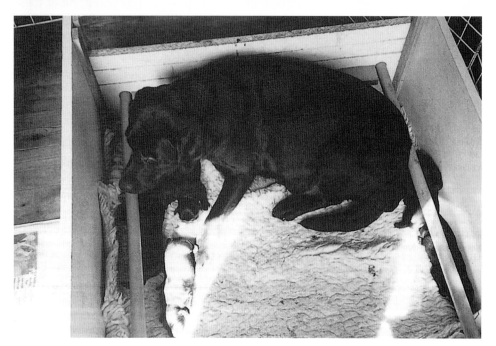

Figure 6.10 Post parturient phase. The bitch settles with her puppies which have been checked for any congenital defects. Vetbed is replaced. Note the creep bars in use.

escape it is more likely to try. Animals will sometimes be easier to move if owners come with them. If this is not appropriate asking the owner to leave the building first will often ensure the animal goes with the nurse more happily. Nervous or aggressive dogs are often best with the lead left on in the kennel as this is easy to get hold of or hook out and avoids a possible confrontation with the animal.

Wherever possible animals should be taught to associate positive experiences with the veterinary practice instead of fearful ones. Do this by ensuring that time is spent with animals during routine procedures and check-ups, such as health clinics or boosters, in reassuring them, by giving titbits, making friends and even having a short but not too overly exciting game. For hospitalised animals the use of 'soothing' pheromones, such as feline facial pheromones ('Feliway') or dog appeasment pheromone (DAP) to ensure a conducive environment, the provision of shoe boxes to hide in or other items, such as familiar smelling toys or towels to increase animal confidence level, are also worthwhile practices (see Figure 6.11).

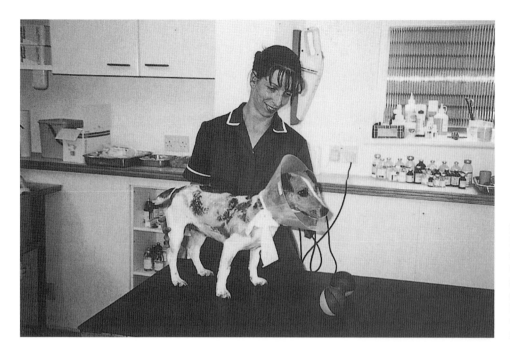

Figure 6.11 This badly burnt dog requires minimal restraint but the provision of a favourite toy and daily games helps to keep his attention away from the Elizabethan collar he must wear to prevent self-mutilation.

General considerations

The aims are to enable:

- safety of handler/restrainer
- safety of the person examining or treating the animal
- security and avoidance of injury to the restrained animal
- reduction of anxiety in the restrained animal
- reduction of anxiety and creation of confidence by owners or others witnessing the procedure
- prevention of the animal learning to avoid the restraining procedure in the future
- operator to examine or treat specific parts/areas of the animal
- lowest level of restraint possible in order to achieve these aims.

Preparation

Personal preparation
1. Hair tied back to prevent contamination and obscuring of animal or site to be examined.
2. Jewellery removed to prevent animal catching claws, limbs or teeth in it.
3. Correct protective clothing worn and fastened properly. It should be of a sensible fit and length to prevent riding up or splitting and to retain flexibility of restrainer. Frightened or nervous animals may evacuate, therefore disposable aprons are sometimes necessary.

4. Ensure in advance the procedures to be carried out, so that a suitable restraint position can be adopted (see Figs 6.12–6.18).
5. Arrange help as necessary to lift or restrain heavy or difficult animals correctly (see Figs 6.19 and 6.20).
6. Find out any information from the owner or the animal's record card regarding any previous difficulties in handling or restraining the animal.

General preparation
1. Prepare and check the condition of any restraining or transport equipment that may be necessary (see Table 6.12).
2. Ensure complete familiarity with use of any restraint equipment required (see Figure 6.21).
3. Ensure any equipment the veterinary surgeon may need to examine or treat the animal is ready, so that the time required for restraint is reduced to a minimum.
4. Check that all gates, doors and windows are closed and secure.
5. Ascertain the temperament, mood and condition of the animal by talking to it in a soothing but confident voice whilst observing its body language and posture (see Figs 6.22 and 6.23)
6. Ensure correct lifting procedures are carried out to avoid injury to the handler (see Figs 6.19 and 6.20).

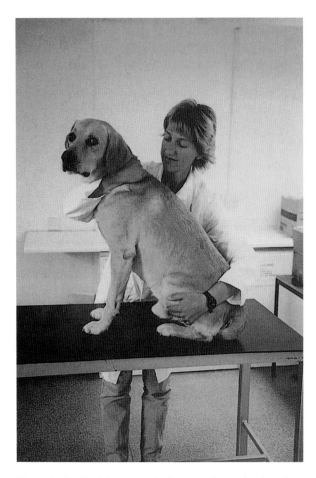

Figure 6.12 Body hug restraint for general examination of a dog. The handler's right arm can be moved close to the dog's head and by pulling the dog into her body she can gain even more control of this area. The left hand can be used to hold up the front leg for examination or intravenous injection.

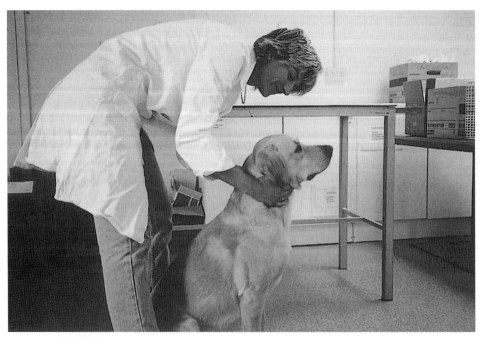

Figure 6.13 Using the collar to steady the dog's head and standing astride the body for examination of the head and front. For photographic reasons, the handler's head is nearer to the dog's head than normal.

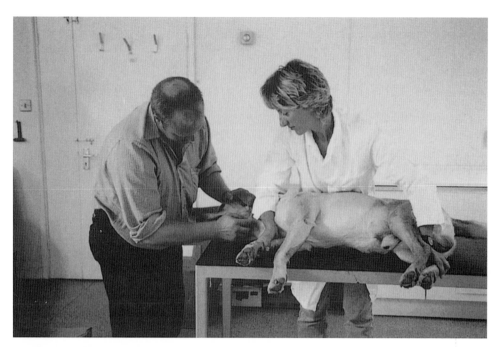

Figure 6.14 Lateral recumbency restraint. Where there is no abdominal conditions or injury the handler's left arm can be positioned in front of the upper hind leg and downward pressure on the dog's body will give even more control.

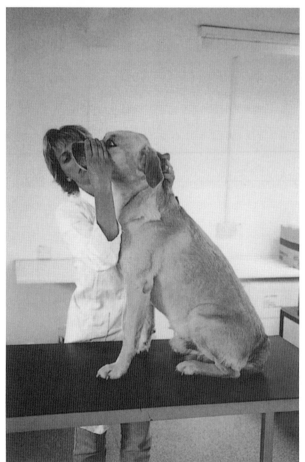

Figure 6.15 Restraint of the dog to allow examination of the eyes or ears. A muzzle could be applied if necessary and a second person could be used to steady the rump and prevent the dog pulling away backwards.

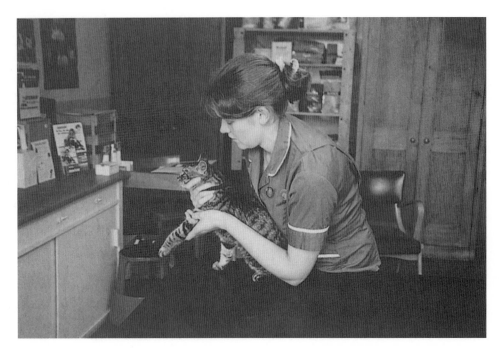

Figure 6.16 General restraint of a cat for intravenous injection. Stroking under the chin with a finger whilst restraining can relax the cat. The scruff can be held as an alternative in difficult cats. The cat can be held flat on the table with the other foreleg over the table edge to prevent scratching.

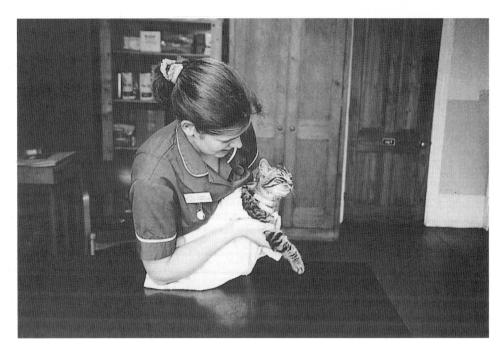

Figure 6.17 Using a towel to wrap up the body and legs of a more difficult cat. A cat bag could be used as an alternative.

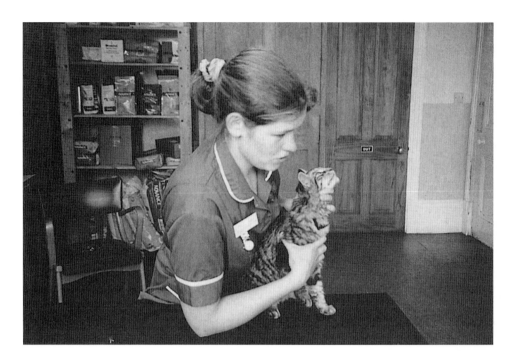

Figure 6.18 General restraint for jugular intravenous injection or collection.

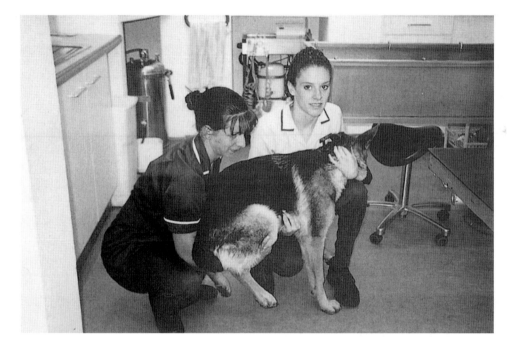

Figure 6.19 Lifting of a big dog. Bending from the knees with back straight.

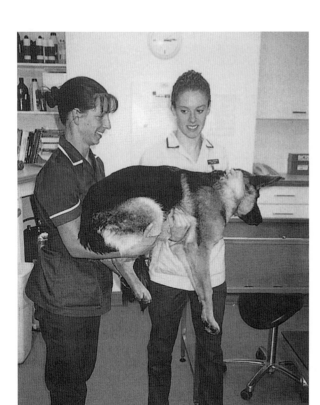

Figure 6.20 Animals should never be lifted under the soft abdomen.

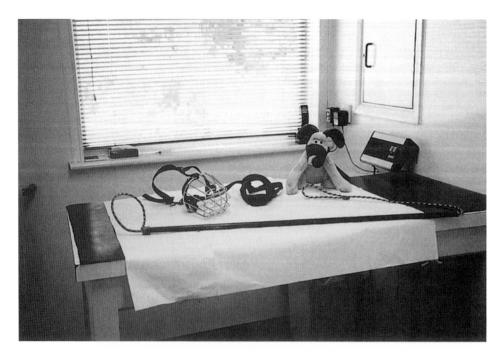

Figure 6.21 Restraint equipment. Front: dog or cat catcher. Back left: muzzle which allows panting and drinking. Centre and right: tight-fit muzzles for short-term use only.

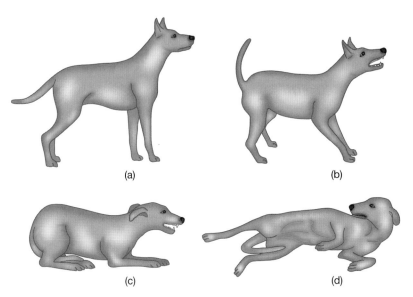

Figure 6.22   Canine body language. (a) A confident dog – ears pricked, no piloerection (hair standing up), tail level and still or gently wagging. (b) An aggressive dog – ears pricked, head high, neck stiff, tail high, may or may not be stiffly wagging or vibrating, piloerection along neck and dorsum (back), leaning into squared forequarters, hind quarters broadly set tense and ready to spring. (c) A fearful dog – piloerection but mostly over shoulders and hips, tail goes lower as fear increases, the head is in line with the plane of the back, feet closer together and legs lower to the ground. (d) A submissive dog – feet and limbs flexed, tail tucked, neck haunched and belly exposed, may urinate and salivate. **Notes:** dogs (b) and (c) will bite if approached or cornered. Also, dog d would normally only be sniffed by other dogs, so if handled may sometimes try to bite. These pictures represent the average dog. However, some long-coated breeds are unable to demonstrate piloerection and hair can conceal their body language. Docked dogs and brachycephalic breeds may also present difficulties when interpreting their body language.

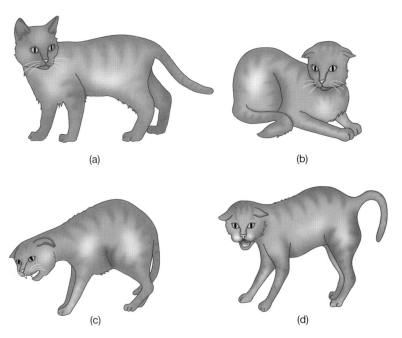

Figure 6.23   Feline body language. (a) A confident cat examining the environment. (b) A rather withdrawn cat with back arched, ears flat – may become fearfully aroused if provoked. (c) A non-confident cat provoked into defensive aggression. The ears are flat, the back is arched and the tail down, although the tail may rise as the cat becomes more aroused. (d) A more confident cat likely to stage an attack. The ears are pulled back but the body is more in line with the level of the head, the hind legs are extended, the tail piloerected and may be carried straight down.

Table 6.12	
Advantages	Disadvantages
Collars and leads	
1. Many designs and sizes available. 2. Easy to put on. 3. Dog and owner acceptance level high. 4. Can enable secure control.	1. Owners often put collars on too loosely so they slip off (2 fingers only should be able to be inserted under the collar, pull forward to ensure no slippage over the head). 2. Easy for dogs to pull on them. 3. Some breeds e.g. Bull Terriers slip out of them because of head shape and need much wider fitting. 4. Push down spring action lead clips can get caught on dogs leading to injury. Pull back action is preferable.
Check chains and slip leads	
1. Easy to buy and slip on. 2. Variety of materials: metal, nylon and cord available (some softer/kinder than others). 3. Comfortable for dogs which walk to heel well. 4. Owner acceptance high. 5. Can reduce pulling if used correctly.	1. Owners often put them on upside down. 2. Difficult for non experts to use correctly. 3. Often results in owners jerking or constantly pulling on the dog's neck which can lead to permanent traumatic damage. 4. Dogs can slip out of them if slack (a stop should be attached) or strangle themselves if they get caught up.
Harnesses	
1. Variety of designs and materials. 2. The best designs can reduce pulling. 3. Well tolerated by dogs. 4. Usually secure control.	1. Can be difficult to put on. 2. Can be difficult to ensure proper fitting and size. 3. Can cause chaffing if incorrect fit or design for dog. 4. Some designs loosen when lead is relaxed, allowing dog to step out of them.
Headcollars	
1. Can dramatically reduce pulling. 2. Can be used in conjunction with traditional collar and lead for extra control. 3. Easy for owners to control dog's head 4. Can prevent dog from biting/barking if used correctly. 5. Dogs will often paw at them so cannot always be left on unattended.	1. Can be difficult to find right design for differing dogs' heads. 2. Needs fitting by someone experienced as initial tolerance by dogs is low and positive reinforcement techniques are required. 3. Some dogs can slip out of them. 4. Owner tolerance can be low.
Flexi leads	
1. Allows some controlled freedom for dogs. 2. Can be stopped at short or longer lengths. 3. Useful training aid. 4. Can be used with collars, headcollars or harnesses.	1. Owners need to be shown how to check rather than haul dogs in. 2. Dogs/owners can get tangled in them. 3. Large dogs can pull owners off their feet. 4. Control mechanism can fail and rope burn can result if handle not held. 5. Handle can clank and frighten dog.

Common types of restraint equipment for difficult animals:

Cats
- crush cages
- restraining bags
- muzzles
- grabbers.

Dogs
- catchers
- muzzles

- quick muzzles made from a length of bandage.

Muzzles should never be left on unsupervised as dogs may vomit and asphyxiate. Never let dogs paw at them and get them off as they may learn this trick making future use very difficult.

Brachycephalic breeds such as boxers and bulldogs are difficult to muzzle and should not be held by the scruff of the neck because of the risk of eyeball prolapse. Wrapping a rolled-up towel or blanket around the dog's neck will prevent it from turning round to bite.

Further reading

Breeding of Dogs Act (2000) HMSO, London.

Dallas, S. (1999) Manual of Veterinary Care. British Small Mammal Veterinary Association.

England, G. (1996) Normal parturition in the bitch. Veterinary Nursing Journal 11:39–44.

Hewitt, D., England, G. (1999) Sexual development and puberty in the bitch. Veterinary Nursing Journal 14:131–135.

Lane, D.R., Cooper, B. (eds) (1999) Veterinary Nursing. Butterworth-Heinemann, Oxford.

Simpson, G. (1998) Manual of Small Animal Reproduction and Neonatology. British Small Animal Veterinary Association.

Venturi Rose, J. (1999) Dog breeding, managing the mating. Veterinary Nursing Journal 14:18–23.

Responsibilities and legalities

Helen Dingle

Chapter objectives

This chapter gives an introduction to:

- Responsibilities of pet owners
- Charitable organisations
- Pet insurance
- Identification and dog registration
- Dangerous Dogs Act
- Pets and society
- Quarantine
- Pet Travel Scheme

RESPONSIBILITY OF PET OWNERS

Deciding to take responsibility for an animal is the first step of many years of good husbandry. The animal owner has a duty to members of the public and to other animals by keeping their pet under controlled supervision at all times. Their animals should not present a health risk to other animals or people and basic hygiene precautions should be practised at all times.

Toilet training is foremost and should commence as soon as the animal is introduced into its home. Dogs can be trained to toilet at home and cats should be litter trained to prevent soiling in the garden. Excitement, car journeys and illness can result in your animal fouling land when out for a walk so be prepared and carry a poop scoop or alternative and promote responsible dog ownership.

Elementary obedience should also be taught from an early age, enabling the handler to gain respect from the pet also.

Guidelines for responsible pet ownership

- Obedience train your animal
- Ensure your dog wears a collar with an identity tag
- Train your dog (and cat) to toilet at home
- Always carry a poop scoop for emergencies!
- Ensure regular vaccinations are given
- Administer parasiticides as a preventative measure
- Offer a balanced nutritional diet
- Provide adequate exercise
- Prevent unwanted offspring by getting your pet neutered
- Do NOT let your pet be a nuisance to neighbours, especially with excessive noise
- Do NOT allow your dog to enter food halls (unless they have special access, e.g. Guide Dogs)
- Prevent access to farm land; livestock worrying is an offence and can result in the shooting or compulsory euthanasia of your pet
- Ensure you provide enough TLC!

There are various current legislations to cover 'responsible pet ownership' and the following Acts are of particular significance:

- **Dog fouling of Land Act 1996 and Dog fouling bylaws.** These state that it is an offence to allow your animal to foul a public highway without clearing it up.
- **Animals Act 1971 (not applicable to Scotland).** This will provide the defence if an animal is injured or killed as part of the protection of livestock.
- **Protection of Animals Acts 1911–1988.** If there is known cruelty to an animal, then disqualification can follow. Cruelty can cover beating, kicking, administration of poisons (including known drugs), fighting or baiting.
- **Abandonment of Animals Act 1960** states that it is an offence for any one to knowingly abandon an animal without good reason.
- **Dangerous Dogs Act 1991.** This Act prohibits the breeding, selling, exchanging or parting as a gift of certain breeds of dog, often kept for the intention of fighting. Animals listed under this Act have additional requirements with reference to

identification and access to public land. The breeds named by this Act are:

Pit Bull Terrier
Japanese Tosa
Dogo Argentino
Fila Braziliero.

Any dog that is a cross breed or shows any resemblance to the listed breeds has to comply with the strict regulations or face prosecution.

Each animal has to be permanently identified, neutered and covered by third party insurance and, when on public land, must be muzzled and secured by a person over the age of 16 years.

▪ **Dangerous Wild Animals Act 1976.** This controls the ownership of a wild dangerous animal by stating that no-one is to keep one without being in receipt of a licence by the local authority.

The companion animal is normally well loved and enjoyed by its owner, but circumstances can change; neglect sometimes occurs. When the animal is originally purchased, there may be all good intentions to care for it, but financial pressures or relationship breakdowns can result in the animal's future becoming uncertain. Abandonment is not an option and is illegal, but re-homing via an animal charity is a choice that can be adopted without the animal suffering from neglect or welfare issues.

There are many animal welfare organisations and they have a responsibility to ensure and regulate the control and welfare of animals. The Dog Warden, Police Constable and RSPCA Inspectors are all involved with animals mistreated in the community; they enforce local bylaws and aim to educate the public on responsible pet ownership. Certified charities rely on public support and therefore run through contributions collected during fund raising programmes and donations. They do not receive government funding and are primarily involved with the care and re-homing of such animals.

The facilities remain open all year round to received unwanted pets.

▪ **Wildlife and Countryside Act 1981.** This Act gives protection to wild and game birds and some wild creatures. Under this Act, species are listed as schedules which read as follows:

Schedule 1 – Birds which are protected by special penalties
Schedule 2 – Birds that may be killed or taken
Schedule 3 – Birds that may be sold
Schedule 4 – Birds which must be registered and ringed if kept in captivity
Schedule 5 – Animals that are not protected
Schedule 6 – Animals that may not be killed or taken by certain methods
Schedule 4 – Protects the most endangered species of British bird. Any bird kept legally in captivity has to be licensed, ringed and registered with the

---

Wildlife and Countryside Act 1981, Birds included on Schedule 4

• Bunting, cirl	• Fish-eagle, Madagascar	• Kestrel, Mauritius	• Shorelark
• Bunting, Lapland	• Forest-falcon, plumbeous	• Kite, red	• Shrike, red-backed
• Bunting, snow	• Goshawk	• Merlin	• Sparrowhawk, New Britain
• Buzzard, honey	• Harrier, hen	• Oriole, golden	• Sparrowhawk, Gundlach's
• Eagle, Adalbert's	• Harrier, marsh	• Osprey	• Sparrowhawk, small
• Eagle, golden	• Harrier, Montagu's	• Redstart, black	• Tit, bearded
• Eagle, great Philippine	• Hawk, Galapagos	• Redwing	• Tit, crested
• Eagle, imperial	• Hawk, grey-backed	• Sea-eagle, Pallas'	• Warbler, Cetti's
• Eagle, New Guinea	• Hawk, Hawaiian	• Sea-eagle, Steiler's	• Warbler, Dartford
• Eagle, white-tailed	• Hawk, Ridguùay's	• Serin	• Warbler, marsh
• Chough	• Hawk, white-necked	• Serpent-eagle, Andaman	• Warbler, Savi's
• Crossbills (all species)	• Hawk-eagle, Wallace's	• Serpent-eagle, Madagascar	• Woodlark
• Falcon, Barbary	• Hobby	• Sparrowhawk, imitator	• Wryneck
• Falcon, gyr	• Honey-buzzard, black	• Serpent-eagle, Mountain	
• Falcon, peregrine	• Kestrel, lesse		
• Fieldfare			
• Firecrest			

Any bird, one of whose parents or other lineal ancestor was a bird of a kind specified in the above list.
All birds of prey in the world with the exception of vultures and condors.

Table 7.1 Management of common wild life species

Animal	Handling	Housing	Diet	Zoonotic potential	Release
Hedgehog	Wear gloves Place inside a box to transport Gentle rocking may assist the animal to unroll but anaesthesia usually required	Newspaper lining (not shredded to prevent encircling the legs) Clean towel (to hide under) Nest box	Dog/cat food (especially Canine Maintenance dry or feline growth dry) Worms Snails Water (not milk which is difficult to digest)	None in the UK	Not territorial so can be released in a suitable habitat if origin is unknown
Birds	Encase whole body (to include wings) and support the head to prevent pecking	Quiet area of practice Away from predator species Newspaper lining (assists with cleaning and faecal observation) Natural wood perch	Herbivores: Seed, poultry food, grains Carnivores: Mice, chicks, road kills, worms (important to offer food the bird can recognise)	*Chlamydia psittici*	Depends on species

Department of the Environment, Transport and Regions (DETRI) now reconfigured as DEFRA. As these closed rings are applied over the foot of the birds whilst they are in the nest as chicks an absence may indicate a bird being kept illegally. The veterinary surgeon in receipt of a Schedule 4 bird may treat it for up to 6 weeks without the need for registering with DETRI (DEFRA) but must keep records of any such occurrence. A full list of birds within this schedule can be seen (see Box on facing page).

Wildlife casualties (Table 7.1)

First aid can be applied as an interim method, but it is the Veterinary Surgeon's responsibility to examine and treat wildlife that have been brought to the surgery as a casualty. The decision whether to treat or euthanase the animal must be made immediately to reduce any unnecessary pain or suffering, and with the aim of releasing the animal back to the wild as soon as is practically possible. It is important to acknowledge that the patient will experience pain like their domestic counterpart and will attempt to attack the handler as a method of protection. By utilising the correct handling procedures injuries can be prevented and unnecessary stress reduced in an unfamiliar environment. In addition safe housing should be provided during its temporary hospitalisation until it can be transferred to a Licensed Rehabilitation Keeper or released back to the wild (see Chapter 11).

CHARITABLE ORGANISATIONS
RSPCA and SSPCA

The Royal Society for the Prevention of Cruelty to Animals and the Scottish equivalent (The Scottish Society for the Prevention of Cruelty to Animals) find new homes for 70 000 animals annually and answer one telephone call on their cruelty line every 25 seconds. The 323 uniformed RSPCA Inspectors and 146 Animal Collection Officers (ACOs) are involved with rescue and rehabilitation of animals and with Veterinary Hospitals and animal care centres around the UK. They provide information on the care and welfare of animals to the general public and schools, and to society generally. The four main areas of welfare concerning the RSCPA include:

- Animal experimentation
- Farming
- Wildlife
- Pet ownership.

PDSA

The People's Dispensary for Sick Animals (PDSA) provides free treatment for animals whose owners are genuinely unable to afford the treatment and can provide evidence of state benefits. Each Veterinary Centre has a geographical band stating which areas it serves.

PDSA hospitals are used as training centres for Veterinary Nurses and the organisation employs many hundreds of staff, including animal carers and kennel maids.

Blue Cross

Staff of the Blue Cross care for domestic and equine animals via their veterinary hospitals and clinics around the UK. Volunteers are available to walk and groom the patients and carry out fund raising activities to continue the rescue mission of ill-treated pets.

Dogs' Trust

Dogs' Trust exists to protect and defend all dogs from abuse, cruelty, abandonment and from any form of mistreatment. The organisation also promotes responsible dog ownership.

CPL

The Cats' Protection League is a nationally recognised charity which specialises in the care of unwanted and stray felines.

As a method of population control, all charities neuter, or assist towards the cost of the operation. The aim is to prevent unwanted offspring. Charities also microchip animals and check potential homes to ensure the new owners can offer the correct care.

There are some specialised organisations which train dogs to assist the owner who has a disability, e.g.

Guide Dogs for the Blind Association (GDBA)
Hearing Dogs for the Deaf
Support Dogs
Dogs for the Disabled.

PET INSURANCE

Unfortunately there is no equivalent to the National Health Service for the domestic pet and therefore owners must take responsibility for veterinary services that are required throughout their pet's life. A new owner should be advised and anticipate that, like humans, their pet will not necessarily remain healthy and medical assistance will need to be sought. To help prepare the owners for expenses incurred during illness or accident, there are insurance policies that can be accessed. Charities may be able to assist with a percentage of the final amount, but as previously mentioned they rely on public support and are in receipt of a limited budget.

Routine vaccinations, elective surgery and invoices not reaching the excess threshold cannot be claimed from the insurer and these expenses should be taken into account when deciding on a species and breed of pet.

Pet insurance is now regulated by The Financial Services Authority (FSA) who are an independent non-governmental body whose objective is to protect the consumer and reduce financial crime. Under FSA rules, veterinary practices can display insurance leaflets and point out the basics of pet insurance, but not compare individual companies and their differing policies. Practices can become registered with a specific insurance company and act as an Appointed Representative Practice or Introducer Appointed Representative

to give further advice and guidance again on a non-comparable basis.

IDENTIFICATION AND DOG REGISTRATION

Dog registration was in force for all dogs until the late 1980s. Each dog owner had to purchase a licence that would prove ownership and identity of their animals. Any dog over the age of 6 months had to have a licence and they expired on 31 December each year. A fine was issued for those who failed to register and purchase a document for their pet.

The last licences were issued in 1988 and owners are now advised to provide a method of identification on their pet at all times.

Although it is compulsory for listed breeds under the Dangerous Dogs Act, it is also a legal requirement under the Control of Dogs Order 1930 (consolidated in the Animal Health Act 1981) and requires that dogs are to wear identity discs in public places. Dogs that are seized and have no identity can be impounded by the Dog Warden and the owner, once informed, will have to pay a fee consisting of boarding costs, vaccinations etc., and be advised on responsible pet ownership before being allowed to have their pet returned.

As discussed, identification is a method of retrieval if your pet goes missing. Without it, the pet could be a permanent stray, be re-homed or destroyed. There are various straightforward methods and procedures that can be undertaken, the most common and relatively inexpensive being the collar and tag.

Alternative methods include:

- Photographs
- Micro-chipping
- Tattooing
- Leg rings for birds.

Photographs are useful where there are distinguishable features and can assist friends and neighbours in recognising a lost pet.

Microchips are becoming increasingly popular, especially with the new Pet Travel Scheme, and are a permanent and effective method of identification. Most chips are ISO regulated and can therefore be read by most hand-held scanners. All animal charities, Dog Wardens and similar animal welfare based organisations have access to these scanners and can reunite pet and owner in as few as two phone calls.

The process involves the painless injection of a tiny microchip implant under the skin, between the two scapulae (shoulder blades), away from normal injection sites. The implant is normally encapsulated within 24 hours and migration throughout the tissue is rare.

Weighing less that 1/100th of an ounce, the micro-electronic device is encased in a bio-glass capsule. It will only release information when a corresponding scanner is applied to the area of insertion and the data retrieved. Throughout this process, the animal does not feel a thing and is unaware of the procedure.

Tattooing is another method of permanent identification and all owners of tattooed animals are advised to register the pet with the 'National Dog Tattoo Register' which holds the relevant information in preparation for retrieval. The tattoos are placed in a relatively hairless area of the body, e.g. the inside of the ear pinnae and the medial aspect of the proximal femur.

Leg rings are used in birds and are placed over a bird's foot between the ages of 8 to 10 days. They come in a variety of sizes to suit each breed and are used in a similar way to that of a car registration plate. Each number, as with tattoos and microchips, is unique and can be identified by the bird fancier and records can be adjusted as appropriate.

▪ **Dangerous Dogs Act 1991 (amended 1997).**
   Animals listed under this Act have additional
   requirements with reference to identification
   and access to public land. This Act prohibits the
   breeding, selling, exchanging or parting as a gift of
   certain breeds of dog, often kept for the intention
   of fighting.

The breeds named are:

Pit Bull Terrier
Japanese Tosa
Dogo Argentino
Fila Braziliero.

Any dog that is cross bred or has any resemblance to the above breeds has to comply with the regulations or its owners may face prosecution. Each animal has to be permanently identified, neutered and covered by third party insurance and, when on public land, must be muzzled and on a lead secured by a person over the age of 16 years.

PETS AND SOCIETY
Benefits provided by pets

Pet ownership is becoming increasingly popular with the majority of households owning at least one, if not more animals. These are not only dogs and cats. The influence of television documentaries and publications relating to animal care and veterinary work have made a considerable contribution to the pet world and also to the variety of species there are available to purchase.

Why people decide to own a pet relates to individual needs, but they are normally a source of comfort, security and companionship.

Pet ownership is an emotional bond between two living beings and extensive thought must be put into deciding on a purchase and how you plan to look after the animal during the time it is in your care. They provide health benefits by reducing stress and anxiety, a common disorder of today's lifestyle.

Although allergies and sensitivities, especially amongst children, are on the increase, there are breeds that can be owned by sufferers that will have minimal to nil effects when handled. Medical advice should always be sought to prevent illness or disappointment.

Animals are also used to support disabilities or medical disorders, e.g. diabetes. The animals complete an extensive and specialised training programme, allowing them to open and close doors, switch lights on and off, assist with dressing changes, warn their owners they are to suffer from a seizure and aiding their handlers across the road. These pets are working animals but are also an invaluable source of independence and comfort for the owner.

Pets that develop alongside children are often more tolerant. The child benefits from the responsibility and education a living creature presents when correct handling and care is offered.

Buying and choosing a pet

Prior to making a purchase on an expensive piece of equipment for their home, the home owner would compile a list of qualities required then compare them to the goods on offer. It is normally a lengthy process covering reasons why the equipment is required, how often it would be used, how often would it require servicing, would it take up too much room and would it fit in with the decor! Although inanimate objects require care, animals require much more attention and similar questions should be asked when advising the owner on which pet to purchase.

Small mammals such as rabbits, guinea pigs and rodents still remain popular with the younger generation as they are compact, relatively easy to handle and take up little space, but other species within the 'exotics' group are gaining rapid approval with many households, possibly without essential knowledge on their specialised husbandry. Always be prepared and be practical when dealing with customers who require your knowledge on animals. Compile a list of questions that need to be asked, even design a 'which pet' questionnaire which can be a fun process as well as a serious learning exercise.

Involve the following questions:

Reasons for owning a pet
Companionship
Necessity (GDBA, Dogs for Disabled)
Aid change of lifestyle for owner
Working – Gundog, Security

Size of house/garden
Exercise requirements
Accommodation
Access to fresh grass
Storage area for feed/cleaning materials
Restrictions by landlord/Council?

Lifestyle
Working shifts
Part-time
Working away from home
Frequent holidays
Age (elderly/young)
Health (allergies/disabled)
Weekend/holiday cover for animals kept in schools and colleges

Previous experience
Multi household
Beginner's pet

Financial implications
Initial outlay
Daily costs
Routine vaccinations and treatment
Insurance option available?

Species
Check temperament
Any specialised equipment required?
Any special dietary requirements?

Breed
Size
Colour
Coat
Medical problems
Restrictions
Pet insurance availability.

Once the decision on the choice of pet has been decided, a suitable outlet needs to be sought. Animals can be obtained from various sources ranging from the big pet supermarkets to the smaller, relatively unknown, hobby breeders. Animals bred and sold in large shipments are not necessarily the most healthy and the client should be advised to visit various suppliers before acquiring their pet.

Any breeding establishment that has two or more breeding bitches must be licensed under the **Breeding of Dogs Act 1973**. Pet shops are controlled by the **Pet Animals Act 1951** and this legislation prohibits the selling of animals in a street or public place. It also controls the selling of animals to children under 12 years of age.

If purchasing a pedigree animal, check that documents are available and that the sire and dam have been tested against some of the more common hereditary diseases such as hip dysplasia in dogs.

Unfortunately some pet sale outlets do little to assist and prepare the owner with their choice and whether it will be suitable to fit in with their modern lifestyle. The pet is taken away to a new, relatively unprepared environment. Leaflets provided at some larger stores for the owner to take home and view should, ideally, be complemented with a verbal discussion with an experienced and knowledgeable member of staff.

Alternative sources for finding a pet are the Veterinary Practice and Charity organisations that temporarily house strays and unwanted pets. These shelters employ staff who perform 'home checks' and gain relevant information about the family before allowing the animals to be re-homed, ensuring the pet and owner are a suitable match. Owning animals from an early age can provide you with invaluable knowledge that is often not gained through reading books or leaflets.

Honest advice is the best advice to offer and, on occasions, the owner will realise that they need to re-evaluate their plans and concentrate on another species that may be a more suitable companion.

QUARANTINE

Isolation is the segregation of one animal from another
Quarantine is compulsory isolation.

The British Isles have used quarantine as a method of disease control since the early 1900s. Its strict rules and guidelines have controlled, and eventually, eradicated, some contagious and possibly zoonotic disease from the UK. All imported warm-blooded mammals and birds are placed into isolation to allow their bodies to incubate a disease, if infected, and show symptoms or 'clinical signs' that can be clearly diagnosed and controlled without placing any immediate danger to other animals or the public.

The most significant threat from imported animals is from rabies, and **The Rabies (Importation of Dogs, Cats and Other Mammals) Order 1974** requires that imported dogs and cats stay in a quarantine kennel for 6 calendar months.

For birds, including poultry, the **Importation of Birds, Poultry and Hatching Eggs Order 1979**, is referred to, to prevent unwanted outbreaks of foreign disease within the avian community.

Rabies is a potential killer and this section will review the legislation and control methods adopted by the UK to prevent an outbreak.

Quarantine kennels

Animals staying at a quarantine kennel are housed separately, with the exception being two animals of the same species and from the same household sharing a compartment. There are various Department of the Environment, Food and Rural Affairs (DEFRA) approved quarantine kennels throughout the UK and they are privately owned but authorised by the DEFRA and each have their own Veterinary Superintendent who visits the kennels and checks the animals every day, excluding Sunday, unless requested.

The choice of kennel, with respect to its location, is made by the owner and the decision normally reflects the visiting accessibility, with the owner choosing an establishment close to their family home as opposed to the point of entry into the UK. The animal is transported from the dock or airport to the kennels via an approved carrier and is vaccinated against rabies within 48 hours. Owners cannot visit their pet for the first 14 days of their stay, but these restrictions are then relaxed, allowing the owner to arrange appointments with the kennel owner to see their pet.

DEFRA can supply a list of kennels but will not specify in which kennel the animal must reside nor pass comment on the differing services offered.

Each kennel has to meet certain criteria on height, width and length, allowing the animal room to defecate, urinate and exercise comfortably whilst still within its allocated space (Table 7.2).

Basic requirements also cover the providence of fresh air and visual stimuli to prevent boredom and depression, especially in those housed on their own. Cats should be provided with sleeping boxes and scratching posts with additional toys if required. No contact with the other boarders is allowed, and breech of these guidelines could result in a further stay of 6 months.

The building material used must be impervious and hardwearing, making them easy to clean and disinfect routinely. Any cleaning materials used must meet DEFRA guidelines to ensure strict hygiene and disease control methods are adhered to and are successful. An extensive list of approved disinfectants can again be sought from the local DEFRA office or website.

All costs accrued by the quarantined animal during its stay are met by the owner. This includes the transportation from the point of entry into the UK to the kennels, veterinary services, daily boarding fees and any material (e.g. bedding, bowls, litter trays etc.) that are used during its segregation period.

The approximate cost of quarantining an animal in 2004 was £350 per month. Bedding, bowls etc. used by the animal have to be disposed of by incineration on site, following discharge of the pet.

There are alternatives to quarantine. One option is the **Balai Directive**, which has been in operation since July 1992 and works in conjunction with the **Rabies (Importation of Dogs, Cats and Other Mammals) Order 1974**. It allows commercially traded dogs and cats to enter the UK from other Member States (not the Republic of Ireland) without the quarantine requirement, as long as they conform to the following criteria:

(i) The animal was born on a registered holding and has remained there since birth, having no contact with wild animals susceptible to rabies
(ii) It has been vaccinated against rabies with an inactivated vaccine when at least three months of age and at least six months before export
(iii) It has been blood tested after vaccination to show that this had resulted in an adequate level of protective antibodies against rabies
(iv) It is accompanied by a veterinary health certificate and vaccination record
(v) It is individually identified by an implanted microchip
(vi) Details of movement into the UK have been notified to one of the Agriculture departments in the UK at least 24 hours in advance (MAFF 1997).

Table 7.2 Quarantine kennels			
	Small dogs Less than 12 kg (26 lb)	Medium dogs 12–30 kg (26–66 lb)	Large dogs 30 kg (66 lb)
Sleeping compartment area	Not less than 1.1 m^2	Not less than 1.4 m^2	Not less than 4 m^2
Width and length	Not less than 0.9 m	1.2 m	1.2 m
Exercise run area	Not less than 3.7 m^2	5.5 m^2	7.4 m^2
Width	Not less than 0.9 m	1.2 m	1.2 m
Height of unit	Not less than 1.8 m	1.8 m	1.8 m
Source: MAFF Publications PB 2109. Cats: Sleeping compartment and exercise area must have total minimum floor area of 1.4 m^2, width and length not less than 0.9 m.			

The second option is the new Pet Travel Scheme, also known as the acronym, PETS. This is a new system that piloted in February 2000 with a small collection of UK resident animals and owners travelling abroad and returning to the UK without the need for quarantine.

In order for a dog or cat to qualify under the PETS agreement, they must also meet set criteria and have proof of doing so.

The basic requirement is for the animal to be UK resident (UK is rabies free); additional requirements are listed below and must be in the following order. The animal must:

(i) be fitted with a microchip implant
(ii) be vaccinated against rabies using an approved inactivated vaccine
(iii) be blood tested to show that the vaccine has worked and the animal has produced antibodies
(iv) be issued with an official PETS certificate
(v) be treated against ticks and tapeworms before arriving back in the UK.

Although this system is in use in the UK, quarantine has NOT been abolished. Additional information can be obtained from a Veterinary Surgeon or by obtaining a DEFRA fact sheet.

It is important that the microchips implanted before the vaccine is given, as it will be the animals permanent method of identification. A microchip that conforms to ISO (International Standards Organisation) standard 11784 or to Annex A of ISO standards 11785 is thoroughly recommended as most scanners will be able to read the data on the chip. Alternative microchips will require a different type of hand-held scanner and this must be provided by the owner whenever the microchip is to be read for identification purposes.

The blood tests are performed in a DEFRA approved laboratory and the British Isles offers this test in laboratories. Laboratories receive blood samples taken from animals vaccinated with the rabies vaccine 30 days previous to sampling. Any correspondence with the laboratory should be left to the Veterinary Surgeon.

Treatment against foreign ticks and tapeworms before returning to the UK are to control potential zoonotic disease.

Rabies

This is a virus that affects the central nervous system (CNS) of all mammals. The disease is transmitted via penetration of the skin (depositing the virus-laden saliva) or, in the cases of bats, via aerosol droplets invading the oral/nasal mucosa. The rabies virus can be present in an animal's saliva for up to 14 days before clinical signs are shown, demonstrating how important close observation of the quarantined animal is justified.

The incubation period has a wide range, depending on the site of inoculation. A bite to the distal limb would have a longer incubation period compared to one on the head region as the muscle tissue is closer to the brain and spinal cord.

The virus is labile and like all viruses, cannot survive for long off the host. Strict hygiene precautions and the correct use of disinfectants are used as prophylaxis to an outbreak.

When the virus is still within the muscle tissue, a vaccine preparation can be administered and antibodies formed giving the animal a chance of survival. Unfortunately, once the virus has reached the nervous tissue, death is imminent.

Vaccination

Inactivated vaccines are used routinely in many rabies-affected countries and until the recent introduction of the new PETS importation scheme, vaccines could only be obtained following DEFRA authorisation and administered only when documentation concerning the export of animals was complete. Strict guidelines on their supply have now been reviewed. Humans in 'high risk' areas can receive rabies vaccine if required.

Suspect cases

When an animal is suspected of being rabid, the DEFRA must be contacted immediately and the animal isolated. This circumstance will be seen in quarantine kennels more readily than a veterinary practice, but staff must be prepared for this type of emergency.

Additional contacts would be:

- A local authority animal health inspector
- A police constable.

Action to be taken in the case of suspected rabies

1. Contact DEFRA, Police Constable and local health inspector
2. Confine animal (and people present)
3. Vet must stay with the animal at all times
4. DEFRA will set-up a 20 mile radius isolation area
5. Animal is euthanased
6. Head and brain are taken, via the DEFRA to the diagnostic lab
7. If personnel are bitten – wounds should be washed with soap and water. Follow with copious amounts of water. Apply iodine (or quaternary ammonium compound). Seek medical help ASAP.

Basic veterinary nursing

Microbiology and parasitology

Jo Masters

MICROBIOLOGY AND PARASITOLOGY

Microbiology

Microbiology is the study of micro-organisms (or microbes) such as:

Viruses, Bacteria, Fungi, Protozoa.

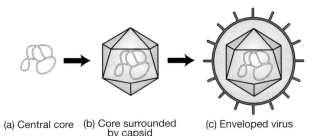

(a) Central core (b) Core surrounded by capsid (c) Enveloped virus

Figure 8.1 Structure of a virus.

If a micro-organism causes disease to cells it is known as a **pathogen**.

If this disease can be spread from animals to humans it is known as a **zoonotic disease**.

Micro-organisms range greatly in size from a large fungi to a microscopic virus, and they are measured using micrometres (microns) which are one thousandth of a millimetre in size.

Viruses

The study of viruses is known as **Virology**. A virus can only be viewed under an electron microscope, a row of a million viruses would only be around 5 millimetres long!

A virus is a relatively simple structure (Figure 8.1), which has a central core containing one of two types of nucleic acid:

▨ Deoxyribonucleic acid (DNA)
▨ Ribonucleic acid (RNA).

It will depend on the type of virus as to which of the nucleic acids are found in the central core. The nucleic acid in the core holds all the genetic material, or information required for the virus to multiply. This core is then surrounded by a protein coat called a capsid, and some viruses have a further protective layer called an envelope.

Animal viruses replicate by invading host cells. The nucleic acid will take over the metabolism of the host cell and direct it to form new virus material, after which the host cell will rupture and be destroyed. Therefore viruses are always parasitic, i.e. they always require a host cell in which to replicate (Figure 8.2).

Many viruses will invade the body cells with no apparent ill effect, it is only when a number of host cells have been destroyed that disease symptoms occur.

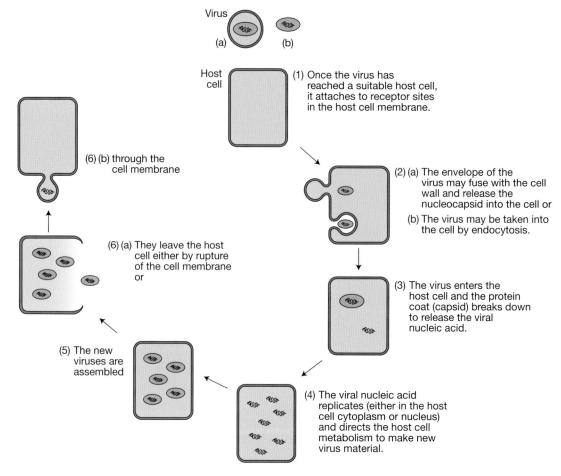

Figure 8.2 Replication of a virus.

Transmission of viruses

As previously discussed, viruses require entry into the host cell in order to replicate, and it will depend on the type of virus concerned as to how it will be transmitted from one host to another.

Most viral diseases are contagious, i.e. they spread from one animal host to another. This is done either by **direct contact**, where animals are in close proximity, e.g.

- housed together
- biting one another
- having sexual contact
- grooming one another.

or by **indirect contact**, where the host sheds virus into the environment to be picked up by another animal. Body fluids such as urine, faeces, and saliva are usually responsible, but sometimes the contaminated item can be an inanimate object such as a food bowl or bedding.

If the virus is found on an animate item, such as urine or faeces the item is known as a **vector**. If it is found on an inanimate object the object is known as a **fomite**.

Some animals carry disease without showing any symptoms. These animals are known as **carriers**, and can be very difficult to isolate due to the lack of clinical signs.

When a virus enters the new host it will eventually travel to its target organ and symptoms will occur. The animal's immune response will be acting against the virus and therefore will be depleted. As a result, bacteria gain easy access to the host animal causing a secondary bacterial infection, often causing more problems than the viral infection itself. (See Tables 8.1, 8.2 and 8.3.)

Bacteria

The study of bacteria is known as **Bacteriology**. A bacterial cell includes the following structures (Figure 8.3):

- Cell wall – maintains cell shape
- Nucleus – the brain of the cell, contains chromosomes
- Slime layer – protects cell
- Plasma or cell membrane – controls passage of substances into and out of cell and contains

Table 8.1 Common viral diseases affecting the dog*

Disease name	Common name	Zoonosis	Vaccine	Organ/s under attack	Symptoms	Transmission	Incubation
Canine distemper virus (CDV)	Distemper Hard pad	No	Yes	Central nervous system Respiratory system Gastrointestinal system Skin	Nasal and ocular discharge Coughing Vomiting and diarrhoea Fitting, disorientation Paralysis Hardening of pads	Direct contact (Mucous membranes) Inhalation Body fluids	7–21 days Virus killed by light, heat and disinfecting
Infectious canine hepatitis (ICH)	Hepatitis	No	Yes	Liver Kidneys	Sudden puppy deaths Acute pyrexia Acute abdominal pain Hepatitis Nephritis Clouding of cornea post-infection (Blue eye)	Direct contact Environment Urine and faeces ingestion (can be transmitted by foxes)	5–9 days Can survive off host for ≈10 days. Carriers can shed disease for up to six months
Canine parvovirus (CPV)	Parvo	No	Yes	Heart Gastrointestinal system	Myocarditis (puppies) Sudden puppy deaths Gastroenteritis (foul smell) Dehydration Shock Hypothermia Death	Direct contact Environment (faeces)	3–5 days Isolation of patients required
Canine parainfluenza virus (CPIV) Type of canine contagious respiratory disease (CCRD)	Kennel cough (term also includes respiratory disease caused by: *B. bronchiseptica*, Adenovirus CAV2, CDV)	No	Yes	Respiratory system (tracheobronchitis)	Coughing Nasal discharge Depression Self-limiting	Direct contact (inhalation from coughing) Seen where large numbers of dogs are together as in kennels	5–7 days Highly contagious – isolate patient, vaccinate prior to kennelling
Rabies virus	Rabies	Yes	Yes (for animals going to a country where rabies is endemic)	Nervous tissue (Brain and spinal cord)	Three stages: Preclinical: 2–3 days (bite wound, pyrexia) Furious: lasts ≈7 days (aggression, fitting, disorientation) Dumb: lasts ≈7 days (paralysis of pharynx and skeletal muscles – respiratory problems, excess salivation, death) These symptoms may be mixed – not all affected animals show all stages	Direct contact (saliva – bite wounds)	2 weeks–4 months (average 3 weeks)

*Routine vaccination programmes include the main four viral diseases that affect the dog – CDV, ICH, CPV, CPIV.

Table 8.2 Common viral diseases affecting the cat*

Disease name	Common name	Zoonosis	Vaccine	Organ/s under attack	Symptoms	Transmission	Incubation
Feline upper respiratory tract disease (FURD) Two causative viruses: Feline herpes virus 1 (FNV-1) (*Sometimes known as FVR – feline viral rhinotracheitis*) Feline calici virus (RCV)	Cat 'flu	No	Yes	Respiratory tract Conjunctiva Secondary bacterial infection is the cause of most symptoms	Sneezing Ocular and nasal discharge Anorexia, pyrexia Depression Ulceration of mucous membranes Keratitis Complications – chronic infection, bronchopneumonia, chronic rhinitis, carriers of FHV-1, excretors of FCV	Aerosol – sneezing of infected cats	2–10 days Prognosis generally good
Feline panleucopaenia	Feline infectious enteritis	No	Yes	Small intestine Lymphoid tissue Bone marrow Across placenta – brain damage – cerebellar hypoplasia	Sudden deaths in kittens Brain damaged kittens showing disorientation and in-coordination. Depression, anorexia Persistent vomiting Abdominal pain Diarrhoea in later stages – blood stained	Direct or indirect contact – ingestion of body fluids – saliva, vomit, faeces and urine Possibly also carried by fleas	2–10 days Occurs where many cats are housed together
Feline leukaemia virus (FeLV)	FeLV	No	Yes	Lymphatic tissue Cats may become symptomatic and seem to recover but may be carriers Some cats may develop an immunity	Pyrexia Vomiting and diarrhoea Weight loss Splenic enlargement Nephritis Kittens are very susceptible to the virus and may die within 3 years of infection. FeLV related conditions include: Lymphosarcoma Anaemia Other contagious viral diseases This is due to immunosuppression Once symptoms occur the prognosis is extremely poor	Direct contact Shed in body fluids such as saliva, urine, faeces and milk Often passed on during cat fights	Weeks–years Most cats will come across this virus at some stage in their life Commonly diagnosis in areas of high cat population

(*Continued*)

Disease				System affected	Clinical signs	Transmission	Notes
Feline immunodeficiency virus (FIV)	Feline AIDS	No	No	Lymphatic system (immunosuppressive) Many will recover initially, succumbing to immunodeficiency problems later	Pyrexia Generalised lymphadenopathy Secondary infections, conjunctivitis, nasal discharges, stomatitis, gingivitis, diarrhoea, neurological problems. More common in the male cat due to territorial fighting	Saliva – cat bites are thought to be the main route of transmission Sexual transmission	Weeks–years Frequent bouts of illness
Feline pneumonitis Causative agent is *Chlamydia psittaci* a virus-like microbe that lives within cells	Chlamydiosis	No	Yes	Conjunctiva Possibly reproductive tract	Conjunctivitis Pyrexia Diarrhoea in kittens Possible abortion or infertility	Direct contact with carrier cats – discharges from the mucous membranes; eyes, nose, gastrointestinal or genital tract. Carriers can shed the disease from several weeks post-recovery from symptoms	2–3 weeks Easily destroyed by disinfectants
Feline infectious anaemia (FIA) Causative agent is a blood parasite called *Haemobartonella felis*	FIA	No	No	Red blood cells	Cats may be exposed without exhibiting any clinical signs and become carriers Anaemia Pallor Dyspnoea Anorexia Pyrexia Weight loss Possible death	Cat bites Flea infestation In utero transmission At lactation	50 days
Feline infectious peritonitis (FIP)	FIP	No	No	Peritoneum	Pyrexia Weight loss Inappetance Diarrhoea Vomiting Peritonitis – leading to distended fluid-filled abdomen	Virus shed in urine and faeces Passes across placenta	Carriers may shed the virus for years before showing any symptoms

(Continued)

Table 8.2 (Continued)

Disease name	Common name	Zoonosis	Vaccine	Organ/s under attack	Symptoms	Transmission	Incubation
					Neurological signs There are two forms of the disease: Wet – fluid-filled cavities Dry– tumour type lesions on organs		
Rabies virus	Rabies	Yes	See Common viral diseases of the dog	See Common viral diseases of the dog	See Common viral diseases of the dog. Cats are much more resistant to this disease than dogs	See Common viral diseases of the dog	See Common viral diseases of the dog

*Routine vaccination programmes include the three major viral diseases that affect the cat – FURD, FIE, FeLV.

Table 8.3 Common viral diseases affecting the rabbit*

Disease name	Common name	Zoonosis	Vaccine	Organ/s under attack	Symptoms	Transmission	Incubation
Myxomatosis	Myxi	No	Yes	Mucous membranes	Conjunctivitis Blepharitis Anorexia, listlessness Orchitis Swelling of vulva and anus Death	Rabbit flea is the common vector	5–14 days
Haemorrhagic viral disease (HVD)	HVD	No	Yes	Liver Vascular system	Only in rabbits over 6 weeks. Hepatitis Anorexia, lethargy Dyspnoea Epistaxis Death	Direct contact in body fluids. Indirect contact – insects, birds, fomites Virus can survive for ≈3 months off of host	1–3 days

*Routine vaccination programmes include the two major viral diseases that affect the rabbit – myxomatosis and HVD.

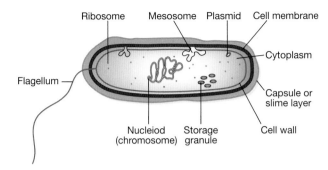

Figure 8.3 Structure of a bacterial cell.

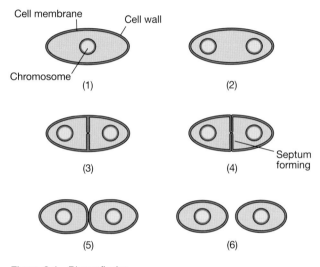

Figure 8.4 Binary fission.

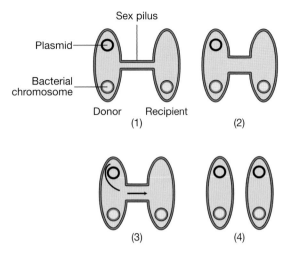

Figure 8.5 Conjugation.

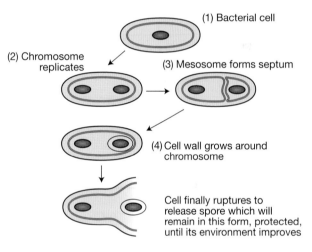

Figure 8.6 Production of bacterial spores.

mesosomes which are responsible for cell respiration and division
▨ Cytoplasm – site of protein synthesis
▨ Flagella – enable movement
▨ Fimbrae – attaches cell to other cells.

Types of bacteria are described by the way in which they live:

▨ Saprophytes – live and feed off of dead organic matter
▨ Commensals – live in harmony with other organisms
▨ Mutualistics – benefit the organism
▨ Pathogenic – damage the organism – causing disease.

Replication of bacteria
Bacteria will only replicate once they have grown to an appropriate size and if the conditions are right, i.e.

▨ Temperature is correct: 37–39°C
▨ Nutrients are available
▨ Oxygen is available if required – some bacteria require oxygen (**aerobic**) and some do not (**anaerobic**)
▨ Correct pH – alkaline.

The majority of bacteria reproduce using **binary fission** (Figure 8.4) where one cell simply divides into two, but some use a process known as **conjugation** where genetic information is passed from a donor bacteria to a recipient (Figure 8.5).

If, however, conditions are unfavourable for replication some bacteria ensure survival by producing spores (Figure 8.6) which can survive in the environment until conditions are right for bacterial growth and replication (see Table 8.4).

Fungi
The study of fungi is known as **Mycology**. Fungi are either parasites or saprophytes as they cannot live without a constant food source. Fungi are classed in a kingdom of their own.

Table 8.4 Infectious bacterial diseases affecting the dog

Disease name	Common name	Zoonosis	Vaccine	Organ/s under attack	Symptoms	Transmission	Incubation
Canine leptospirosis Causative bacteria are of two types: (i) *Leptospira canicola* (ii) *Leptospira icterohaemorrhagiae*	Leptospirosis	Yes – common name in man is Weil's disease	Yes	Liver Kidney	Pyrexia Anorexia Jaundice Haemorrhagic diarrhoea Petechial haemorrhages Oliguria Dehydration Death	Direct contact with the urine of affected dogs – through the mucous membranes or through a skin wound. Can infect through intact skin. Across the placenta from dam to pups. (Rats are thought to be a key factor in the spread of this disease as they can be carriers and excrete the bacteria in their urine.)	7–21 days
Bordetella bronchiseptica	Kennel cough term also includes respiratory disease caused by: CPIV, CAV2 and CDV	No	Yes – intranasal	Respiratory system (tracheobronchitis)	Coughing Nasal discharge Depression Self-limiting	Direct contact (See CPIV)	5–7 days (See CPIV)

Types range from microscopic forms such as *Candida albicans* to large multicellular forms such as mushrooms.

Yeasts

Yeasts are forms of microscopic fungi which are unicellular. An example of a yeast that can be pathogenic is *Candida albicans*, which is normally found in the gastrointestinal tract. When the host resistance is low, the yeast will flourish and spread to other organs.

Yeast's reproduce **asexually** by a process called 'budding'. This involves the cell developing a 'bud' or projection at one end which eventually breaks free and becomes another yeast cell.

Moulds

A mould is another form of microscopic fungi which is multicellular and composed of long filaments called

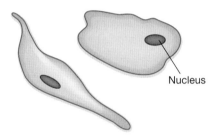

Nucleus

Figure 8.7   Structure of a protozoan.

hyphae. They can reproduce either **sexually** or **asexually** by producing spores.

A common example of a disease caused by a fungal mould is ringworm or **dermatophytosis**. Dermatophytes are the type of mould that causes ringworm and they are of zoonotic importance.

Ringworm is highly contagious as it can be passed both by using direct and indirect contact. Spores can remain infective on fomites and carrier animals for years. However the disease is self-limiting and apart from dermatitis with some alopecia it has no other detrimental effects.

Protozoa

Protozoa are classed as the most simple form of animal life – one single cell (Figure 8.7). Many are free living and do not cause disease but others are parasites of mammals and birds.

Protozoa reproduce **asexually** by binary fission and live off of organic material found in their environment. Movement is controlled by the cell flagella and cilia.

Toxoplasmosis

This disease is caused by the protozoan parasite *Toxoplasma gondii*. The cat is the final host of this parasite, but it uses other species such as sheep, rodents, dogs and man as intermediate hosts during its lifecycle (Figure 8.8).

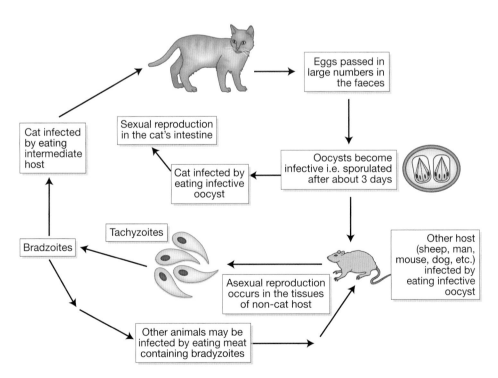

Figure 8.8   Life-cycle of toxoplasmosis.

Once the parasite enters the intermediate host it multiplies in various tissues before forming cysts often in muscles. These cysts now await ingestion by the final host. Obviously, this outcome is unlikely if the intermediate host is a sheep or man and the life-cycle ends.

Zoonotic implications

The zoonotic implications associated with man becoming the intermediate host are extremely dangerous for pregnant women, causing abortion or foetal brain damage. Pregnant women should avoid any contact with cat faeces including cleaning out litter trays and gardening without gloves.

In the cat, the final host, the parasite rarely causes symptoms as a strong immunity is present. Cats can spread the eggs or **oocysts** for 7 days post-infection.

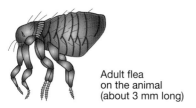

Adult flea
on the animal
(about 3 mm long)

Figure 8.9 *Ctenocephalides felis.*

Parasitology

Ectoparasites

An **ectoparasite** is a parasite which lives externally, e.g. on the animal's skin. Examples of ectoparasites are fleas, lice, ticks and mites.

The flea (Figure 8.9)
Ctenocephalides felis or the cat flea is by far the most commonly diagnosed ectoparasite in practice. A cat flea is more likely to be found on a dog than *Ctenocephalides canis* or the dog flea. Fleas are **macroscopic**, i.e. they can be seen with the naked eye and are often diagnosed by the presence of flea **dirts** or dried blood droppings.

C. felis eggs are found in the environment from where they will hatch into larvae when conditions are appropriate (Figure 8.10). The adult flea feeds by biting the host and injecting saliva containing an anti-coagulant enabling it to suck blood. Some animals and humans are highly sensitive to flea saliva, developing **pruritus** resulting in a flea allergic dermatitis (FAD).

There are many products available in the practice to treat for flea infestation, the main aims are to treat both the animal and its environment, encompassing both the adult fleas and their larvae.

Fleas are the intermediate hosts of the tapeworm *Dipilydium caninum*.

The louse (Figure 8.11)
Lice are host-specific parasites, i.e. they only live on one species – each animal species has its own louse

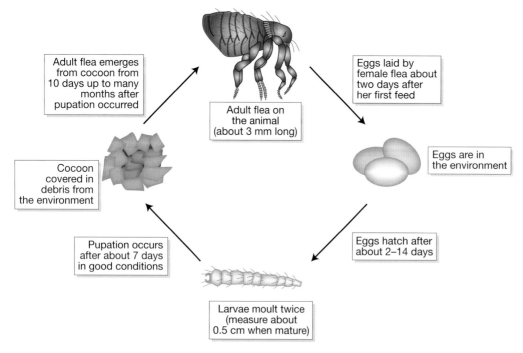

Adult flea emerges from cocoon from 10 days up to many months after pupation occurred

Adult flea on the animal (about 3 mm long)

Eggs laid by female flea about two days after her first feed

Eggs are in the environment

Cocoon covered in debris from the environment

Eggs hatch after about 2–14 days

Pupation occurs after about 7 days in good conditions

Larvae moult twice (measure about 0.5 cm when mature)

Figure 8.10 Life-cycle of the flea.

type. Lice complete the whole of their lifecycle on the host, cementing their eggs onto the hair shafts. Louse eggs are known commonly as **nits**. Bad infestations can lead to **anaemia,** and often indicate some underlying disease as lice will spread when the animal's immune system is depressed.

There are two types of louse species found on the dog:

- *Trichodectes canis* – the canine biting louse
- *Lingonathus setosus* – the canine sucking louse.

Lice are macroscopic and infestations will usually result in pruritus and *alopecia*. Most modern insecticides will treat for lice if used at the correct intervals. *Trichodectes canis* can also be an intermediate host of *Dipylidium caninum*.

The tick (Figure 8.12)
Ticks are temporary parasites spending relatively short periods on the host, and require more than one host to complete their lifecycle. All mammals and birds can be hosts of ticks. Ticks feed by sucking blood from the host and as a result can cause an anaemia. Bite wounds can become infected and ticks can transmit blood-borne disease from one host to another.

When engorged with blood ticks are easily spotted with the naked eye. They can cause a pruritus leading to alopecia.

The most commonly diagnosed species of tick seen in practice is the *Ixodes* spp.:

- *Ixodes ricinus* – sheep tick – will live on a variety of hosts – common

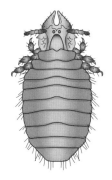

Figure 8.11 *Trichodectes canis.*

Figure 8.12 *Ixodes* – the tick.

- *Ixodes hexagonus* – hedgehog tick – will live on a variety of hosts – common
- *Ixodes canisuga* – dog tick – will only use the dog as a host.

Ixodes can be found on a variety of hosts and is recognised as a problem in kennels where it is capable of surviving in crevices and cracks on floors and walls.

Mites
The ear mite (Figure 8.13)
Otodectes cynotis, the ear mite, is the most common type of mite found in practice. It lives in the ear canal of the cat and dog causing a pruritus often leading to *otitis*, and sometimes *aural haematomas* due to shaking of the head.

It is thought that the majority of infections are spread by cats, which often show no clinical signs. Mites can be seen on the skin surface of the ear canal using an auroscope. Treatment often includes the use of antibiotic ear preparations to treat secondary bacterial infection.

Rabbits also suffer from ear mites, a species called *Psoroptes cuniculi*. Infestation with this mite will lead to pruritus and otitis and will sometimes spread to other regions such as the head. *Psoroptes cuniculi* is shown in Figure 8.14.

Cheyletiella (Figure 8.15)
Another type of surface mite, *Cheyletiella*, can be found all over the body. It lives off of dead skin and carries it around the skin surface, earning it the name 'walking dandruff'. It will cause a dermatitis with some pruritus, and is treated with insecticidal shampoos.

It does present a zoonotic problem as it is highly contagious and can penetrate clothing causing an intense pruritus in humans.

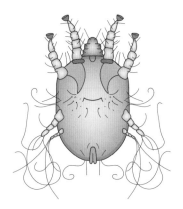

Figure 8.13 *Otodectes cyanotis.*

The three main species of *Cheyletiella* seen in small animal practice are:

- *Cheyletiella yasguri* – canine species
- *Cheyletiella blakei* – feline species
- *Cheyletiella parasitivorax* – rabbit/cavy species.

Demodex canis (Figure 8.16)

Demodex canis is a subsurface mite, i.e. a mite that burrows under the skin surface, found in the dog. It is microscopic, cigar-shaped, and can live on the dog without causing any problem. However, if the animal's immunity is suppressed in some way demodex can multiply and begin to cause a mild alopecia on the face and forelimbs along with skin thickening.

Sometimes this 'demodectic mange' or **demodecosis** can spread over the whole body, where it can range from being dry and fairly mild to infected with secondary bacteria leading to severe disfigurements for survivors.

Demodex is treated using topical insecticides.

In the cavy a mite known as *Trixacarus caviae* can cause similar problems.

Sarcoptes scabiei (Figure 8.17a)

Another subsurface mite, *Sarcoptes scabiei*, burrows into the upper layers of the skin, collecting around the ears, muzzle, face and elbows – areas where there is little hair growth. It can cause an intense pruritus leading to self-mutilation, alopecia, and pustule formation – known as sarcoptic mange.

Sarcoptes is highly contagious and if left untreated the whole skin surface may become involved, with the host becoming progressively weaker. Treatment consists of appropriate shampoos/dips at regular intervals. All affected animals should be isolated.

Sarcoptes scabiei can be of some zoonotic risk, causing a mild dermatitis in man. Humans have their own species of *Sarcoptes* which is the causative agent of **scabies**.

Endoparasites

An **endoparasite** is a parasite which lives internally, e.g. inside the alimentary tract. Examples of endoparasites include roundworms and tapeworms (Table 8.5).

Nematodes (roundworms) (Figure 8.18)

The two types of roundworm most commonly seen are:

- *Toxocara canis* – affecting the canine
- *Toxocara cati* – affecting the feline.

Another common nematode which affects the canine is *Trichuris vulpis*, commonly known as the 'whipworm'.

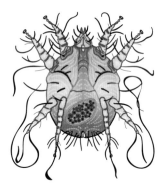

Figure 8.14 *Psoroptes* mite.

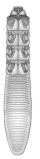

Figure 8.16 *Demodex.*

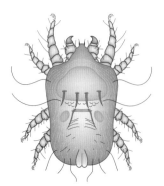

Figure 8.15 *Cheyletiella.*

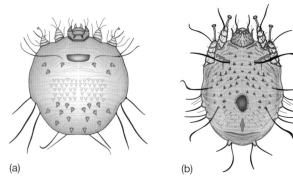

(a)   (b)

Figure 8.17 (a) *Sarcoptes scabiei*, (b) *Trixacarus caviae.*

All species of roundworm develop from infective eggs to adults worms by means of a series of moults (Figure 8.18). During these stages of growth they are known as *larvae*. Adult worms in the host animal produce eggs that pass in the faeces into the environment where they develop to an infective stage.

It is at this infective stage that *Toxocara canis* can be of zoonotic importance. Infective larvae can be ingested by humans, commonly children, and migrate through body tissues until they find a resting place. This condition is known as **visceral larval migrans** or **toxocariasis**. In rare cases the larvae can come to rest in the eye and blindness can result. Sometimes the larvae will cause damage to the tissue they are migrating through, but more often migration will take place without exhibiting any clinical signs.

Cestodes (tapeworms) (Figure 8.19)

Dipilydium caninum is the most common cestode treated in small animal practice. All cestodes use an **intermediate host**, i.e. a host in which they develop to the next stage in their lifecycle. *D. caninum* uses the flea (Ctenocephalides) and the canine biting louse (Trichodectes) as its intermediate hosts.

Table 8.5   Differences between nematodes and cestodes

Nematodes	Cestodes
Round in cross section	Flat and rectangular in cross section
Common to see the whole worm	Often will just see segments appearing around the anus
Worm is a whole organism with an alimentary tract and is either male or female	Both sex organs are present in each segment
May or may not migrate	Always migrate at some stage in their life cycle
May or may not use an intermediate host	Always use an intermediate host

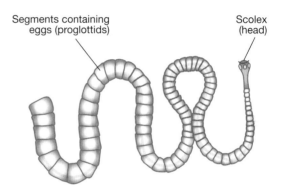

Figure 8.19   Cestode.

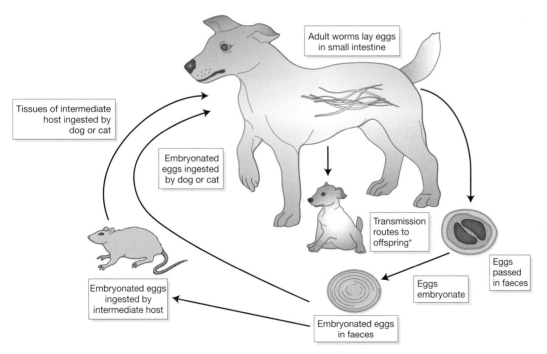

Figure 8.18   Life-cycle of *Toxocara canis*.

Clinical signs of endoparasite infection may include:

- Polyphagia
- Pot bellied appearance
- Vomiting/diarrhoea – with a heavy worm burden
- Dull coat
- Sightings of parasites – whole worms in faeces or vomit (nematodes), segments around the anus (cestodes)
- 'Scooting' anal irritation.

Control of endoparasites

- Regular use of **anthelmintics** – wormers as per manufacturer's instructions
- Ectoparasite control (flea and louse)
- Removal and disposal of dog faeces
- Encourage personal hygiene, i.e. do not allow animal to lick face, wash hands before eating, wash animal bowls separately
- Routinely examine animal for signs of infestation.

SPREAD OF INFECTION
Infectious diseases

An infectious disease is a disease produced by pathogens such as:

- Bacteria
- Viruses
- Fungi
- Protozoa
- Parasites.

It may or may not be **contagious**. A contagious disease can be transmitted from one host to another, e.g. parvovirus; a non-contagious disease cannot, e.g. an abscess.

Routes of disease transmission

Pathogens can transfer from one host to another in a variety of ways:

- Direct contact – one animal to another
- Indirect contact – fomites
- Aerosol route – sneezing or coughing droplets into the air
- Contaminated food or water
- Carrier hosts.

To gain entry to the new host the pathogen will use the following routes:

- Orally – ingestion of contaminated food/water/ faecal matter/urine/intermediate hosts
- By inhalation – through the respiratory tract – droplets/dust

- Through the skin surface – wounds, bites, scratches, penetration by parasite, penetration by infected equipment, e.g. needles
- Congenitally – e.g. pass from the dam to the foetus through the placenta
- Sexually – during coitus
- Through mucous membranes.

Once the pathogen has entered the new host there will be a period of time before clinical signs may appear. This is known as the **incubation period**.

Host resistance to the pathogen will depend on a number of factors including age and nutrition, as well as vaccination status and immune response.

Control of infection

Methods for controlling the spread of infection include:

- **Isolation** – segregation of infected or potentially infective animals from those not infected. A separate kennel area should be used for this purpose, and each isolation cage should have its own equipment, e.g. bowls and bedding. Quarantine is a type of isolation used for animals coming in from abroad.
- **Immunisation** – Vaccines are given to stimulate antibody production and prevent infection of specific diseases. Hyperimmune serums which already contain antibodies are usually only given when there is a high risk of the disease having already been transmitted.
- **Hygiene** – high standards of hygiene, including disinfection regimes for all animal areas and equipment, is extremely important.
- **Client education** – especially in the areas of vaccination and worming.
- **Treatment of infected animals** – should be treated as soon as possible with effective therapies.
- **Immunity** (Figure 8.20). The immunity of the host is its ability to resist disease. There are three ways in which the animal can develop immunity to disease:
  - **Inherent immunity** – genetically some species are immune to certain diseases, e.g. cats to leptospirosis.
  - **Active immunity** – the animal produces its own antibodies to disease, e.g. vaccination, or post-disease.
  - **Passive immunity** – the animal is given antibodies to a specific disease, e.g. via placenta, or by anti-serum.

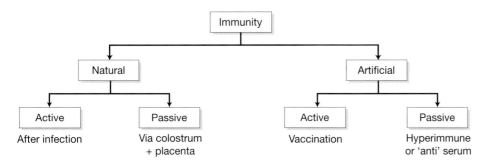

Figure 8.20   Types of immunity.

Vaccines stimulate the immune response to produce **antibodies**, which are then able to fight the disease should infection occur. Booster vaccinations keep this immunity stimulated.

Vaccination protocols for puppies and kittens are aimed to begin when maternal immunity starts to diminish – usually between 6–9 weeks of age.

Prevention of zoonotic infection

Protecting yourself against possible zoonotic infection whilst in the practice is a high priority. Protection measures should include:

- Wearing of protective clothing; such as disposable gloves, aprons, shoe covers, masks etc. as applicable
- Dispose of all animal waste immediately and correctly
- Ensure that animal utensils are washed separately from utensils intended for human use
- Confine eating and drinking to the staff areas
- Wash hands after handling patients.

Advise your clients about the dangers of zoonotic infection and encourage them to:

- Regularly worm and vaccinate
- Have any signs of disease checked by a Veterinary Surgeon
- Not to feed pets from household crockery
- Wash hands after handling pets
- Collect and properly dispose of faeces on a daily basis
- Not to allow pets to lick children's faces.

References/Further reading
Lane, D.R., Cooper, B. (2004) Veterinary Nursing. Butterworth-Heinemann, London.

Dallas, S. (2001) Animal Biology and Care. Blackwell Science, Oxford.

General hospital care

Jenny Smith

ANTISEPTICS AND DISINFECTANTS

What is a disinfectant? A disinfectant is a chemical substance that kills bacteria, viruses, fungi and fungal spores, i.e. disease causing organisms/pathogens. They either kill bacteria (bactericidal) or inhibit their growth (bacteriostatic). Disinfectants however do vary in their ability to kill viruses and fungi and most do not kill bacterial spores. Disinfectants are generally too toxic to be applied directly to living tissues and are therefore only used for hard surfaces, equipment, instruments and apparatus. Therefore disinfection is the process of killing pathogenic (disease causing) organisms.

What is an antiseptic? An antiseptic (also called a skin disinfectant) is a chemical substance that kills or prevents the growth and reproduction of the above pathogens. Antiseptics are non-toxic and can be used on living tissues. They are applied to skin before a surgical operation or to broken skin to treat, for example, wounds or burns. Antisepsis is the prevention of infection in living tissues.

What is sterilisation? Sterilisation is a method that produces an object, e.g. a surgical instrument, which is free from all living organisms. Disinfectants are unreliable as sterilising agents because they are not efficient in killing bacterial spores.

Types of disinfectant

All products can be placed into categories. These main categories are shown in Table 9.1.

Table 9.1 Chemicals and examples of trade names

Chemical	Examples of Trade Names
Halogens	
Hypochlorite (bleach)	Chloros, Domestos, Milton
NaDCC (sodium dichloroisocyanurate)	Presept, Vetaclean Parvo, Halamid
Halogenated tertiary amine	Trigene
Iodine	Pevidine, Betadine, Phoraid
Peroxides	
Peracetic acid	Oxykill, Vetcide 2000, Sorgene 5
Powdered peroxygen compounds	Virkon
Phenolic compounds: (a) Clear soluble phenolics (b) Black/white fluids (c) Chloroxylenol	Hycolin, Stericol, Clearsol Jeyes Fluid, Lysol and Izal Dettol
QACs (quaternary ammonium compounds)	Cetavlon, Sanivet, Roccal Conc, Vetaclean
Glutaraldehyde/aldehyde	Cidex, Formula-H, Gigasept, Parvocide, Vetcide, Formalin
Alcohols	Surgical Spirit, Methylated Spirit
Chlorhexadine	Hibiscrub, Hibitane, Savlon
Triclosan	Mediscrub

Properties and potential hazards

There are a variety of factors that influence the activity of disinfectants:

- Organic matter, e.g. faeces, blood and pus – some disinfectants are neutralised; others are unable to penetrate through the material.
- Incompatibility with other detergents.

Table 9.2 Chemicals and their properties	
Glutaraldehyde/aldehyde	Slow acting Toxic to personnel causing skin and eye sensitivities; respiratory problems (sinusitis/rhinitis/asthma) Proteins are fixed onto instruments and equipment, therefore needing cleaning before disinfection Instruments of different metals immersed together may corrode Wide range of bactericidal, virucidal, and fungicidal activity Slow activity on bacterial spores
Hypochlorite	Fast acting Rapidly inactivated by organic matter Irritant and unpleasant to use Corrosive to metal and textiles Suitable for surface disinfectant Wide range of bactericidal, virucidal, and fungicidal activity Sporicidal particularly if buffered at pH 7.6
NaDCC	Fast acting Inactivated by organic matter Irritant/unpleasant to use Corrosive to metal and textiles Suitable for surface disinfectant Wide range of bactericidal, virucidal, and fungicidal activity Sporicidal, particularly if buffered at pH 7.6
Quaternary ammonium compounds	Readily inactivated by hard water and organic matter Poor environmental profile – bacteriostatic action affects sewage treatment plants Suitable only for low level disinfection of surfaces Good bactericidal and fungicidal activity Variable virucidal activity No sporicidal activity
Phenolics	Toxic to cats Not readily inactivated by organic matter Absorbed by rubber and plastics Incompatible with cationic detergents Cheap Wide range of bactericidal activity Good fungicidal activity Variable virucidal activity No sporicidal activity
Peracetic acids	Active in the presence of organic matter Relatively environmentally friendly Can cause corrosion problems Handle concentrates with care Has a distinctive 'vinegar' odour Wide range of bactericidal, virucidal, and fungicidal activity Good sporicidal activity
Peroxygen compounds	Active in the presence of organic matter Environmentally friendly Powder irritant In-use dilution non-toxic and non-irritant Continued use may lead to corrosion of metal surfaces Wide range of bactericidal, virucidal, and fungicidal activity Variable sporicidal activity
Halogenated tertiary amines	Bactericidal, virucidal, fungicidal and sporicidal Active in the presence of organic matter Environmentally friendly (biodegradable) No health risks, non-irritant and non-toxic

(Continued)

Table 9.2 *(Continued)*

Alcohols	Fast acting Skin and objects need to be thoroughly cleaned before application because alcohol cannot penetrate organic matter Dries and irritates the skin Flammable Suitable only for instruments and skin. Poor surface disinfectant activity Good bactericide and fungicide Variable virucidal activity No sporicidal activity
Chlorhexadine	Low toxicity and irritancy Inactivated by soap Antiseptic Good bactericidal though more active against Gram-positive than Gram-negative bacteria Good fungicidal activity Limited activity against viruses and no activity against spores
Iodine	Inactivated by organic matter May corrode metals Non irritant Antiseptic Wide range of bactericidal, virucidal and fungicidal activity Some activity against spores
Triclosan	Non-toxic Good residual effect on skin Antiseptic More active against Gram-positive than Gram-negative bacteria Little activity against other micro-organisms

- Hard water – affects the efficiency of some disinfectants.
- Material such as cork, rubber and plastic – can neutralise and/or absorb disinfectant.

Selection and use of a disinfectant

The selection should be based on the properties of the disinfectant and the job that it has to do. The choice should ensure disease control is maintained at the lowest risk to patients and personnel.

When choosing a disinfectant the following properties should be taken into account:

- Wide range of activity against viruses, bacteria, fungi and spores.
- Efficiency and speed of action (slow or fast).
- Whether organic matter affects it.
- Safety – toxicity of concentrate and in-use dilution.
- Corrosion effects – particularly with metals.
- Effect on the environment and ease of disposal.
- Cost.

Some manufacturers recommend different dilution rates for their disinfectants – it will depend on where the disinfectant is to be used and the type of organism to be killed. Often there is one rate for general and routine use and a stronger solution for the more resistant bacteria

and viruses. For example, one manufacturer recommends for their disinfectant 10 mL per litre (1:100) as a general cleaner, 20 mL per litre (1:50) for broad spectrum activity with the exception of parvovirus and 40 mL per litre (1:25) including parvovirus.

Areas such as offices, corridors, reception areas and unoccupied kennels require a general strength solution of a disinfectant. This should be easy to use, does not create pungent odours and combines cleaning with disinfectant activity.

Areas such as theatres, wards, runs, consulting room tables and waiting rooms require a stronger solution, that is fast acting, broad-spectrum, and is not affected by organic matter.

Cleaning of the environment

Physical cleaning by mechanical methods, such as removing solids, mopping up fluids, then scrubbing and rinsing with lots of water before disinfecting is extremely important for several reasons:

- A large percentage of micro-organisms are removed this way.
- Organic matter affects the efficiency of disinfectants.
- The disinfectant has direct contact with the surfaces, maximising the disinfecting qualities.

Cleaning kennels

- Remove patient and put in a secure place, either another (clean) kennel or run.
- Remove bedding and other equipment, toys and bowls, these should be cleaned or laundered.
- Remove any faeces and dispose of in suitable clinical waste bin.
- Disposable bedding, e.g. newspaper should also be placed in a clinical waste bin.
- Remove dust and hair with a vacuum or broom.
- With a bucket of correctly diluted disinfectant vigorously scrub the walls and floor of kennel and allow a suitable contact time.
- Rinse with clean water.
- Dry kennel with a squeegee or clean mop so that no residue remains.
- Replace bedding and water bowls.
- Replace patient!

If kennel is to be left unoccupied, it should be allowed to air thoroughly before putting in bedding for next patient.

Cleaning runs

- Between patients, faeces should be removed with a shovel and disposed of and urine rinsed away.
- After the exercise regime for each session the runs should be hosed down.
- Buckets of correctly diluted disinfectant should be distributed around the run.
- The area is vigorously scrubbed.
- Rinse thoroughly and allow to dry.

Cleaning theatre

- Every morning before the operating list starts, all horizontal surfaces should be damp dusted with a disinfectant and clean cloth to remove any dust that has settled overnight.
- Any areas that are contaminated during the operation should be spot cleaned with a disinfectant solution and clean cloth between patients.
- At the end of the day all surfaces and equipment should be wiped with disinfectant solution or a spray bottle on squirt (not mist) setting is useful for this.
- Hair and debris should be removed taking care not to create any airborne dust particles before cleaning the floors thoroughly with disinfectant.

Cleaning waiting rooms

- 'Accidents' should be cleaned up as soon as they occur.
- At the end of the day or a particularly busy consulting session the floors should be vacuumed and, depending on floor surface, mopped with disinfectant and rinsed.

Antiseptics

Antiseptics can be used either for cleaning patient's skin and the surgeon's hands before a surgical operation or for cleaning wounds. Surgical scrubs of chlorhexadine (Hibiscrub, Schering-Plough) or povidone iodine (Pevidine Surgical Scrub, C-Vet) contain a detergent and should only be used on unbroken skin and not on mucous membranes.

Antiseptic solutions of chlorhexadine (Hibitane Conc, Schering-Plough) and povidone iodine (Pevidine antiseptic solution, C-Vet) do not contain detergents and are suitable for use on mucous membranes and wounds. Care must be taken when cleaning wounds with antiseptics because it is easy to damage delicate tissues and cause delay in the healing process. They must be used at the correct dilution 0.04% chlorhexadine and 1% povidone iodine.

Health and safety

The Control of Substances Hazardous to Health Regulations 2002 (COSHH) is the most recent safety legislation to affect the way that disinfectants are selected and used. The handling and use of the chemicals as well as the substances themselves are all assessed under these regulations.

Substances are harmful to health through:

- inhalation – breathing in vapour or powder when mixing with water ready for use.
- ingestion – accidental swallowing
- absorption through skin or eyes – splashing of chemical.

Safe handling suggestions

1. Always read manufacturer's instructions.
2. Wear protective clothing, e.g. gloves, aprons, safety glasses.
3. Use correct dilution using manufacturer's instructions. Strong solutions are wasteful, may be corrosive and are irritant to the patients. Weak solutions are ineffective and bacteria will grow in them.
4. Fill container with the correct amount of water before adding disinfectant, to avoid breathing in vapour.
5. Concentrated solutions/powders can be harmful, therefore handle with great care and store carefully, keep away from animals and children.
6. Keep solutions in their original container with the lid secured tightly.

7. Do not mix chemicals, this can be potentially dangerous because harmful gasses can be given off or the mixture can become toxic or corrosive.
8. Minimise splashes to the skin, if an accident does occur wash with lots of water and consult manufacturer's instructions.
9. Only use product as required to avoid introducing unused material into the sewage system, this is also uneconomical.
10. Wash hands thoroughly after use especially before eating.

Examination of an animal (Table 9.3)

While performing a clinical examination it is important to know the normal parameters – anything that is abnormal should be reported to the veterinary surgeon. It is therefore important to know what is normal for individual breeds and species. A Greyhound appears to be emaciated (very thin) compared with the St Bernard for instance, but each could be within the normal range for that particular breed. Age must also be taken into consideration. A healthy but aged Labrador is very different from a healthy Labrador puppy; its coat is not so glossy, its eyes not so bright and alert and of course the older dog is less energetic.

Clinical history
The patient's clinical history taken either from the owner or if an in-patient, from observation is important. It can reveal abnormalities:

- Urine should be passed easily, and without pain. It should be clear and pale yellow in colour and not contain blood or sediments.
- Faeces should be passed without pain or straining (tenesmus) and should be firm and brown in colour. Loose faeces (diarrhoea) should be noted along with its colour, consistency and the presence of any obvious blood or mucus.
- The patient should be interested in food and able to eat and drink normally.
- Any vomiting should be noted, along with the amount, how often and the contents (i.e. regurgitated food with or without bile or blood).
- Any coughing is abnormal.

While performing a clinical examination adopt a logical approach, start from the head and work towards the tail, that way nothing will be missed accidentally.

Table 9.3	Diagnostic table	
Normal		**Abnormal**
Nose	Moist clear orifices	Hot and dry, discharge
Mouth	Pink mucous membranes	Pale, yellow or congested (dark pink/red) mucous membranes, bad breath
Teeth	Clean and even	Tartar, loose teeth
Eyes	Clear and bright	Dull, discharge, yellow or reddish colour of mucus membranes or white of eye (sclera)
Ears	Clean, odour free	Discharge, smell, inflammation
Lymph nodes	Cannot be felt	Enlarged nodes
Coat	Glossy and clean	Dull, parasites, hair loss
Skin	Clean and supple	Parasites, lumps, lesions, dandruff, cuts and wounds, pruritus (itching)
Limbs/joints	Free movement	Uneven gait, pain, or stiffness, swelling
Paws	Even sized	Swelling of toes, cuts and abrasions
Nails	Correct length	Long nails especially dew claw, broken or shredded
Mammary glands	Present in both sexes	Hard lumps around nipples, discharge from nipples
Rectum	Healthy pink skin	Inflammation, lumps
Sheath/vulva	Healthy pink skin 'in season'	Swelling, discharge
Weight	Normal for breed	Obesity, thin, muscle wastage

Temperature, pulse and respiration (Tables 9.4 and 9.5)

Taking an animal's temperature

There are two types of clinical thermometer, mercury and digital. Mercury thermometers are calibrated in degrees Fahrenheit or Centigrade or both, they are however, quite difficult to read and easily broken. Digital thermometers are easier to read more accurately. In conscious animals the normal route for taking the temperature is via the rectum.

- Have the patient properly restrained.
- If using a mercury thermometer, it is important to shake the level of the mercury to below the scale.
- The thermometer (either digital or mercury) needs to be disinfected with an antiseptic solution and lubricated with petroleum jelly, or other water soluble lubricant.
- Hold the thermometer between the tips of fingers and thumb and gently insert the thermometer a couple of centimeters into the rectum with a gentle rotating action.
- Hold the thermometer within the rectum for 1 minute, do not let go of it or it can disappear into the rectum.
- Remove the thermometer taking care not to touch the end with your fingers because this may alter the reading.
- Wipe clean with a dry swab.
- Take the reading and record on the animal's notes.

Reasons for temperature change
- **High temperature**
  Infection
  Heat stroke
  Convulsions
  Pain
  Excitement and exercise
  Some poisons
- **Low temperature**
  Prolonged exposure to cold
  Shock
  Metabolic disorders, e.g. uraemia

Circulatory collapse
Impending parturition
Some poisons.

Taking an animal's pulse rate

The pulse can be felt at any point where an artery runs near the surface, these include:

- Femoral (this is the easiest). It is located on the inside of the thigh in the groin.
- Digital. This is located at the back of the paw between the 'stopper' (carpal) pad and the metacarpal pad.
- Coccygeal located on the underside of the tail near the base.
- Lingual (only on anaesthetised patients) located on the underside of the tongue.

Gently locate the artery with the fingers (not thumb), apply firm pressure taking care not to occlude the artery, and count the number of beats in one minute (or

Table 9.5	Terminology
Temperature	
Hyperthermia	Higher than normal body temperature
Hypothermia	Low body temperature
Normothermia	Normal body temperature
Pyrexia	Fever
Pulse	
Bradycardia	Slow heart rate
Tachycardia	Abnormally rapid heart rate
Respiration	
Apnoea	Temporary absence of breathing
Bradypnoea	Slow breathing, as in sleep
Cheyne–Stokes	Alternating breathing pattern fast and slow
Cyanosis	Bluish discolouration of mucus membranes
Dyspnoea	Difficulty in breathing
Tachypnoea	Rapid breathing

Table 9.4	Normal parameters		
Species	Temperature	Pulse (beats/min)	Respiration rate (breaths/min)
Dog	38.3–38.7°C	60–140 (small breeds nearer higher end)	10–30 (small breeds nearer higher end)
Cat	38.0–38.5°C	110–180	20–30
Rabbit	38.5°C	180–300	30–60

count the number of beats in 15 seconds and multiply by four, but this method is less accurate). Also note the nature of the pulse, is it strong and regular or weak and thready.

Reasons for variations in pulse rates

- **Increase in pulse rate**
  Stress
  Pain
  Pyrexia
  Early shock
  Exercise
  Excitement
- **Decrease in pulse rate**
  Unconsciousness
  Debilitating disease
  Sleep
  Hypothermia
- **Strong**
  High blood pressure
  Fear
- **Weak**
  Shock
  Poor cardiac output.

Taking an animal's respiration rate

The patient should be calm and at rest but not sleeping or panting. One breath consists of one inhalation (breath in) and one exhalation (breath out), therefore count each time the chest moves either in *or* out but not both.

Reasons for change in respiratory rate

- **Increase in respiratory rate**
  Excitement
  Pain
  Pyrexia
  Exercise
  Poisons
  Hyperthermia
- **Decrease in respiratory rate**
  Poisons (sleep inducing)
  Trauma to the brain
  Hypothermia
  Sleep
- **Difficulty in breathing – can cause an increase or decrease in respiratory rate**
  Obstruction of the respiratory tract
  Bronchitis and emphysema of the lungs
  Pneumonia or haemorrhage into lungs
  Air or fluid collecting in the chest (pleural space)
  Trauma to the chest
  Diaphragmatic hernia
- Cheyne–Stokes respiratory pattern often occurs just before death.

Chapter 4

Animal first aid

Carole Martin

OBJECTIVES AND LIMITATIONS OF FIRST AID

Introduction

The provision of first aid is an interim measure, designed to preserve life and suffering until a veterinary surgeon is able to attend the animal. This can be provided by any member of a veterinary practice or a lay person (Tables 10.1 and 10.2).

Basic rules

Don't panic

When dealing with a first aid situation one of the most important rules is not to panic! A client requires help

Table 10.1   Definition of first aid
First aid is the immediate treatment of injured animals with the aim of preserving life and alleviating suffering

Table 10.2   Basic rules in first aid
Don't panic
Maintain airway
Control haemorrhage
Contact veterinary surgeon

in an emergency and expects to see a calm, controlled efficient approach to the care of their pet. Anticipation and preparation are essential requisites in order to deal with first aid situations quickly and effectively. It is therefore important to think ahead.

Maintain airway

Maintaining an airway is essential to ensure the patient receives sufficient oxygen for its body requirements. Provision of equipment to supply oxygen to the patient is essential. A few simple pieces of equipment can be prepared in advance such as:

- endotracheal tubes
- face masks
- oxygen supply.

Control haemorrhage

Several methods of controlling haemorrhage can be implemented depending on the nature and severity of haemorrhage. This will be covered later in the haemorrhage section.

Contact the veterinary surgeon

It is essential that the nurse is familiar with the whereabouts of the duty veterinary surgeon and how to contact him/her. The client must be reassured that the veterinary surgeon is easily contactable and on the way to deal with their pet.

Handling telephone calls and the client (Figure 10.1)

On receiving a call from a client regarding a pet that has been involved in an accident or incident there are some important points to follow:

- Listen
- Be calm, patient and sympathetic
- Obtain name, address and telephone number

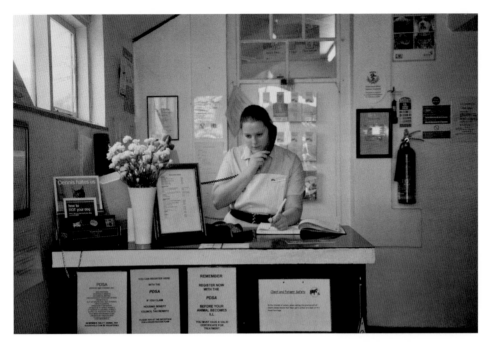

Figure 10.1   Taking accurate details during a telephone call is vital in any emergency situation.

- Obtain animal details
- Obtain brief history of the problem
- Ascertain degree of problem
- Where possible always advise the client to bring the pet to the surgery.

Handling the pet

An animal that has been involved in an accident or emergency needs careful handling to ensure the safety and well-being of all involved. An injured animal will appear confused and sometimes aggressive and these behaviour patterns must be remembered when approaching and handling these animals.

Handling equipment for first aid patients:

- Large towels for cats
- Cat baskets
- Dog muzzle and dog catcher
- Slip leads
- Assistance.

How to handle the first aid patient:

- Talk to the animal
- Approach calmly
- Secure cats in basket or wrap in large towel
- Apply slip lead and muzzle to dog where applicable
- Provide flat firm surface for patient to lie on if spinal injuries are suspected.

Arrival at the surgery

The following points should be followed when the first aid patient arrives at the surgery:

- Obtain full client details
- Obtain full animal details
- Obtain signature on a consent form
- Assess patient's condition (see Table 10.3)
- Contact and report to veterinary surgeon.

Practice policies

It is essential to ascertain who does what in the practice when emergency first aid cases arise. All practices will have policies and it is important that the veterinary nurse is familiar with and understands them (Figures 10.2 and 10.3).

Basic emergency preparation

- Prepare kennel – ensure bedding is absorbent, supportive and comfortable; choose kennel in quiet area with easy access.
- Prewarm kennel – provide ambient temperature of approximately 18–20°C; prepare extra warmth with use of heated pads, hot water bottles wrapped in towel, or examination gloves filled with warm water.
- Prepare oxygen supply – have oxygen supply ready and switched on with delivery mask and tubing or oxygen chamber or incubator.

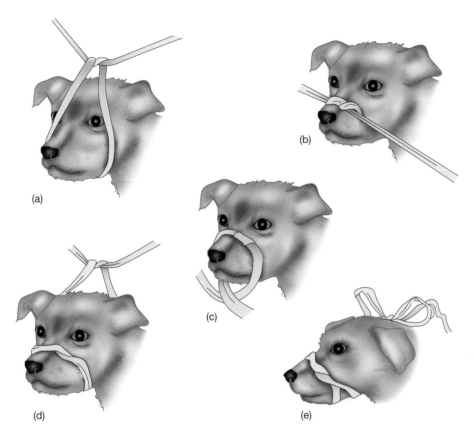

Figure 10.2 Muzzle on dog.

■ Prepare airway equipment – have a supply of endotracheal tubes ready for use.
■ Prepare emergency box – check emergency first aid box is complete and ready for use (see below).

Emergency first aid kit
This should include:

■ Gloves
■ Curved or flat scissors
■ Cotton wool
■ One pair of dressing forceps
■ Skin disinfectant – chlorhexidine or povidine iodine
■ Normal saline
■ Selection of syringes – 1 mL, 2 mL, 5 mL, 10 mL, 20 mL
■ Selection of hypodermic needles – 25 g × 5/8″, 23 g × 5/8″, 21 g × 5/8″
■ Selection of sterile non adherent wound dressings
■ Selection of conforming bandages and cohesive or elastic adhesive bandages
■ Intravenous catheters ×3 (24 g, 22 g, 20 g)
■ Zinc oxide tape or similar 2.5 cm
■ White open weave bandage 2.5 cm and 5 cm
■ Small pot of bicarbonate of soda
■ Small pot of vinegar
■ Muzzle
■ Towel

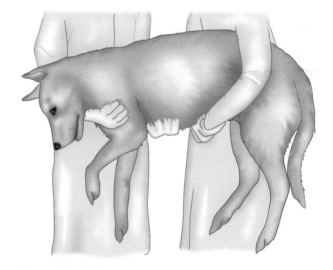

Figure 10.3 Lifting dog.

Examination of the patient

While being restrained by a colleague a thorough examination should be conducted in order to ascertain the site and degree of any injury. This examination needs to be carried out in a methodical manner to ensure that all areas are checked. All findings must be recorded accurately both verbally and in writing. It is essential to make assessments of any life-threatening situations as

Table 10.3	Emergency parameters to check	
Airway	Check airway is clear and patent; check for any blood, mucus, vomit or excess saliva. Check colour of mucous membranes, these should be salmon pink in colour indicating good oxygenation levels in the circulating blood	ACTION – Clear any mucus or discharges away. Prepare equipment to provide patent airway such as endotracheal tube, mask and oxygen supply
Breathing	Check for clear respiratory noises. Any noisy or laboured breathing may indicate injury to the lungs or surrounding structures; assess respiratory rate (normal see Table 10.5)	ACTION – If breathing laboured clear any obstructions and provide oxygen supply and keep patient as quiet and unstressed as possible
Circulation	Check the pulse rate on the femoral or tarsal arteries and/or listen for heart sounds; assess rate and character of pulse (see Table 10.5). Check capillary refill time on gums which should be less than 2 seconds indicating good circulatory blood volume. Check body temperature by feeling extremities and taking using rectal thermometer readings (normal see Table 10.5). Any marked changes from normal may indicate circulatory problems and shock	ACTION – If any pulse deficits of slow capillary refill time check for any external haemorrhage and control appropriately. Prepare fluid therapy equipment to support circulation. If hypothermic provide warmth gradually with blankets and heated pads or similar. If hyperthermic/heat stroke detected by temperature reading being off the scale cool body rapidly with hosing or bathing in cold water, check temperature regularly and stop once temperature drops to 39°C
Consciousness	Check general demeanour of patient; alertness; responsiveness to noise, ability to stand; panicking or calm	ACTION – If dull and unresponsive, prepare supportive oxygen and fluid therapy, keep warm and monitor responses regularly

identified in Table 10.3 before commencing the head to tail check as outlined later.

Head to tail examination

Once the life-threatening parameters have been checked it is now important to work down through the body and record all findings accordingly. This check can be simplified by use of a form where you can tick the areas checked and add comments on your findings (Tables 10.4 and 10.5).

WOUNDS

A wound is described as a break in the skin and surrounding soft tissues. Wounds can be divided into two main groups – open and closed.

An open wound is where an injury causes a break in the covering of the body surface. A closed wound is where an injury does not cause a break in the covering of the body but causes damage to underlying tissues resulting in bruising for example.

Classification of open and closed wounds can be seen in Table 10.6 and in Figure 10.4.

Open wounds

- **Incised** – An incised wound has clean, straight and clearly defined edges. A sharp instrument such as glass, slate, knife, and scalpel blade may cause this type of wound. These wounds tend to heal quickly providing the edges are closely apposed, resulting in little if any scar formation.

- **Lacerated** – These wounds have jagged uneven edges and are irregular in shape. They may be caused by road traffic accidents, barbed wire tears and dog bites. Healing tends to be slow due to the irregularity of the wound's edges and surface area involved. Scar formation is likely.

- **Punctured** – This wound usually has a small entrance site but the wound usually penetrates deeper into the surrounding tissue. A long sharp instrument such as a nail, thorn or stake may cause this.

- **Abrasion** – This wound is best described as a graze. It does not involve the full skin thickness but can cover a considerable area. This type of wound may occur due to friction or dragging part of the body against a rough surface.

First aid treatment of open wounds

- Treat for shock (see section on shock)
- Control haemorrhage (see section on haemorrhage)
- Remove causal agent (if applicable)
- Clip hair (take care to avoid contamination of wound with hair)
- Lavage wound with normal saline
- Dress the wound (Figure 10.5)
- Provide analgesics and antibiotics as prescribed by the veterinary surgeon.

Reasons for dressing the wound:

- to prevent further contamination
- to prevent damage to tissue

Table 10.4 Head to tail examination check list

Area	What to check	Checked ✓	Comments
Skull	Feel for any swellings, abnormal shape, wounds or pain		
Nose	Check nostrils for any haemorrhage or discharge		
Eyes	Check both eyes for any discharges, bruising or discolouration of the corneas. Check pupil sizes are equal and check for any flickering of eyeballs. Check eyelids for swellings or redness or wounds		
Ears	Check pinnas for swellings, heat, wounds or pain. Check ear canals for any discharges		
Mouth	Check mucous membrane colour and capillary refill time as in Table 10.5. Check upper and lower jaw for any swelling, pain or deformity. Check mouth for any haemorrhage. Check any odour in case of poisoning. Check teeth and tongue for any injury		
Neck	Check for any pain, haemorrhage or wounds around whole circumference		
Thorax	Feel along the vertebral column and down rib cage for any swelling, wounds, haemorrhage or pain and continue check of whole thoracic area		
Abdomen	Feel whole area including vertebral column to detect any haemorrhage, wounds, pain or discomfort		
Limbs	Methodically palpate each limb checking for any pain, swelling, deformity, wound and/or haemorrhage. Check patient is weight bearing on each limb normally		
Pelvis	Feel pelvic area for any swelling, pain or deformity		
External genitalia and perineal region	Check for any haemorrhage, discharge, pain or swelling		
Tail	Check for any wounds or discomfort and assess if patient able to move it voluntarily		
General condition	Assess if under or over weight or normal for individual. Check coat condition and check for parasites. Check skin for any signs of inflammation or discomfort		
General demeanour	Assess alertness and responsiveness to voice and handling		

Table 10.5 Normal range of vital signs

	Cat	Dog
Temperature	38.0–38.5°C	38.3–38.7°C
Pulse	110–180 beats per minute	60–180 beats per minute
Respiration	20–30 breaths per minute	10–30 breaths per minute
Capillary refill time	Less than 2 seconds	Less than 2 seconds
Mucous membrane colour	Pink	Pink

Table 10.6 Wound classification
Open
Incised
Lacerated
Punctured
Abrasion
Closed
Contusion
Haematoma

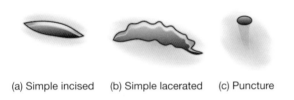

(a) Simple incised   (b) Simple lacerated   (c) Puncture

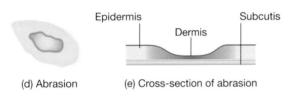

(d) Abrasion   (e) Cross-section of abrasion

Figure 10.4 Wound classification.

- to prevent self mutilation
- to restrict movement
- to absorb wound discharge
- to provide comfort and support.

Principles of wound dressing and bandaging
- Wash hands and wear gloves
- Ensure the area is clean
- Pad between toes if they are to be included in the bandage
- Apply a sterile non-adherent wound dressing
- Apply a layer of padding over the wound dressing
- Secure padding and dressing in place with conforming bandage
- Apply an outer/tertiary layer for support and protect
- Never apply cotton wool directly to a wound.

Closed wounds

- **Contusion** – This is also known as a bruise. This type of injury results from pressure or a blow with a blunt instrument. Capillaries beneath the skin surface are ruptured and the blood disperses over the injured area. The skin area becomes swollen, warm to touch and there is discoloration to the skin.
- **Haematoma** – This is a blood-filled swelling that results after damage to a blood vessel within a

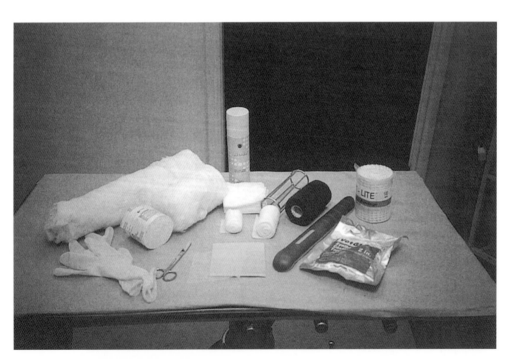

Figure 10.5 Dressing and bandaging equipment.

Table 10.7   Basic wound dressing and bandaging equipment
Curved or flat scissors
Gloves
Normal saline
Range of wound dressings – non-adherent
Conforming bandages
Padding – cotton wool, gamgee or synthetic padding
Elastic adhesive or cohesive bandages

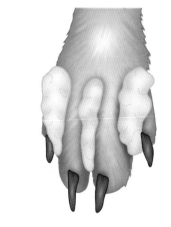

(a)

pocket of connective tissue. Back pressure within the site affected arrests haemorrhage. A common site for this type of injury is the pinnae of dogs and cats.

Treatment of closed wounds (Table 10.7 and Figure 10.6)

- **Cold compresses** – These will help to reduce blood flow to the area by constricting the capillaries.
- **Support and bandaging** – This will help to produce back pressure and help control haemorrhage. By providing support the nerve endings will be protected and therefore the patient will be more comfortable.

Burns and scalds

These injuries do not fall into the remit of open and closed wound classification but nevertheless need including within injuries to the skin surface.

A burn is an injury caused by dry heat, electrical current, excessive cold or chemicals. A scald is an injury caused by moist heat such as boiling water or oil.

Treatment

The severity of the injury depends on the depth and size of the area affected. Consideration needs to be given for the provision of fluid replacement and non-adherent dressings to the injury sites to prevent and control further fluid loss. Painkillers are essential with these types of injuries as the nerve endings are exposed.

- Treat for shock
- Cool the affected area with water
- Keep the areas moist
- Dress the wounds with non-adherent dressings covered with warm saline soaked swabs (do not allow them to become dry)
- Prepare intravenous infusion equipment
- Provide analgesia as prescribed by the veterinary surgeon.

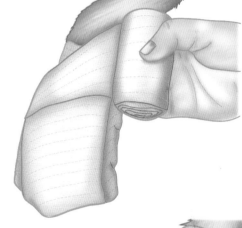

(b)

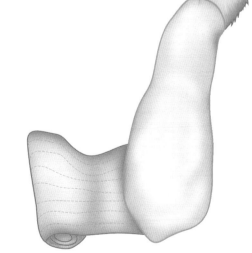

(c)

Figure 10.6   Basic bandaging.

Insect stings

Wasp and bee stings are the commonest form of insect stings seen in dogs and cats. They rarely pose a serious problem unless the site of the sting is involving the airways. If there is any fear that the airway has been involved the patient must be monitored closely for signs of swelling and the veterinary surgeon contacted.

Basic first aid treatment is as follows:

Bee stings – Remove the sting if visible, and bathe the area in bicarbonate of soda and water.

Wasp stings – Remove the sting if visible, and bathe the area with diluted vinegar.

HAEMORRHAGE

Haemorrhage is the escape of blood from a ruptured vessel. It can arise due to the damage of any blood vessel. External haemorrhage can be classified and identified as follows (Figure 10.7 and Table 10.8):

- Arterial – pumping and bright red and spurting
- Venous – flowing and dark red
- Capillary – general ooze
- Mixed – two or more of the above.

Arresting haemorrhage

This can be achieved in a number of ways:

- Direct digital pressure
- Pad or bandage
- Use of pressure points
- Tourniquet.

Direct digital pressure

Direct digital pressure can be applied directly to the bleeding vessel. Hands must be clean and the fingers used to apply pressure to the vessel and immediate surrounding tissue.

Pad or pressure bandage

A non-adherent dressing can be applied directly to the wound and a pad of gauze swabs, gamgee or cotton wool can be overlaid to apply direct pressure to the area. The padded area can then be kept in place with an outer layer of bandage. If haemorrhage seeps through the bandage, apply additional layers on top of original bandage. Do not remove or disturb first bandage as this could disturb any clotting process already taking place.

Pressure points (Figure 10.8)

Pressure points are sites on the body where an artery can have pressure applied against the body thereby preventing blood flow.

- **Brachial artery** – Located approximately 3 cm below the elbow on the medial aspect of the lower

Artery

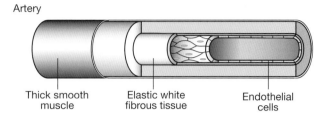

Thick smooth muscle   Elastic white fibrous tissue   Endothelial cells

Vein

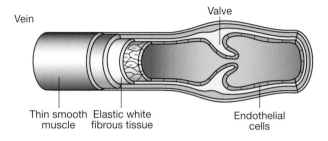

Valve

Thin smooth muscle   Elastic white fibrous tissue   Endothelial cells

Capillary

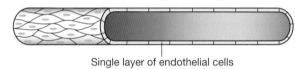

Single layer of endothelial cells

Figure 10.7   Blood vessels.

Table 10.8   Clinical signs of haemorrhage
External haemorrhage
Pale mucous membranes
Rapid and weak pulse
Shallow, rapid respirations
Cold extremities
Low body temperature
Dull, listless patient

third of the humerus. Pressure applied to this area will control haemorrhage below the elbow.

- **Femoral artery** – Located on the medial aspect of the femur at the site where the pulse can be taken. This will control haemorrhage below the stifle.
- **Coccygeal artery** – Located on the ventral aspect of the proximal tail. This will control haemorrhage of the tail only.

SHOCK (Tables 10.9, 10.10 and 10.11)

Classifications of shock

- **Pending** – Shock is pending; the history of the patient is known and shock is expected to follow but clinical signs are not yet evident. Interception of shock treatment at this point will have a

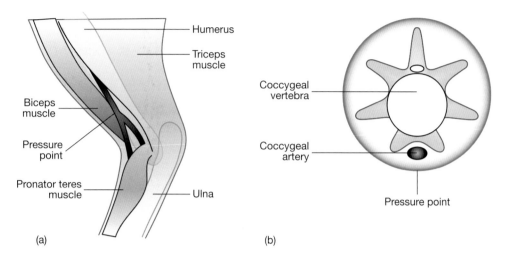

Figure 10.8   Pressure points. (a) Elbow; (b) tail base.

Table 10.9   Definition of shock
Shock is a state of circulatory failure in which cardiac output is insufficient at meeting the needs of the body tissues for oxygen and nutrients and removal of waste products

Table 10.10   Clinical signs of shock
Weak, rapid pulse
Increased heart rate
Pale mucous membrane
Slow capillary refill time
Rapid, shallow respiration
Cold extremities
Subnormal rectal temperature
Decreased level of consciousness
Reduced urine output
Dry mucous membranes
Dilated pupils
Poor skin turgor

favourable effect in preventing deterioration of the patient.

- **Established** – Shock is already established; the patient is showing clinical signs of shock and treatment is essential. With effective supportive treatment the result should be favourable, providing further complications do not arise.
- **Irreversible** – Shock is irreversible; the patient has been suffering from shock for a considerable time and despite supportive treatment efforts the patient is likely to deteriorate further.

Hypovolaemic shock

This is the commonest type of shock seen in veterinary practice. It results from an inadequate circulating blood volume. This can be as a result of:

- haemorrhage (external or internal)
- loss of body water and electrolytes due to water depletion or starvation
- loss of tissue fluid due to severe or prolonged vomiting and diarrhoea.

First aid measures for shock

- Control and prevent further haemorrhage – see haemorrhage section.
- Restore body temperature – provide insulation with blankets and towels by wrapping them around the patient. The use of hot water bottles and heat pads is acceptable providing they are covered and the patient's state of recumbency is monitored to avoid contact burns due to persistent and excessive heat in one place.
- Provide a comfortable kennel – It is essential that the patient is comfortable to avoid further damage to itself. The provision of subdued lighting and avoidance of excessive noise will help to calm the patient, therefore aiding recovery.
- Provision of intravenous access equipment (Figures 10.9 and 10.10) – Preparation of equipment necessary to permit intravenous access and fluid administration is essential in a patient with shock. Blood or fluid losses may be replaced and emergency drugs required in shock can be administered via this route.

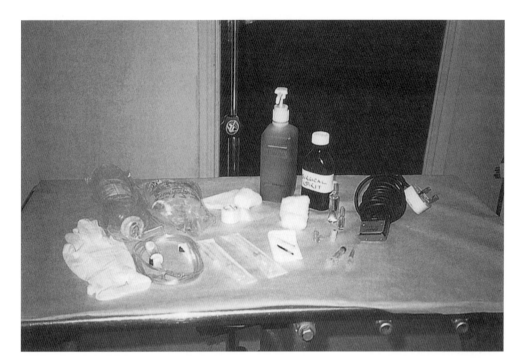

Figure 10.9 Intravenous access and infusion equipment.

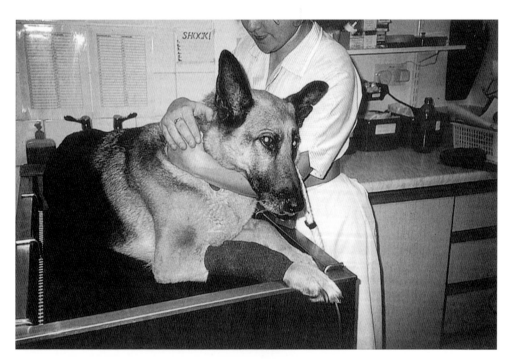

Figure 10.10 A patient with intravenous catheter in place.

■ Maintain constant observation – This is essential as the condition of the patient may deteriorate rapidly and immediate actions may be necessary. Record baseline parameters every 5–10 minutes on a kennel chart.

■ Comfort the patient – Reassure the patient with voice and touch. Tender loving care in these cases should not be overlooked.

■ Provision of analgesics and painkillers as directed by the veterinary surgeon.

FRACTURES AND DISLOCATIONS
(Tables 10.12–10.18; Figures 10.12–10.17)

Fractures

Fractures can be described in relation to the degree of damage to the bone:

- **Simple** – The bone has broken cleanly into two pieces.
- **Compound** – The bone has a communicating wound leading to the fracture site. This type of fracture has an increased risk of infection.
- **Complicated** – Other vital structures such as nerves and blood vessels are involved in the fracture site.

First aid treatment

- Handle the fracture site as little as possible – This will help reduce the risk of the fracture becoming compound or complicated and avoid unnecessary pain perception of the patient.
- Provide support – This can be provided most appropriately in limb fractures. Support should be applied above and below the fracture site making sure the joints above and below the fracture are included in the dressing. In providing support the fracture is stabilised, the nerve ending cushioned and patient made comfortable. Application of a Robert Jones bandage or splint can be performed to provide this support.
- Control haemorrhage (see haemorrhage section).
- Treat for shock (see shock section).
- Provide analgesia – Fractures are acutely painful and therefore the patient will require some form of analgesia as prescribed by the veterinary surgeon.

Limb support methods

Splint application (Table 10.14)
1. Ensure any open wounds are dressed and covered
2. Choose a splint of the correct length to include the joint above and below the fracture
3. Apply padding evenly to the whole limb
4. Apply the splint to the limb
5. Apply outer bandage layer to hold splint in place.

Robert Jones bandage application (Table 10.15)
1. Pad between the toes with cotton wool strips
2. Ensure any open wounds are dressed and covered
3. Apply two stay tapes of zinc oxide to apposing side of limb extending approximately 5 cm from the toes
4. Use cotton wool or synthetic padding to roll around entire limb evenly. Ensure two central toes are visible
5. Repeat with at least three layers of padding
6. Start to compress the padding with conforming bandage evenly
7. Reflect stay tapes up onto bandage

Table 10.11 First aid equipment for shock
Warm, darkened kennel
Blankets and towels
Oxygen supply
Wound dressing and bandaging equipment
Intravenous catheter
Infusion set
Pre-warmed infusion fluid
Thermometer
Curved or flat scissors
Record sheet
Drugs for shock (as per practice policy)

Table 10.12 Definition of a fracture
A fracture is a break in the continuity of a bone

Table 10.13 Clinical signs of a fracture
Pain at the site
Deformity of the limb
Crepitus
Loss of function
Unnatural mobility

Table 10.14 Splints
Wooden
Metal
Plastic gutter
Inflatable airbags
Plaster or resin

Table 10.15 Equipment for Robert Jones bandage
An assistant
Curved or flat scissors
Zinc oxide tape
Conforming bandage
Cotton wool
Wound dressing
Synthetic padding
Cohesive or elastic adhesive bandage

Table 10.16 Transport and handling of spinal fractures

In the case of a suspected spinal fracture the patient must be handled with caution
Provide a flat firm surface
Gently and slowly move the patient onto the board
Have an assistant to reassure the patient while in transit
If a board is not available gently move the patient onto a large strong blanket or towel
Have at least two assistants to carry the blanket or towel evenly

Table 10.17 Definition of dislocation

A dislocation is a displacement of the articular surfaces of bones within a joint. It can be partial or complete

Table 10.18 Dislocation – clinical signs

Pain on manipulation
Swelling of the joint
Deformity
Limited movement
Crepitus

8. Apply a further layer of bandage
9. Apply an outer layer for protection and support.

Dislocations

Common sites for dislocation

- carpus
- tarsus
- hip joint
- patella.

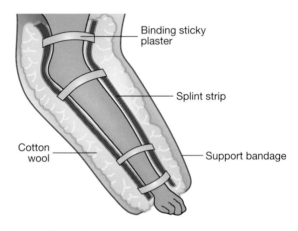

Figure 10.12 Splint and bandage equipment.

Binding sticky plaster

Splint strip

Cotton wool

Support bandage

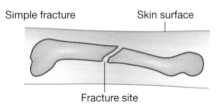

Simple fracture   Skin surface

Fracture site

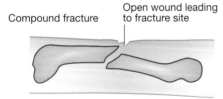

Compound fracture   Open wound leading to fracture site

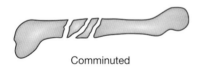

Comminuted

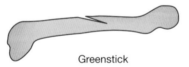

Greenstick

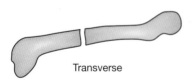

Transverse

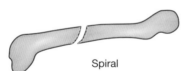

Spiral

Figure 10.11 Fracture classifications.

First aid treatment

- Do not attempt to reduce the dislocation.
- Avoid bandaging the area – the bones will be displaced within the joint cavity and any bandage application to this area may encourage them to remain in the incorrect alignment.

- Apply cold compresses to swollen joints – this will help to reduce blood flow by vasoconstriction and therefore help reduce swelling and pressure on nerve endings.
- Provide analgesia as directed by the veterinary surgeon.
- Restrict movement – This will help to reduce discomfort of the patient.

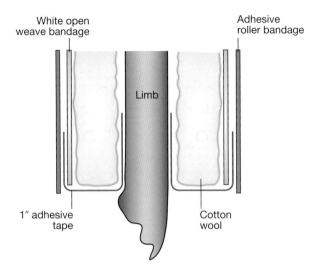

Figure 10.13   Splint and bandage equipment.

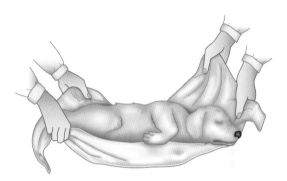

Figure 10.15   Handling spinal injuries.

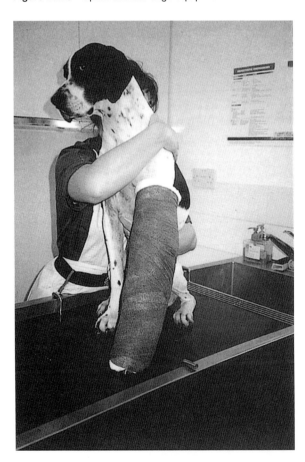

Figure 10.14   Robert Jones application.

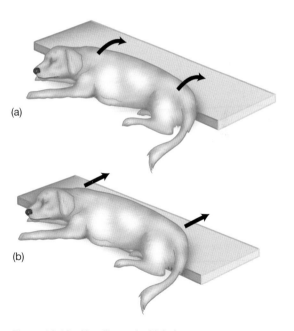

Figure 10.16   Handling spinal injuries.

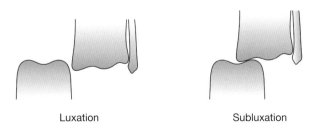

Figure 10.17   Example of a dislocation.

UNCONSCIOUSNESS

First aid measures for the unconscious patient (Tables 10.19–10.24; Figures 10.18–10.22)

- Ascertain cause of unconsciousness
- Maintain a patent airway – equipment for endotracheal intubation should be prepared in case of deterioration
- Provide oxygen supplementation
- Provide warmth – the patient will be unable to regulate its own body temperature
- Provide comfort – the patient will be recumbent and may require extra padding
- Provide intravenous access equipment in order to support circulation
- Monitor the vital signs and record every 5–10 minutes.

Table 10.19   Definition of unconsciousness
Unconsciousness is a state of deep sleep-like unawareness of surroundings with a much-reduced response to external stimuli

Table 10.20   Signs of unconsciousness
Heart and pulse rate are regular but slow
Respiration is deep and regular
The eyeball remains in a fixed position, the palpebral reflex may be weakened but will be dependent on degree of brain damage
Pupillary light response present (level dependent on degree of brain damage)
Flaccid muscles

Table 10.21   Signs of death
Absence of heart beat
Absence of pulse
Absence of respiration
Dilatation of pupil
Loss of corneal reflex
Glazing of cornea
Cool body and rigor mortis

Causes of unconsciousness

Causes of unconsciousness may be primary or secondary. Primary causes are those causing unconsciousness as an immediate result of an injury or incident. Secondary causes are those causing unconsciousness because of another organ failure.

Table 10.22   Monitoring of vital signs
Temperature – core and peripheral
Pulse rate and quality
Heart rate
Respiration rate and quality
Colour of mucous membranes
Capillary refill time
Urine output
Palpebral reflex – eyelids should close when finger tapped on medial aspect of eye
Pupillary reflex – pupils should constrict when light shone into eyes
Demeanour
Response to noise
Response to movement
Continually refer to Table 10.5. Normal clinical parameters

Table 10.23 Causes and treatments of unconsciousness		
Causes	Condition	Treatment
Primary	Epilepsy	Control with medication/sedation
	Brain trauma	Remove cause, relieve pressure, stabilise fracture
	Poisons	If non-corrosive perform gastric lavage. Administer specific antidote
		Treat for shock and control any seizures
Secondary	Airway	Unblock airway and maintain obstruction patency; provide oxygen supplementation and intermittent positive pressure ventilation (IPPV)
	Shock	Establish cause of shock, control haemorrhage and support circulation

(Continued)

Causes	Condition	Treatment
Table 10.23 (*Continued*)		
	Cardiac failure	Ensure patent airway and continue IPPV. Perform external cardiac massage and prepare for internal cardiac massage.
	Hypoglycaemia	Administer glucose orally immediately
	Hypocalcaemia	Prepare for intravenous administration of calcium
	Uraemia	Fluid therapy. May require euthanasia
	Electric shock	Turn off electricity supply before touching animal. Perform cardiac massage and IPPV
	Hypothermia	Warm patient gradually, evenly and effectively with insulation and high ambient temperature
	Hyperthermia	Remove patient from the cause. Cool immediately with cold water baths, ice packs, etc
	Drug overdose	Prepare for administration of reversal agent if appropriate

Clinical signs	Death	Unconsciousness
Table 10.24 Comparison between death and unconsciousness		
Heartbeat present	No	Yes
Respiration present	No	Yes
Palpebral reflex present	No	Yes
Pupillary reflex present	No	Yes (varied)
Corneal reflex present	No	Yes
Muscle tone present	No	Yes
Constant body temperature	No	Yes
Rigor mortis present	Yes	No

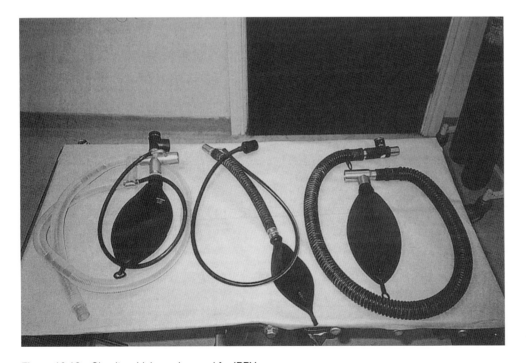

Figure 10.18   Circuits which can be used for IPPV.

Figure 10.19 Assessing heart rate.

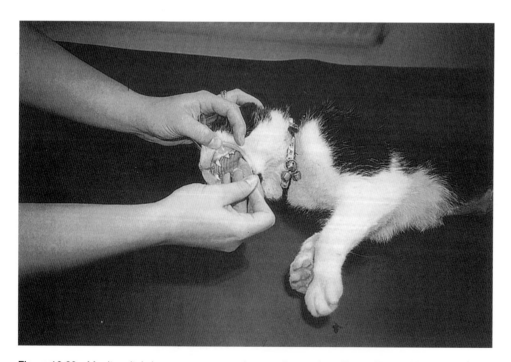

Figure 10.20 Monitor vital signs – mucous membrane colour and capillary refill time (CRT).

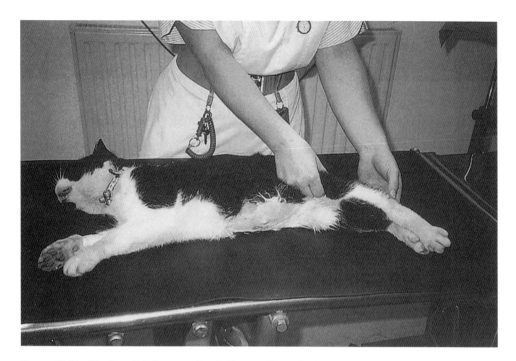

Figure 10.21   Monitor vital signs – pulse rhythm, quality and rate.

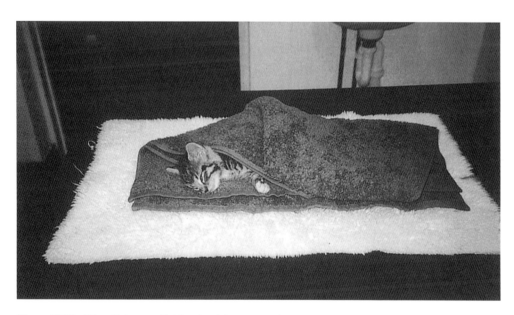

Figure 10.22   Warmth is essential for circulatory support.

Basic nursing skills

Ross D. White

Chapter objectives

This chapter describes:

- Veterinary terminology
- Hospitalisation of domestic pets
- Wild birds and animals brought to the surgery
- Theatre work
- Sterilisation
- Instrumentation

VETERINARY TERMINOLOGY

Many words and terms and conditions are combinations of suffixes, prefixes and anatomical structures.

Some commonly used prefixes and suffixes

A prefix is the first few letters of a word that precedes the main word:

acou – hearing	anastomos – come together
aqua – water	arthr – joint
basal – base	bi – two
brady – slow	cata – down
cephal – head	contra – against
dys – difficult, faulty, painful	endo – within
pulmo – lung	pyo – pus
retro – backward	thromb – clot

A suffix is the last few letters of the main word:

cide – to kill	emia – condition of the blood
logy – the study of	pathy – disease
plasty – reconstruction of a part	stomy – establishment of an opening
tomy – to cut	

Examples:

Bradycardia – slow heart beat
Arthroplasty – reconstruction of a joint

Some commonly used words and their definitions

Anatomy: This is the science dealing with the form and structure of living organisms.
Histology: The study of the microscopic structure of tissue.
Physiology: The science of the functions of the living organism and its components, and the physical and chemical processes involved.
Pathology: The study of disease and its cause.

HOSPITALISATION

Hospitalisation is the admission of the patient to the Veterinary Surgery. The admission of animals to the Veterinary Hospital prior to an operation is often the responsibility of the Veterinary Nurse.

Kennels and cages should be prepared in advance of the admission of routine surgical cases to enable a smooth admission process. Owners may not fully listen to you because they are concerned about their pet, but it is essential that certain information is obtained before they leave the premises.

Essential information required:

- The time the patient last ate (stress to the owner this includes tit bits and treats too).
- The time the patient last drank.
- A contact telephone number.
- A consent form, signed by the owner or representative over 18 years of age (Figure 11.1).
- Confirm the scheduled procedure (this should include a simple explanation of what the procedure

involves). Ensure the procedure and associated complications and anaesthetic risks have been explained by the consulting vet and understood by the owner.

- A contact name and convenient time for the owner to telephone the practice for a progress report.
- Estimation of fees by the consulting vet.
- Ask the owner to check that their own and their pet's details are correct.

- Ask the owner if there are any other simple procedures they would like carried out whilst their pets is anaesthetized, e.g. nail clipping.
- Check that the patient's vaccination history is correct, if they use another practice for vaccination ask a vet to speak to them.
- Postoperative care and special requirements for the patient can also be discussed with the owner during admission, and written postoperative instructions can be handed out.

Form of Consent
Please take time to read this form carefully before signing
Please ask if you have any questions.

Animal Name	Owner's Name	Case Number

I agree to entrust to this veterinary practice the animal described above for examination and treatment on the understanding and condition that reasonable care and attention will be given. Neither the veterinary practice nor any individual member of staff shall be liable for the loss of, or any damage or injury to such animal whether resulting from treatment, care or otherwise.

I hereby give full permission for the animal above to undergo the operation or procedure of:

....

....

....

or for such further or alternative measures or procedures as may be found necessary.

I hereby give permission for the animal described above to be given a sedative, an analgesic, a local or general anaesthetic, or a combination of the aforementioned, or any further or alternative measures as may be considered necessary. I also give my consent for the use of drugs that are not licensed for veterinary use and for which there are no veterinary licensed equivalents, if it is considered necessary by the veterinary surgeon.

I understand that all procedures and anaesthetic techniques involve some risk to the animal, and that these risks may be higher in some animals and some procedures. These risks have been explained to me.

I understand that I will be charged for the service provided by the veterinary practice and that the initial estimation cost for consultation, investigative procedures, treatments and care of my animal will be approximately _____. It has been explained to me that this is an estimate and not a quotation and that the final charge may be greater. (Prices exclude VAT which will be added to the final charge).

I understand that signing this form does not affect my statutory rights.

Signature of owner or agent   Date

....

Name and address of owner

....   Hospital clinician ....

....   Telephone No. ....

....   Contact time ....

Figure 11.1 An example of a consent form.

Hospitalisation of the patient

Once admitted to the hospital it is essential to provide suitable accommodation to minimise the stress encountered by the patient. The individual accommodation will depend on several factors:

- Species of the patient
- Size of the patient
- Operation to be performed (or condition with which the patient is suffering)
- Age of the patient
- Special equipment needs (fluid therapy, electrocardiogram or oxygen therapy).

Once housed in appropriate accommodation the cage should be labelled using a hospital sheet which will incorporate all appropriate details for its care. This will include the following:

- Species
- Operation to be performed (or condition with which the patient is suffering)
- Age
- Name
- Date admitted
- Veterinary Surgeon in charge of the case
- Special requirements and treatment plan.

The hospital sheet should also provide spaces for monitoring the following (Figure 11.2):

- Temperature of the patient
- Pulse of the patient
- Respiration of the patient
- Food intake
- Water intake
- Urination
- Defecation
- Vomiting or diarrhoea
- Administration of any prescribed medication
- Any other relevant comments e.g. demeanour of animal.

Detailed recording of these clinical details is important to allow information to be interpreted by other nurses or Veterinary Surgeons in the practice at a glance, and allow a clinical judgement to be made.

The monitoring of the patient's condition is both a vital and rewarding task. The ward nurse is more likely to be able to assess subtle changes in demeanour than a busy Veterinary Surgeon.

Any subtle changes should be recorded onto the hospital sheet and if urgent reported to a Veterinary Surgeon immediately.

Individual accommodation for patients will depend greatly on the species, size and condition of the patient but the following properties should be considered. (Table 11.1).

The maintenance of hygiene

Several different materials are commonly used for the construction of the accommodation. Each has different properties.

Cleaning of the accommodation

The accommodation must be suitable to undergo daily cleaning with disinfectants. The design should ensure all corners, bars and doors can be thoroughly cleaned.

The facility to disassemble the accommodation which will allow cleaning of all parts is particularly useful.

The kennel should be designed in such a way that any urine and other fluids will drain away from the patient.

Suitable substrates for the patient

Various substrates are available and the ultimate suitability of each will depend on the individual patient's needs. The most commonly used substrates are shown in Table 11.2.

Environmental control

Adequate and controllable heating and ventilation should be provided to allow for the needs of each individual patient.

Natural light should also be provided and supplemented with artificial light during the day with provision for darkness during the night so as not to disorientate the patient's body clock.

Heating of the accommodation

The ward area must be a comfortable temperature for both patients and staff. The recommended temperature for a hospital kennel should not fall below 15°C, and ideal average being around 20°C.

There are various methods of heating the hospital wards that are suitable:

- **Central heating.** This is the most common form of heating used because it has many positive properties. These include:
  - Cost efficiency to install and run
  - A clean form of heating
  - A thermostat to provide a controllable temperature.
- **Underfloor or wall heating.** This form of heating is used in larger purpose built hospitals. If built into the design of a new hospital, wall or floor heating has all the advantages of central heating without unsightly radiators. Provides warmth where the patient is lying.

The individual patient may need additional warmth dependent on its condition. Great care must be taken when arranging direct heating for a patient. Some patients may not be able to move around or be suffering from circulatory shock. Both these conditions will increase the chances of burns to the skin.

Kennel Chart

Animal	Owner	Case Number
Species	Clinician	Student
Breed	Clinical Summary	
Colour		
Sex		
Age		

Date	Day No.	Date	Day No.
Weight	Diet	Weight	Diet

	AM	PM		AM	PM
Temp			Temp		
Pulse			Pulse		
Resp			Resp		
Fed			Fed		
Ate			Ate		
Drank			Drank		

Taken Out				Taken Out			
Urine				Urine			
Faeces				Faeces			

MEDICATION		MEDICATION	
PROCEDURES		PROCEDURES	
COMMENTS		COMMENTS	

Figure 11.2   Example of a kennel chart.

Table 11.1   Accommodation

Type of accommodation	Advantages	Disadvantages
Stainless steel cages	Long lasting, look professional, easy to clean and indestructible	Initially very expensive to purchase; tend to be cold
Brick built kennels with tiled walls	Easy to clean and long lasting	Tiles occasionally become dislodged and grouting may harbour micro-organisms
Wooden kennels	Ease of construction	Will become scratched which may cause injury to patients and can not be easily disinfected
Glass tank	The only suitable accommodation for fish and very useful for rodents	Great care must be taken when moving to avoid breakage

Table 11.2   Substrates

Type of substrate	Advantages	Disadvantages
Newspaper	Often used to line cages under the bedding material. It is readily available, absorbent and easily disposed of	Will offer little warmth or padding and may leave stains on the patient's coat
Straw, wood chippings and sawdust	Readily available, absorbent and warm	May cause allergies in some patients. Very time consuming to clear up afterwards
Vet Bed	Warm, comfortable, easy to wash, hardwearing	Initially expensive and occasionally puppies will rip bits off and ingest them

There are several methods of heating the individual patient:

- **Infrared heating lamp.** These are heating lamps which are usually suspended from the ceiling using a chain. They will provide a localised area of heat but it is essential to remember recumbent patients can easily become over heated and even burned if unable to move from directly under the lamp.
- **Electric heating mat.** These are placed on the floor of the kennel and the patient bedding is put on top. It is an effective, clean and localised form of heating. Great care must be taken if used with a recumbent patient who is not able to move away from the heat. Care should be taken to ensure the patient is not able to chew the electric cable.
- **Hot water bottles.** These should be covered to prevent intense heat coming into direct contact with the patient. Hot water bottles are convenient as they can be positioned next to the patient. Once the temperature of the water falls below body temperature however, the patient will become even colder.
- **Corn heating pads.** These pads are placed in a microwave to heat them through. They must also be covered; however unlike hot water bottles they will not take heat from the patient.
- **Bair Hugger blanket.** This is a system that blows warm air through a type of bag with holes in one side directly over the patient. Excellent for use on patients recovering from and under anaesthesia. Can be expensive to purchase.

A safe and stress-free environment

It is the responsibility of the nurse to ensure a safe environment is provided for the patient to prevent injury whilst at the hospital. Points that should be considered when evaluating the safety of accommodation are as follows:

- Are there any sharp edges which the patient could hurt themselves on?
- Are the bars of the cages adequately spaced to prevent escape or entrapment of limbs?
- Is the substrate suitable to prevent ingestion or slippage resulting in injury?
- Can the patient escape?

The provision for keeping stress levels to a minimum is of particular importance, as stress is a physiological condition with many detrimental effects. These include:

- Increased metabolic needs
- Immunosupression
- Prolonged recovery times
- A poor induction of anaesthesia
- An erratic recovery from anaesthesia
- Restless patients
- Increased risk of injury to both personnel and patient.

Remember a comfortable, safe, happy and stress free patient will recover more quickly than a restless patient.

The individual need of each species must be considered but some rules will apply to all animals:

- Consider the temperature of the accommodation
- Offer the patient an area where they can hide away if applicable
- Keep noise levels to a minimum – ideally have a separated dog and cat ward
- Ensure natural light is available and darkness at night
- Monitoring of the hospitalised animal.

Patients in the ward can be broadly divided into the following five categories depending on their condition:

1. Preoperative surgical patient
2. Postoperative anaesthesia patient
3. Postoperative surgical patient
4. Medical conditions (such as diabetes)
5. Infectious diseases (such as parvovirus).

Preoperative surgical patients

Surgical patients can be divided into the following groups:

- Elective
- Emergency
- Other.

These patients should be prepared prior to surgery, which may include bathing, grooming and the withholding of food and water.

The patient recovering from anaesthesia

These patients have special needs during the recovery period. These include:

- A swollen larynx which will need constant monitoring after extubation to ensure they can maintain their own airway.
- Environment must be stress free to allow a smooth recovery from anaesthesia.
- Accommodation must be well padded to prevent self-injury.
- Patient will be cold and therefore additional heating may be necessary.
- Patients recovering from anaesthesia occasionally vomit, while they are still drowsy and this results in an increased risk of choking – constant monitoring is vital.
- Check for bleeding around the surgical wound – if there is anything more than a small ooze tell the surgeon immediately.
- Temperature, pulse and respiration parameters should be regularly checked as part of routine postoperative care.

The patient recovering from a surgical procedure

These patients will have a surgical wound and it is vital that the wound is kept as clean as possible to prevent post operative wound infection.

The kennel area should also be kept disinfected and these patients should be cleaned out before others suspected of infection.

Postsurgical patients will invariably be in some degree of pain. When the nurse is observing the patient a pain assessment should be made. Observations such as vocalisation, shivering, gait, and mucous membrane colour will help indicate the amount of pain being suffered.

Pain relief may be prescribed by the Veterinary Surgeon in the form of analgesics; however basic nursing skills can also help provide pain relief:

- Provide soft bedding
- Don't move patient excessively
- Immobilisation of local wound area if possible – such as fracture support
- Reduce stress to the animal to a minimum.

These patients may have a wound or internal tissue which will need to heal, therefore will have greater metabolic requirements than most. Particular attention should be paid to providing a high quality energy dense protein diet.

Many patients recovering from surgery may be recumbent and will need regular turning and possibly physiotherapy.

The patient with a medical condition

These patients may have additional nursing requirements such as:

- maintenance of an intravenous drip
- additional monitoring requirements
- special dietary requirements.

There are many different types of medical condition and it is particularly important the patient's individual requirements are discussed with the vet.

The infectious patient

An infectious disease can be defined as a disease due to organisms which may be contagious in origin.

There are a number of conditions which may be described as infectious, these include:

- Parvovirus
- Kennel cough
- Leptospirosis
- Cat flu and enteritis.

Thought must be given to ward routines to prevent the spread of infection to other animals in the hospital.

Ideally the patients with infectious conditions should be isolated from others.

The isolation facility

This is an important part of any ward. When entering an isolation facility, precautions should be undertaken to prevent the spread of disease to other areas.

Specialised protective clothing for members of staff working with these cases should include:

- Disposable gloves
- Disposable mask
- Wellington boots or disposable shoe covers
- Disposable apron
- Disposable cap
- Some practices may use a boiler suit which will cover the entire nurse's uniform.

The facility should be fitted out with its own:

- Sink and washing area
- Food and medicine preparation areas
- Clinical waste and sharps disposal containers
- Stock of bedding materials
- Cleaning and disinfection areas.

Potentially infective material should be carefully monitored and contaminated bedding should not leave the isolation facility before being adequately rinsed and disinfected. Wherever possible a nurse should be specially designated to work with patients in isolation. This nurse should not have contact with other patients.

Barrier nursing

Barrier nursing is the nursing of a patient in the general hospital ward taking great care to avoid cross infection from it to others hospitalised.

The kennel/cage chosen to accommodate the suspected infectious patient should be as far as possible from the other patients, and never opposite where infection could be transmitted in the form of aerosol transfer from coughs and sneezes.

The following principles apply to barrier nursing:

- The staff nursing the patient should not nurse others of the same species if possible and never the young or immunosupressed.
- The infectious patient should be cleaned out after the others.
- Protective clothing should be worn when handling this patient to prevent uniforms from harbouring micro-organisms (a lab coat and disposable gloves would be the minimum).
- The patient should have an individual food bowl, litter tray etc. which is washed separately after others from the ward. Ideally equipment should be sterilisable.
- The protective clothing worn must only be used for this patient.

The special requirements of other species

Pet rodents

These are popular pets particularly amongst children. As a general rule it is preferable to house these rodents in their own cage which the owner should bring into the surgery. This will reduce the stress for the patient. If it is in for a longer stay it will be necessary to thoroughly clean and disinfect the cage at the hospital.

A captive environment for rodents should offer space for exercise and an area for privacy as well as warmth. Food should not be withdrawn before anaesthesia and the patient should be encouraged to eat as soon after the anaesthetic as possible.

Cages should be escape proof and gnaw resistant. Glass or polypropylene tanks are the most suitable and these should incorporate an escape proof and well ventilated lid. Metal cages are not as warm and comfortable and wooden cages soon become gnawed and impossible to clean effectively.

Rodents will need plenty of bedding both to keep them warm and absorb urine. Wood shavings can be used. Man made fibres should be avoided as bedding material as can cause a serious obstruction if ingested.

Feeding of these animals is generally best provided by using a specially designed commercial diet of which there is a large range available.

Rabbits and guinea pigs

Guinea pigs and rabbits can usually be housed in a cat cage without any undue problems. It is preferable to provide a thick towel on the floor, rather than just newspaper, to prevent sore hocks. It should be remembered that some rabbits have been litter trained so the provision of a litter tray may be beneficial. The urine of rabbits is very alkali so cleaning it up regularly will prevent staining of stainless steel hospital cages.

Rabbits tend to be difficult to anaesthetise safely as they can easily become extremely stressed. For this reason it is vital that good stress-free nursing is employed both pre- and postoperatively. Rabbits should be encouraged to eat as soon as possible postoperatively to aid recovery and reduce gut stasis. Various foods can be tried but grated apple or dandelion leaves seem particularly successful.

The hospitalisation of amphibians, reptiles and birds

The treatment and husbandry of these patients can be complicated and constitutes a specialist area. If your practice is not equipped with both adequate equipment and expertise referral should be considered.

Iguana

A large aquarium is a suitable type of accommodation, however if this is not available at the hospital it is possible to improvise using a large cat cage.

It must be considered that the reptile may ingest its substrate material. Newspaper and towels are suitable but monitoring of ingestion should be regularly carried out. Alfalfa pellets can be used as bedding and the iguana may eat this as well. Do not use sand, gravel or wood shavings as these can lead to inpaction and gastric obstruction.

Branches or rocks can be used to provide some environmental enrichment in the cage and an area for the patient to hide. All reptiles are cold blooded and additional heat must be provided. Ideally the cage should be set-up to provide a heat gradient with the heater at one end providing 32–37.7°C and the cooler end being approximately 21–23.8°C. A suitable way of providing this heating is with a 100 Watt incandescent bulb (which should be placed outside the cage).

UV light must be provided if the patient will be spending a prolonged period at the hospital and especially if it is suffering from metabolic bone disease. The UV light should emit light in the UV-B range (290–320 manometers).

Tortoise

The diet provided for tortoises should be plant material with only small quantities of fruit. Acceptable vegetables include mixed greens, cucumber, parsley and other vegetables. Although tortoises are omnivorous, dog and cat food are too rich in vitamin D. Reptile pellets are an acceptable source of proteins.

Again the cage should be set up with a heat gradient between 26°C and 29.4°C at the warmer end and between 15.5°C and 18.3°C at the cooler.

Budgerigar

The budgerigar is the most popular cage bird kept. As with many of the other smaller pets described here, the budgerigar is best hospitalised in its usual cage. The cage however should be a minimum size of 30 × 60 × 60cm to allow the bird to spread its wings fully and obtain some exercise.

Perches should be provided, however it is important the perch is large enough to prevent the claws wrapping themselves all the way round and impaling themselves into the bird own feet. The diameter of the perches should vary and this can be achieved using branches from non-toxic trees. Those from fruit or nut trees, elm or willow are suitable.

The perches and all other furniture should be removed before catching or handling the bird is attempted. The cage should be placed in a quiet and slightly darkened area defiantly not near other natural predators like cats.

Corn snake

A simple vivarium can be used for the housing of smaller snakes. It should be easy to clean and escape proof. A hide box, rock and water bowl can be provided. Newspaper and gravel will make a suitable substrate for the accommodation. A temperature between 28°C and 30°C is suitable for most snakes with one end of the vivarium being warmer than the other.

Wild birds and animals brought to the surgery

Wildlife and Countyside Act 1981. This Act is designed to protect wildlife from cruelty. It is enforced and administrated by The Department for the Environment and Nature Conservancy Council. It is complicated legislation and for the purposes of this chapter the most important points have been highlighted.

Many wild animals have been included in the Act and they have been classified into five Schedules or groups as shown in Table 11.3.

- It is an offence to kill, injure or take any wild bird or to disturb a nesting Schedule 1 bird or its depending young, exempt by special licence in certain circumstances.
- It is an offence to kill, injure or take any Schedule 5 animal intentionally, exempt by licence, or to possess or control such an animal live or dead.
- You are however allowed to take a disabled animal in order to tend and release it, or euthanase it because it was so seriously injured that it has no reasonable chance of recovery or release.
- If the animal is in Schedule 4 you must register it with the Department of the Environment, have a leg ring put on and it should only be treated by a Veterinary Surgeon.
- You will be able to offer emergency first aid to an injured wild animal but after that it should be referred to a Veterinary Surgeon.
- Birds classified under Schedule 4 of the Act may be kept and treated for up to six weeks by a Veterinary Surgeon.
- Wild non-native species such as Canada geese, coypu, mink or grey squirrels should not be released back into the wild. This will cause a dilemma as once these animals are admitted to the veterinary surgery they should not then be released.

The role of the licensed rehabilitation keeper

This is a person who has the experience, facilities and expertise to tend and successfully release birds back into the wild. This person should hold a licence issued by the Department of the Environment. If the bird

Table 11.3   Protected species under the Wildlife and Countryside Act 1981 (revised 1986)

BIRDS

ALL BIRDS, except those listed in Schedule 1, Part II, and in Schedule 2, are fully protected throughout the year, including their nests and eggs.

SCHEDULE *1*, PART *I*: Birds protected by special penalties at all times

*Avocet	*Greenshank	*Sandpiper, Wood
Bee-eater	Gull, little	Scaup
*Bittern	Gull, Mediterranean	*Scoter, common
*Bittern, little	*Harriers (all)	*Scotor, velvet
*Bluethroat	*Heron, purple	*Serin
Brambling	*Hobby	*Shorelark
*Bunting, Cirl	*Hoopoe	*Shrike, red-backed
*Bunting, Lapland	*Kingfisher	*Spoonbill
*Bunting, snow	*Kite, red	*Stilt, black-winged
*Buzzard, honey	*Merlin	*Stint, Temminck's
*Chough	*Oriole, golden	Swan, Bewick's
*Corncrake	*Osprey	Swan, whooper
*Crake, spotted	Owl, barn	*Tern, black
*Crossbills (all)	Owl, snowy	*Tern, little
*Curlew, stone	*Peregrine	*Tern, roseate
*Divers (all)	*Petrel, Leach's	*Tit, bearded
*Dotterel	*Phalarope, Red-necked	*Tit, crested
*Duck, long-tailed	*Plover, Kentish	*Treecreeper Short-toed
*Eagle, golden	*Plover, Little Ringed	*Warbler, Cetti's
*Eagle, White-tailed	*Quail, Common	*Warbler, Dartford
*Falcon, gyr	*Redstart, Black	*Warbler, marsh
*Fieldfare	*Redwing	*Warbler, Savi's
*Firecrest	*Rosefinch, scarlet	*Whimbrel
Garganey	*Ruff	*Woodlark
*Godwit, black-tailed	*Sandpiper, green	*Wryneck
*Goshawk	*Sandpiper, purple	
*Grebe, black-necked		
*Grebe, Slavonian		

*Also SCHEDULE 4 species; must be registered if kept in captivity. Schedule 4 includes all birds of prey except Old World vultures and many other birds as shown here.

SCHEDULE *1*, PART *II*: Birds protected by special penalties during the close season (1st February to 31st August, or 21st February to 31st August below high-water mark) but may be killed or taken outside this period

Golden eye
Goose, greylag (in Outer Hebrides, Caithness, Sutherland and Wester Ross only)
Pintail.

SCHEDULE *2*, PART *I*: Birds protected during the close season but may be killed or taken outside this period

Capercaillie	Goose, Canada	Coot
Goose, greylag	Duck, tufted	Goose, pink-footed
Gadwall	Goose, white-fronted	Goldeneye
Mallard	Moorhen	Snipe, common
Pintail	Teal	Plover, golden
Wigeon	Pochard	Woodcock
Shoveler		

SCHEDULE *2*, PART *II*: Birds which may be killed or taken by authorised persons at all times

Crow	Gull, herring	Sparrow, house
Dove, collared	Jackdaw	Starling
Gull, great black-backed	Jay	Woodpigeon
Gull, lesser black-backed	Magpie	Pigeon, feral
Rook		

SCHEDULE *3*, PART *I*: Birds which may be sold alive at all times if ringed and bred in captivity

Blackbird	Greenfinch	Siskin
Brambling	Jackdaw	Starling
Bullfinch	Jay	Thrush, song

(Continued)

Table 11.3 *(Continued)*		
Bunting, reed	Linnet	Twite
Chaffinch	Magpie	Yellowhammer
Dunnock	Owl, barn	
Goldfinch	Redpoll	
SCHEDULE 3, PART II: Birds which may be sold dead at all times		
Pigeon, feral		
Woodpigeon		
SCHEDULE 3, PART III: Birds which may be sold dead from 1st September to 28th February		
Capercaillie	Pintail	Snipe, common
Coot	Plover, golden	Teal
Duck, tufted	Pochard	Wigeon
Mallard	Shoveler	Woodcock
OTHER ANIMALS		
SCHEDULE 5: It is normally an offence to kill, injure, take, possess or sell any of the following animals, whether alive or dead, or to disturb their place of shelter and protection or to destroy that place		
Adder (sale only)	Otter	
Bats (all species)	Porpoises	
Wild cat	Slow-worm	
Dolphins	Grass snake	
Dormouse	Smooth snake	
Common frog (sale only)	Red squirrel	
Sand lizard	Common toad (sale only)	
Viviparous lizard	Natterjack toad	
Pine marten	Marine turtles	
Great crested or Warty newt	Walrus	
Palmate newt (sale only)	Whales	
Smooth newt (sale only)		
(Also several insects, marine creatures etc.) Extracts taken from Animal Rescue 1989, Ashford, Buchan and Enright.		

cannot be released after six weeks it must be registered with the Department for the Environment and ringed.

Handling wild birds

When catching a large wild bird it should be held from above with both hands, one hand may be sufficient with a smaller bird. The hands should be placed to keep the wings close to the body. Birds should not be held by wings or legs alone.

Accommodation

The accommodation must be large enough to allow the bird to stretch its wings fully. Ideally a free flight aviary should be provided.

Ground-loving birds like quail should be given cover in the form of branches on the ground, and provided with a dust bath.

A variety of perches should be provided.

Most birds will need bathing water in addition to drinking water.

Hedgehogs

Hedgehogs can be kept in a hospital cage with an abundance of straw or shredded newspaper provided. A small cardboard box will also allow the hedgehog a place to hide.

The diet can be varied with tinned dog and cat food being acceptable. If hospitalised for a prolonged period fruit, nuts and dog biscuits should be added to provide a more balanced diet.

THEATRE WORK

Maintaining an aseptic theatre

Theatre work is an integral part of the daily routine of a Veterinary Nurse.

The prevention of pathogenic micro-organisms in the theatre is the priority of the theatre nurse and the term used to describe this is aseptic technique. Asepsis is the removal and destruction of all pathogenic micro-organisms.

Common sources of contamination which will lead to a break in asepsis in the theatre include:

- The patient's skin
- Theatre environment
- Theatre staff
- Theatre equipment
- Surgical technique.

Reducing contamination
The patient
- Ensure the patient has been encouraged to urinate and defecate before entering the preparation room or theatre.
- Bath and groom the patient in the wards to remove gross dirt and soiling from the patient's coat if necessary.
- Adequate clipping of the surgical site.
- Appropriate cleansing of the surgical site with an antiseptic solution such as povidon iodine or hibitane.
- Consider the health status of the patient and its implications for example immunosuppression.

Theatre staff
It is normal that the hair and skin of staff will harbour micro-organisms. Although these will not cause us any harm they may become pathogenic to our patients.

- Wash hands or shower before entering the theatre.
- Change clothing worn during other duties in the hospital before entering the theatre area. This may be in the form of a special lightweight scrub suit kept especially for theatre wear and cleaned daily. At the very least a clean theatre gown should be worn over the top of the normal uniform.
- Change footwear to theatre shoes or covers.
- Cover all hair with a surgeon's cap.
- A facial mask should be worn.

Special clothing worn by the surgeon
Additional to the clothing worn by the theatre team the surgeon should also wear:

- a sterile operating gown
- sterile disposable operating gloves.

The theatre environment
It is essential that the theatre environment be kept as clean as possible to keep the levels of micro-organisms in the theatre to a minimum. The cleaning of a theatre is a continual process with the following protocols.

In the morning before the operating session begins:
Damp dust all surfaces with a cloth soaked in a broad spectrum disinfectant solution.

Particular attention should be paid to the following areas:

- the anaesthetic machine
- operating table
- theatre lights
- instrument trolley
- any other surfaces which may have gathered dust over night.

Between operations:
- clean away any used instruments and soak them in a proprietary instrument cleaning solution
- dispose of any used swabs, suture material, bandages, syringes etc, correctly
- wipe up any spots of blood or other contaminants
- sweep and mop any hair off the floor
- repeat damp dusting.

At the end of an operating session:
- dispose of any waste correctly
- systematically clean all surfaces and floors, using a suitable cleaning and disinfecting regime
- avoid thoroughfare once the area has been cleaned.

Disposal of theatre waste
Most waste from the theatre will be contaminated with blood or other body fluids therefore is classified as clinical waste. It is safe practice to dispose of all theatre waste into specific clinical waste bags which will be collected and incinerated.

Conduct of personnel within the theatre
The theatre staff can be broadly split into two categories:

- **Scrubbed personnel.** These are members of the team who have scrubbed hands and arms aseptically and have donned a sterile gown and gloves. This will include the surgeon and possibly a surgical assistant.
- **Non-scrubbed personnel.** These members of the staff should be wearing a mask, hat and either a special scrub suit or protective clothing over their uniform. They will include the anaesthetist and the theatre nurse. Non-scrubbed personnel should not touch anything which is sterile and in use by the scrubbed personnel as this could cause contamination of the operating site and equipment.

Speaking in the theatre should be kept to a minimum as the moisture will reduce the effectiveness of the surgical mask. Movement should also be kept to a minimum as it will create dust which may contaminate the patient.

Table 11.4 Sterilisation

Principle	Method	Sterilisation times	Suitable indicator	Items for sterilisation
Dry heat	Hot air oven	180° for 60min, glass, non-cutting instruments; 160°C for 120min, powders/oils; 150°C for 180min, cutting instruments	Brownes tube (green dot) Spore tests	Sharp/fine instruments
Moist heat	Boiling	100°C (boiling point) for 30min	None available	Instruments (not sharp edges)
Moist heat	Autoclave	121°C, 15psi, 15min 126°C, 20psi, 10min 134°C, 30psi, 3–3.5min	Brownes tube (yellow dot) Indicator strips Bowie–Dick tape TST strips Spore tests Thermocouples	Instruments Drapes and gowns Plastics/rubber (care) Hand towels
Chemical – gas	Ethylene oxide	12 hours exposure followed by 24h ventilation	Indicator tape (green to red stripes) Spore tests Indicator strips	Drills Endoscopes Plastics/rubber Instruments
Chemical – liquid	Chlorhexidine/alcohol/ gluteraldehydes	Follow manufacturer's guidelines	None available	Instruments (some) endoscopes

Sterilisation of surgical equipment

The instruments used during surgery must be free from all pathogenic micro-organisms, this is essential to prevent intraoperative wound infections.

There are several different methods of sterilisation that are used to provide sterile surgical equipment (see Table 11.4).

Instrument cleaning

Surgical instruments must be carefully looked after to ensure they remain sharp and work properly.

Below is a suggested routine for cleaning instruments manually:

- Remove all sharps (scalpel blades etc.) and dispose of correctly.
- Separate instruments, this is to prevent heavy ones damaging more delicate ones.
- Blood and tissue debris should be cleaned off immediately with cold water. Hot water will cause blood to coagulate on the instrument making it more difficult to clean off.
- Saline solutions should be washed off as soon as possible.
- If available place into ultrasonic cleaner (see below for description).
- Use running water and a soft plastic brush to scrub the instrument.
- Use a recommended instrument cleaner.

- Inspect the instruments to ensure there are no contaminates left especially in the joints or teeth. If there is tissue present remove it with a soft brush.
- Once the recommended soaking time has been reached thoroughly rinse each instrument in lukewarm water.
- Dry each instrument individually in disposable paper towel paying particular attention to joints.

Instrument lubrication

The joints of instruments may become stiff with repeated use. Instruments can be lubricated to prevent this problem. This should be performed after cleaning but before sterilisation.

Only use specialised instrument oil, either as a spray or as a water soluble solution which does not affect sterilisation.

The ultrasonic cleaner

This is a small water bath through which very high frequency sound waves are passed. These sound waves agitate the water and in the process clean off any blood or debris from the instrument. These cleaners have the advantage of dispensing with the process of scrubbing which may possibly cause damage to the instrument. The sound and water waves will reach the inside of the joints which cannot be seen or scrubbed.

The packing of surgical instruments for sterilisation

Surgical instruments can be packed for sterilisation and storage in several ways but the following principles will apply to all different materials used:

- Cover sharp edges (such as orthopaedic pin ends) with a swab or specially purchased rubber cap. This is done to prevent damage to the packing material or the instrument.
- Do no pack too many instruments into the packaging as this may impede sterilisation and cause excessively damp packs after autoclaving.
- Do not remove the packs from the sterilisation chamber until they are completely dry.
- All packs should be labelled with date, staff initials and a description of content.
- All packs should contain a sterilisation indicator.
- Once the dry surgical pack is removed from the autoclave it should be stored in a dry dust free cupboard until required.

Some different types of packing materials commonly used in veterinary practice are listed below:

- peel and seal bags
- autoclave film
- metal sterilisation drums
- paper sterilisation bags
- specially designed cardboard or plastic boxes.

Commonly used surgical instruments

- **Mayo scissors.** These are the most commonly used scissors with strong rounded blades. They are used for all purpose tissue dissection.

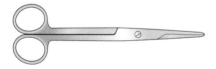

Figure 11.3   Mayo scissors.

- **Metzenbaum scissors.** These are commonly used for more delicate soft tissue surgery. They are a fine lightweight scissors ideal for fine and precession cutting.

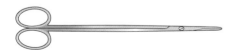

Figure 11.4   Metzenbaum scissors.

- **Gillies needle holders.** These needle holders have a curved thumb piece enabling the user to pass the needle through the skin using a rotation of the wrist. They include scissors for cutting suture material, however they do have the drawback of not having a rack mechanism.

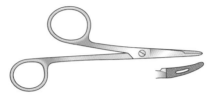

Figure 11.5   Gillies needle holder.

- **Dressing forceps.** These are nontraumatic forceps used for holding tissues with a lumen which must not be punctured such as the uterus. They do have the disadvantage that a firm grip must be used to prevent tissue slippage, this may cause tissue trauma.

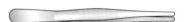

Figure 11.6   Dressing forceps.

- **Rat toothed forceps.** These are the standard tissue forceps used to manipulate tissues such as skin edges. They incorporate teeth at the end to firmly grasp tissue.

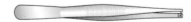

Figure 11.7   Rat-toothed forceps.

- **Allis tissue forceps.** These are the standard tissue forceps with a rach used in veterinary practice. They have small teeth at the ends which will grasp the tissue causing only minimal trauma and hold it firmly while it is clamped in the forceps.

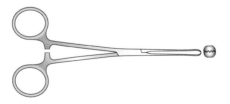

Figure 11.8   Allis tissue forceps.

■ **Artery forceps.** There are a variety of different types of artery forceps the most commonly used being the Spencer Wells. Artery forceps are used for clamping arteries and other vessels in veterinary practice.

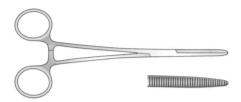

Figure 11.9   Artery forceps.

■ **Towel clips.** These are used to hold surgical drapes in place. There are a variety of different types but the Backhaus towel clips are one of the most commonly used types.

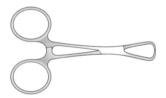

Figure 11.10   Towel clips.

■ **Dental handscalers.** There are two main classification of handscalers – supragingival for use

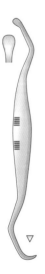

Figure 11.11   Dental handscalers.

above the gum line and subgingival for use below the gum line. Dental scalers are used to remove plaque and dental calculi from the surface of the tooth. They must be used with care as will cause scratching to the surface that must be polished afterwards.

■ **Dental forceps.** These are used to remove teeth. Their tips can be curved or straight depending on what type of tooth is to be removed.

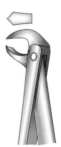

Figure 11.12   Dental forceps.

■ **Peridontal probe.** This is used to measure the depth between the gum line and the tooth attachment and has graduations marked on to it. The depth of the pocket will give the surgeon an indication of the health of the tooth and gum.

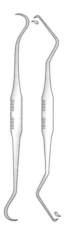

Figure 11.13   Peridontal probe.

■ **Gigli saw (wire).** This is fine barbed wire used to cut bone in difficult to reach places. It should not be confused with embryotomy wire that has much larger serrations and is used to cut soft tissue.

Rongeurs. Used to remove small pieces of bone, as they have a cutting edge at the tip.

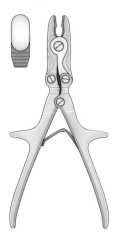

Figure 11.14   Rongeurs.

Bone cutting forceps. Used to cut bone.

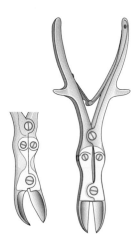

Figure 11.15   Bone cutting forceps.

Bone holding forceps. These are used to hold bone steady whilst fracture repair is undertaken.

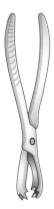

Figure 11.16   Bone holding forceps.

Osteotome. Used for cutting and shaping bone.

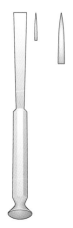

Figure 11.17   Osteotome.

Orthopaedic mallet. Used in conjunction with the osteotome. Some mallets have a copper insert to reduce the impact.

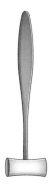

Figure 11.18   Orthopaedic mallet.

Plaster shears. Heavy scissor type instruments used to cut through a limb cast.

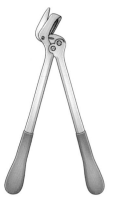

Figure 11.19   Plaster shears.

- **Intramedullary pin.** This is a pin used most often to repair fractures of long bones. It is placed down the medullary cavity of the bone holding both fragments in close proximity.
- **Intramedullary pinchuck/introducer (Jacobs chuck).** Used to hold the intramedullary pin stable whilst it is driven into the bone's medullary cavity.
- **Kirschner wire.** This is very similar to the intramedullary pin however usually much smaller. K wires are used for a variety of fracture fixation purposes and can be easily bent and shaped to suit their function.
- **Putti rasp.** This instrument is used to smooth rough bones to reduce or prevent further soft tissue trauma.
- **Orthopaedic drill.** Their are a variety of drills used in veterinary practice such as air drills, battery powered or hand drills. They are all used to facilitate the placement of pins and screws in fracture fixation.

Further reading and resources

- Alfred Cox Limited, Surgical Instruments.
- Animalcare Limited, Surgery Plus Instrumentation.
- Blood, D.C., Studdert V.P. (1996) Baillière's Comprehensive Veterinary Dictionary. Baillière Tindall, London.
- Cooper, J.E., Hutchison, M.F., Jackson, O.F., Maurice R.J. (1985) Manual of Exotic Pets. British Small Animal Veterinary Association.
- Dennis, M., McCurin, M.S. (2000) Clinical Textbook for Veterinary Technicians, 3rd edn. W.B. Saunders, London.
- Lane, D.R., Cooper, B. (1999) Veterinary Nursing. Butterworth-Heinemann, London.
- Porter, V. (1989) Animal Rescue. Buchan and Enright, Ashford.

Chapter 12

Working safely in practice

Denise Prisk

PHARMACY, DISPENSING AND ADMINISTRATION OF MEDICATION

Classification of medicines

There are different types of legislation that control the use of veterinary medicines. The Veterinary Medicines Regulations 2005 came into force on 30th October 2005. These regulations replaced the Medicines Act 1968. Under the regulations, the groups of veterinary drugs are:

- **Prescription Only Medicine – Veterinarian (POM-V).** Medicines in this group must be prescribed by a veterinary surgeon following clinical assessment of the animal. Clients may choose to have a written prescription or be supplied with the actual product.
- **Prescription Only Medicine – Veterinarian, Pharmacist, Suitably Qualified Person (POM-VPS).** These medicines may be prescribed by a veterinary surgeon, registered pharmacist or registered suitably qualified person. Clinical assessment of the animal is not required. As with POM-V products, clients may choose to have a written prescription or be supplied with the actual product.
- **Non-Food Animal – Veterinarian, Pharmacist, Suitably Qualified Person (NFA-VPS).** These products may be supplied by a veterinary surgeon, registered pharmacist or registered suitably qualified person. Clinical assessment of the animal is not required, nor is a prescription.
- **Authorised Veterinary Medicine – General Sales List (AVM-GSL).** Products in this group can be supplied by any retailer. There are no restrictions as the products generally have a wide safety margin.

The Misuse of Drugs Act 1971

This Act incorporates the Misuse of Drugs Regulations 1985. Its purpose is to prevent the misuse of the drugs of abuse. There are five schedules for categorising Controlled Drugs:

Schedule 1 includes the drugs of addiction, such as LSD and cannabis
Schedule 2 includes morphine and pethidine
Schedule 3 includes pentobarbitone and phenobarbitone
Schedule 4 includes diazepam
Schedule 5 includes some codeine preparations

Drugs in Schedule 1 have the strictest control (although these drugs have no therapeutic use and are not used in general veterinary practice) and those in Schedule 5 have the least control. There are strict regulations that control the purchase, storage, handling and use of drugs in Schedules 2 and 3.

Table 12.1 Drug groups and functions

Group	Function
Analgesic	Relieves pain
Anthelmintic	Acts against parasitic worms (helminths)
Antibiotic	Used to treat or prevent bacterial infections
Anticonvulsant	Prevents convulsions/fits
Anti-emetic	Prevents vomiting
Antihistamine	Used to treat allergies
Antitussive	Suppresses coughing
Diuretic	Increases the amount of urine passed
Ecbolic	Causes the uterus to contract
Emetic	Induces vomiting
Expectorant	Increases the volume of respiratory secretions and makes them less thick
Fungicide	Kills fungi
Hormone	Complex group of chemicals, composed of protein or steroid. They act on various body systems
Laxative	Increases the amount of faeces passed
Narcotic	Induces sleep
Neuroleptanalgesic	Produces analgesia (pain relief) and sedation
Non-steroidal anti-inflammatory drug	Commonly known as NSAID. These drugs reduce pain and inflammation
Parasiticide	Kills parasites. This term is generally used to describe preparations which kill ectoparasites
Sedative	Produces calmness and drowsiness
Tranquilliser	Produces calmness without drowsiness

Table 12.2 Dispensing abbreviations

Abbreviation	Meaning
ad lib	As much as desired, or to appetite
b.i.d.	To be given twice a day
t.i.d.	To be given three times a day
q.i.d.	To be given four times a day
q 4 h	To be given every four hours
s.i.d.	To be given once a day
o.d.	To be given every day

used. Employees should be aware of any such risks and the precautions that should be taken. If in doubt, the drug data sheet should be consulted. It may be necessary to wear gloves when handling some medicines, such as hormones, penicillins, chloramphenicol, griseofulvin and steroid creams. A face mask is also necessary when handling other medicines, such as cytotoxic drugs.

Common abbreviations

Abbreviations of Latin words are used when writing a prescription. Those in regular use are shown in Table 12.2. However, when producing a label for a medicine to be dispensed, the instructions should be written out in full.

Labels should be computer generated. The information which must be shown on a label, by law, is:

- Name and address of veterinary surgeon
- Name and address of owner, or person who has control of the animal
- Date of dispensing
- Warnings: For Animal Treatment Only, Keep out of the reach of children and, if applicable, For External Use Only.

Other information, which is not a legal requirement, but advisable to show:

- Dose/directions for use
- Name and strength of product
- Name of animal.

Medicines are classified according to their use and the way in which they work. There are many different groups of drugs. Some examples of drug groups and their functions are given in Table 12.1.

Dispensing and labelling of medicines

The legal requirements are set out in the Medicines Labelling Regulations. The manufacturer's label should always be consulted before any medicine is handled. The Classification, Packaging and Labelling of Dangerous Substances Regulations 1984 state that all containers of dangerous substances must be clearly labelled. The Control of Substances Hazardous to Health Regulations 2002 require employers to assess the risks created by any work in which a hazardous substance is

It there are any special precautions, these must, of course, be clearly shown, e.g. if the owner should wear gloves when handling the product.

Medicines should be dispensed in an appropriate container. One with solid sides should be used for loose tablets. Pre-packed preparations or small tubes may be placed in a paper envelope or bag and the outer container labelled. Liquids for external use (such as shampoo) should be dispensed in a fluted, or ridged, bottle. Those for internal use (such as cough linctus) should be dispensed in a smooth-sided bottle.

Calculating drug dosages

A dosage is usually shown as a dose rate – weight of drug in milligrams (mg) per weight of animal in kilograms (kg): mg/kg body weight.

Example: If a dog weighing 10 kg needs to be treated with a drug at a dose rate of 5 mg/kg, how many mg of the drug does the dog need?

Dose = Dose rate (mg) × body weight (kg)
5 × 10 = 50 mg

If each tablet or mL of liquid contains 25 mg of the drug, how many tablets/mL does the dog need?

The calculation is the dose required (mg) divided by the strength of tablets/liquid (mg).

50 ÷ 25 = 2 tablets or 2 mL

Administration of medicines

There are various ways in which medicines can be given:

- Oral administration – by mouth
- Topical administration – applied to the body surface
- Parenteral administration – by injection.

Oral administration
Medicines suitable for oral administration are tablets, pills, capsules, liquids, oral powders and pastes.

Tablets, pills and capsules are placed on the back of the tongue, and the mouth held shut until the animal has swallowed. The head should not be tilted too far back as the animal may panic and struggle. Some tablets can be crushed in food to facilitate administration, but the owner must make sure the animal has eaten all its food. Pill poppers are available for use when giving tablets. The instructions for use must be observed, for the medicine to work – i.e. give before or after food, do not break tablet etc.

Liquids are usually given by syringe, into the side of the mouth. Some liquid medicines and nutritional supplements for small animals and exotics can be added to the drinking water. It is not normally crucial that the animal drinks all the water, but it may be necessary or advisable that other animals do not have access to the medicated water.

Oral pastes can be placed directly onto the animal's tongue. Powders are mixed with food.

Topical administration
Medicines given by this route include:

- Shampoo, cream, ointment, lotion, liniment, powder, sprays and 'spot-on' applications, all of which are applied directly to the skin
- Medicines applied to the eyes and ears, such as drops or ointment.

Depending on the type of product, it may be necessary to rub it into the skin (cream or liniment), daub on gently (lotion), apply with an aerosol (spray) or apply drops.

Parenteral administration
Parenteral means giving medicines by any route other than via the gastrointestinal tract, but the term is generally used to describe giving medicines by injection. A sterile syringe and hypodermic needle of suitable size are required.

The most common injection routes are:

- **Subcutaneous (s/c)** – under the skin. Usually the scruff of the neck or loose skin along the back is used.
- **Intramuscular (i/m)** – into a muscle. The quadriceps muscles in front of the femur and the lumbar muscles of the back are the most common sites for i/m injections.
- **Intravenous (i/v)** – into a vein. The most common site for giving an i/v injection is the cephalic vein in the forelimb. The jugular vein in the neck and the saphenous vein in the hind limb can also be used. The ventral tail vein may be used in small mammals, snakes or lizards.

Fluid therapy

Fluid therapy is needed to replace fluid losses from the body. Dehydration may occur because an animal has lost excessive amounts of fluid or because of a lack of fluid intake. Loss of water and electrolytes (salts) occurs in vomiting, diarrhoea, haemorrhage and burns. Water deprivation can occur if the animal is unable to swallow, if it pants excessively, its temperature is very high (pyrexia) or in some medical conditions, such as the hormonal condition diabetes insipidus.

Fluids may be replaced orally, by tube, or by injection. The route chosen will depend on the animal's condition, the type of fluid and the desired speed of effect. Large volumes of fluid are given by intravenous injection, into the cephalic vein on the cranial aspect of the fore limb or the jugular vein, which runs down each side of the ventral neck. The saphenous vein, located on the lateral aspect of the hind limb, just above the hock, can be used if necessary but is often less successful as the vein is mobile. The marginal ear vein or cephalic vein is used to administer intravenous fluids to rabbits. Fluids should be given at body temperature.

Equipment

All equipment should be sterile and in date. The equipment necessary to give i/v fluids:

- **Intravenous catheter** – Over-the-needle or Through-the-needle type. Hypodermic and butterfly needles are less successful than catheters as they tend to move and puncture the wall of the vein.
- **Infusion giving set** – these deliver a specified number of drops per mL – usually 20, although burettes, which are used to give small amounts of fluid to small or young animals, deliver 60 drops/mL, as do paediatric giving sets.

If it is necessary to give whole blood, a blood giving set must be used. This has two chambers and a filter to prevent clots passing into the vein. Blood giving sets usually deliver 15 drops/mL.

Any animal which is receiving i/v fluids must be monitored. The area around the vein should be checked – if the needle or catheter has moved, the fluid will accumulate outside the vein, which is said to 'blow'. If the tubing becomes kinked, the fluid will stop flowing. This may also happen if the animal bends its leg or interferes with the equipment. Fluid infusion pumps deliver a specified volume and rate of fluid. If an infusion pump is not used, the rate of infusion should be closely monitored as either under or over-infusion can be dangerous to the patient. The fluid bag should be suspended from a drip stand, to aid flow by gravity. Any abnormalities must be reported immediately and the fluid disconnected.

LABORATORY PROCEDURES

When performing any type of laboratory procedure a protective coat should be worn. Gloves and a face mask may be necessary, as when performing bacteriology, handling body specimens or using fixative solutions such as formal saline. Long hair should be tied back and jewellery removed.

Microscope (Figure 12.1)

The light microscope is an instrument which uses a system of lenses and mirrors to refract, or bend light, from a given light source, through the object of interest, on to the eyepiece and eye. The strength of the lenses used determines the magnification of the object.

Parts of the microscope are shown in Table 12.3.

Use of the microscope

The microscope is an expensive instrument and must be handled with care. When not in use, it should be switched off and kept in its box or enclosed in a protective cover, to prevent dust settling on it. It should be carried with two hands and placed on a firm surface.

To achieve the best results from the microscope, it should be properly set-up. This involves focusing the condenser and setting the iris diaphragm correctly.

- Set the eyepieces to the correct width and select low power objective lens.
- Turn light intensity to low, switch microscope on, then increase light to a medium setting.
- Raise the substage condenser fully and open the iris diaphragm fully.
- Rack the stage down and place slide in holder on the stage. Make sure the area of interest is centred under the objective lens.
- Rack the stage up until the tip of the objective lens is about 2 mm away from the slide. Most low power lenses will not be long enough to get this close to the slide. In this case, rack the stage up as far as it will go.
- Looking down both eyepieces, slowly lower the stage, using the coarse focus, until the specimen comes into view.
- Adjust the fine focus to bring the specimen sharply into focus.

There are various ways of focusing the condenser and setting the iris diaphragm, depending on the type of microscope, and the manufacturer's instructions should be followed.

Magnification

The total magnification is that of the objective lens multiplied by that of the eyepiece lens, e.g. if the eyepiece lens is ×10 and the objective lens is ×40, the total magnification is ×400. **This is the same whether using a monocular or binocular microscope.**

Table 12.4 shows the use of different objective lenses.

After use, the microscope should be cleaned. The stage should be wiped of any oil or grease, as should the lenses. The eyepiece lenses can be carefully cleaned with a dry lens tissue. It may be necessary to remove these lenses and wipe both ends. Dust can be removed with a soft brush. The objective lenses should also be dusted and wiped clean, paying particular attention to the oil immersion lens. Immersion oil must be removed immediately after use, in case it leaks into the lens. A lens tissue should be used, but if the objective has become sticky it may be necessary to use a

Table 12.3 Parts of the microscope	
Part	**Function**
Foot	The base which supports the microscope
Limb	The main backbone of the microscope
Body and body tube	Area at the top of the limb which extends from the eyepiece to the nosepiece
Stage	A flat platform to hold the microscope slide. A mechanical stage is one with stage motion controls, which allow movement in horizontal and vertical directions
Vernier scales	Found on the mechanical stage, these are two scales, at right angles to each other. They are used to identify the position of a specimen so it can be relocated. The microscope slide is positioned in the slide holder, attached to the Vernier plates, one end of which is spring-loaded. Older microscopes, which do not have a mechanical stage, have two spring clips to secure the slide, which must then be moved manually, to examine the specimen
Substage condenser	This is a lens under the stage, which can be moved towards the stage or away from it. It allows the light source to be focused on the object
Iris diaphragm	Found beneath the condenser, this device has a lever which controls the amount of light passing up the microscope
Light source	An internal light source is incorporated into the base of modern microscopes. There is also provision to adjust the intensity of the light, by means of a lever or dial. Older microscopes require an external light source, which is reflected by a mirror under the stage
Coarse and fine focus	The coarse focus control moves, or 'racks' the stage up and down, and is used to find the object. The fine focus control is used when the object has been found, to give clear detail and to focus to the individual's requirements
Nosepiece	Found at the end of the body, this is a rotating device which holds the objective lenses
Objective lenses	These are the lenses nearest the specimen. They give varying magnifications, such as ×4, ×10, ×40 and ×90/100. The strength is shown on the side of the lens
Eyepiece and eyepiece lens	The eyepiece tube holds the eyepiece lens(es) which have a magnification of ×6, ×8 or ×10. A monocular microscope has one eyepiece and therefore, one eyepiece lens. A binocular microscope has two eyepieces and two eyepiece lenses

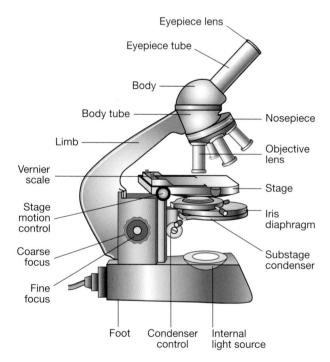

Figure 12.1   A light microscope.

small amount of microscope lens cleaning fluid such as Citroclear.

It is advisable to have the microscope regularly serviced by a qualified technician.

Postage and packing of pathological samples

All pathological samples which are sent in the post are governed by the Postal Regulations. According to these, the only people who are permitted to post pathological specimens are:

■ Recognised laboratories or institutions
■ Qualified medical or veterinary practitioners
■ Registered dentists
■ Osteopaths
■ Nurses.

Members of the public are only permitted to post pathological specimens at the specific request of one of the above and with written permission from the post office. The person making the request should supply appropriate packaging.

Table 12.4 Use of different objective lenses			
Low power ×4	Low power ×10	High power	Oil immersion ×90 or 100
Scanning the slide and initial examination to locate the area of interest	Ectoparasites Hair and skin Urine deposits Worm eggs Faecal smears Blood cell counts	More detail of objects examined under low power Dry preparation of urine Red blood cell counts (easier to count under HP)	Smears: Blood smears for a differential white cell count, or to look for blood parasites Bacterial smears to examine bacteria Vaginal smears

Most commercial laboratories supply the veterinary practice with containers for packaging. The postal regulations state that:

- The specimen must be placed in a securely sealed, leak-proof container, not exceeding 50 mL or 50 grams.
- There must be enough absorbent material to absorb all possible leakage.
- The specimen is then placed in a leak-proof plastic bag. If two or more samples are sent, separate containers and additional absorbent padding will be required.
- An outer, strong container is used to enclose the previously packed sample, such as a light metal container, a strong cardboard box or a two-piece polystyrene box filled with absorbent material and the two halves fixed together with tape.
- The complete package should then be placed in a padded bag and labelled with the words PATHOLOGICAL SPECIMEN – FRAGILE – WITH CARE. The sender's name and address must be shown.
- If large samples are to be sent in the post, or if non-standard packaging is used, the practitioner must first seek approval from the Royal Mail.
- Samples must be sent by first class mail and should not be posted over a weekend or bank holiday, unless laboratory personnel are able to receive them.

RADIOGRAPHY

All ionising radiations present a hazard, but with good safety precautions, exposure to radiation can be limited. Living cells which are exposed to radiation can be damaged or killed. Those which are most susceptible are rapidly dividing cells, such as gonads, cells of young animals or people and tumour cells.

Damage from radiation may be cumulative – exposure to repeated small doses over a long period of time can be as serious as a single exposure to a high dose, as in some cases of leukaemia in people. In addition to damaging cell structure, genes of reproductive cells can also be harmed, causing the genes to mutate. The effects of this may not be obvious until some time later. The box below shows some of the harmful effects of radiation.

Harmful effects of radiation

- Inflammation
- Blood disorders
- Death of tissue
- Death or mutation of developing foetus
- Damage to gonads
- Infertility
- The production of tumours

The main beam which is produced when making an exposure is called the primary beam. This represents the biggest hazard to personnel, although no part of the operator's body should ever be exposed to the primary beam.

Secondary radiation, or 'scatter', is produced when particles of energy from the primary beam hit a surface (such as tissues, or inanimate surfaces) and cause the production of lower energy particles. These low energy particles 'bounce' off the surface at random, and whilst this secondary radiation, like X-rays, only travels in straight lines, it also represents a hazard to personnel. The hazardous properties of X-rays are summarised in the box below.

Hazardous properties of X-rays

X-rays:
- penetrate matter
- can be absorbed by tissues
- affect living cells
- can 'scatter' and cause secondary radiation

Everyone who is involved in radiography must be protected from its dangers.

The Ionising Radiations Regulations 1999 is a document which covers the use of radiation by all medical and research establishments. In 1988, a document specifically for veterinary radiation was produced, called the Guidance notes for the Protection of Persons against Ionising Radiations arising from Veterinary Use.

Any person who has and uses an X-ray machine must notify the Health and Safety Executive (HSE), who can check that the Regulations are being complied with. A summary of the Regulations is shown in the box below.

Summary of the Ionising Radiations Regulations 1999

- The use of radiation must be justified
- The number of people involved should be kept to a minimum
- No dose limit should be exceeded
- All equipment must be in good order
- Protective clothing must be worn and maintained in good repair
- No part of the body must ever be in the primary beam
- Animals should not be manually restrained unless absolutely necessary. It is illegal to hold an animal during radiography unless the use of anaesthesia or sedation and positioning aids may endanger its life
- Personal dosemeters must be worn
- The primary beam should be collimated
- Good radiographic and processing techniques should be employed, to avoid the necessity of repeat exposures
- The machine must be switched off when not in use
- The local rules should be displayed and observed by all personnel
- A Radiation Protection Adviser (RPA) and Radiation Protection Supervisor (RPS) must be appointed

---

Radiation Protection Adviser (RPA)

An RPA is a specialist who possesses the necessary qualifications and experience, as stated in the Approved Code of Practice for the Protection of Persons against Ionising Radiations arising from any Work Activity. This is a document which was published at the same time as the Ionising Radiations Regulations. The role of the RPA is to give advice on all aspects of ionising radiations, including radiation protection. The HSE should be notified of the appointment of the RPA.

Radiation Protection Supervisor (RPS)

This is a senior member of staff (partner or principal) who is familiar with the legislation and ensures that it is observed and all procedures are carried out safely.

Controlled area

This is an area around the primary beam in which a person *might* receive a dose of radiation which exceeds the limit stated in the Regulations. The RPA should advise on the extent of the controlled area, but usually the area extends to a radius of 2 metres of the X-ray beam. The controlled area must be demarcated and labelled, and generally the controlled area is the entire X-ray room. Entry into the room should be restricted and a warning sign and the radiation symbol displayed (see Figure 12.2). There should also be an automatic signal indicating when the X-ray machine is in use, such as a red light. After use, the machine should be switched off and disconnected from the power. The room will then become accessible to others.

Designated persons

This term applies to those people aged 18 and over who are exposed to radiation during the course of their work. Designated persons should be provided with a personal dosemeter. Members of the public, pregnant women, people under the age of 18 and those who have exceeded the maximum permissible dose of radiation are not allowed in the controlled area.

Local rules

These are drawn up in consultation with the RPA and are essentially a set of procedures to be followed when performing radiography. The local rules should be displayed in the X-ray room and a copy should be available for everyone who is involved in radiography. They should be reviewed at least once a year. The local rules contain details of legislation, the RPS, the controlled area, equipment, protective clothing, methods of restraint and the precautions to be taken if a patient has to be restrained manually. They also include a list of designated persons. A Written System of Work is incorporated into the local rules and describes some procedures in more detail, such as the estimated personal doses of radiation which may be received.

Protective clothing

It is important to realise that any protective clothing only provides protection against secondary radiation and not against the primary beam. Aprons, gloves and mittens, sleeves, and thyroid protectors are available. They are made of plastic or rubber which is impregnated with lead (Figure 12.3).

Aprons may be single or double sided (double-sided aprons give better protection) and should be long enough to reach mid-thigh level. They should be worn by anyone remaining in the controlled area during radiography, even if the person stands behind a lead screen.

Gloves and sleeves are designed to cover the hands and forearms and should be worn when manual restraint is necessary. However, even when wearing gloves and sleeves, the hands must never be in the primary beam (Figure 12.4).

Protective clothing should be checked regularly for cracks and replaced if necessary. Correct storage can prevent cracking of the lead. Aprons should be hung up and no lead clothing should ever be folded.

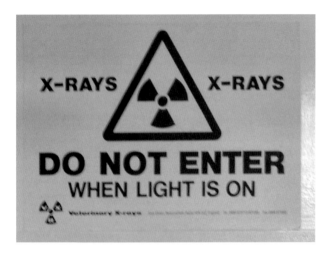

Figure 12.2   Radiation warning sign.

Dosemeters

A dosemeter records the amount of radiation received by an individual. It should be positioned under the apron, at chest or waist level and sent to a dosimetry service (such as the National Radiological Protection Board – NRPB) every month, to be read. Practices which have a low radiography caseload may be able to have their dosemeters read every 2–3 months, but this would have to be approved by the NRPB and the RPA. The practice principal must keep records of doses received for at least two years.

Maximum permissible dose (MPD)

This is the dose of radiation that can be received by the body, or a specific part of it, without causing harm.

Restraint of animal for radiography

As previously stated, it is illegal to manually restrain an animal for radiography unless its condition is such that anaesthesia or the use of sedation and positioning aids may be life-threatening. The animal should be positioned correctly and the position maintained with aids, e.g. for thoracic or abdominal radiography, left or right lateral recumbency may be required, as may dorsoventral or ventrodorsal positions. Once the

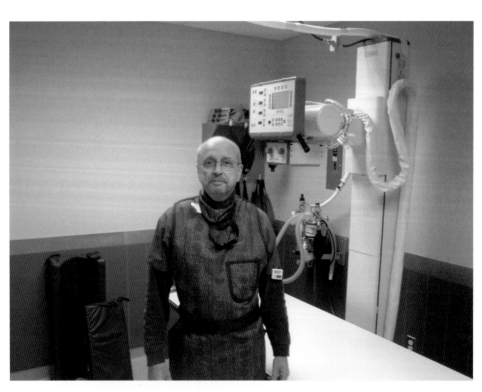

Figure 12.3   Lead apron with thyroid protector.

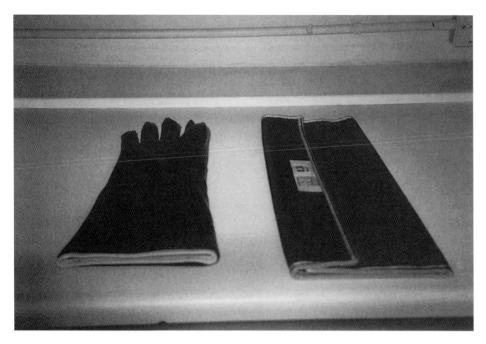

Figure 12.4   A lead glove and sleeve.

Table 12.5 Positioning aids used in radiography	
Positioning aid	**Description and use**
Ties	Long ropes or tapes to hold limbs of unconscious patients in position
Sandbags	Loosely filled bags of various lengths and sizes. Used to restrain limbs or other parts of the body They must be flexible and they should not be placed in the primary beam as they will show on the finished radiograph and they may cause secondary radiation
Troughs and inflatable supports	Used to keep the animal on its back (dorsal recumbency)
Foam wedges	Used in areas where padding or support is needed. They can easily be made into various shapes and can be placed in the primary beam
Sticky tape	May be used to aid positioning, e.g. taping the stifles together for HD radiography or taping digits to the cassette

animal is secure in its position, all personnel should leave the room (or stand behind a lead screen) before the exposure is made. Table 12.5 shows some positioning aids which are commonly used in veterinary radiography. Positioning aids should be cleaned after use as they may be a source of contamination.

Identification and labelling of radiographs

Information can be recorded at any time, but the earlier the better, and the less likely the risk of mistakes occurring. In some cases it is a legal requirement to record information before exposure.

The information that should be appear on the radiograph is:

- Identity of the patient
- Date of radiograph
- Left/Right marker to indicate a limb or side of patient.

Other relevant details, such as time, when performing contrast media studies, and kennel club number for hip or elbow dysplasia scoring. Note: the name of the client and animal must not be shown on radiographs to be submitted for hip or elbow dysplasia scoring.

Table 12.6 shows the various methods used to label radiographs.

All details of radiographs taken should be recorded:

- Client identification
- Patient identification and details
- Date radiograph taken
- Area
- View
- Exposures used.

Table 12.6	Methods of labelling radiographs
Identification before exposure	1. X-rite tape. This allows details to be written on tape which is then fixed to the cassette (in an area covered by the primary beam). Details show up on the radiograph 2. Lead letters or numbers – placed on the cassette, in an exposed area 3. Left/Right marker – placed on the cassette, in an exposed area
Identification in the darkroom	In the dark room, a light marker (a device which uses white light) can be used to imprint details which have been written on paper, onto the film. A corner of the film must be blocked off by an area of lead incorporated into the cassette
Identification of the dry film	This is the least efficient way of recording information. White ink can be used to write on the dry film. It is easy to make mistakes or to forge details, and for this reason, films used in legal cases or to be submitted for hip/elbow scoring cannot be labelled this way. Similarly, it is unacceptable to place the film in an envelope which is labelled

Basic radiographic positioning (Figures 12.5–12.10)

The basic principles of positioning a patient for radiography are as follows:

- Ensure the primary X-ray beam is centred over the main area of interest
- Ensure the primary beam is collimated to include the margins of the area if interest
- Ensure the primary X-ray beam is perpendicular to the X-ray film
- Ensure positioning aids are placed to decrease any risk of obscuring natural position of organs within area of interest.

Positioning for the thorax

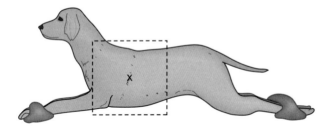

Lateral

x   Centre of X-ray beam
----   Collimation areas

Figure 12.5 Lateral positioning for thoracic radiographs.

Lateral

- Place patient in lateral recumbency
- Support forelegs cranially with sandbags
- Support hind legs caudally with sandbags
- Place foam pad under sternum to prevent rotation
- Centre X-ray beam at caudal border of scapula, midway between sternum and spine
- Collimate to include cranial border of scapula and last rib and just beyond skin margins dorsally and ventrally.

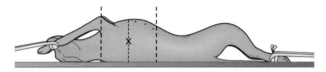

Ventrodorsal

x   Centre of X-ray beam
----   Collimation areas

Figure 12.6 Ventrodorsal positioning for thoracic radiographs.

Ventrodorsal

- Place patient in dorsal recumbency
- Tie forelegs cranially
- Tie hind legs caudally
- Centre mid sternum
- Collimate to include manubrium and last rib and just beyond skin margins laterally.

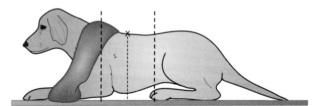

Dorsoventral

x   Centre of X-ray beam
----   Collimation areas

Figure 12.7 Dorsoventral positioning for thoracic radiographs.

Dorsoventral

- Place patient in sternal recumbency
- Support forelegs cranially with sandbag
- Allow hind legs to assume natural position
- Centre on caudal border scapula and thoracic vertebra
- Collimate to manubrium and last rib and just beyond skin edges laterally.

Positioning for the abdomen

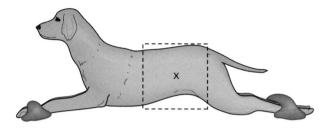

Lateral

x   Centre of X-ray beam
---- Collimation areas

Figure 12.8   Lateral positioning for abdominal radiographs.

Lateral
- Place patient in lateral recumbency
- Support forelegs cranially with sandbags
- Support hindlegs caudally with sandbags
- Place foam pad under sternum and between hind legs to prevent rotation
- Centre X-ray beam at last rib midway between dorsal and ventral skin margins
- Collimate to include umbilicus and cranial border of femur and just beyond skin margins dorsally and ventrally.

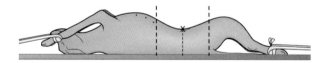

Ventrodorsal

x   Centre of X-ray beam
---- Collimation areas

Figure 12.9   Ventrodorsal positioning for abdominal radiographs.

Ventrodorsal
- Place patient in dorsal recumbency
- Tie forelegs cranially
- Tie hind legs caudally

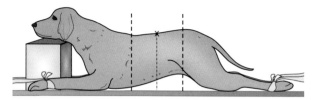

Dorsoventral

x   Centre of X-ray beam
---- Collimation areas

Figure 12.10   Dorsoventral positioning for abdominal radiographs.

- Centre on umbilicus
- Collimate to include xiphosternum and pubic symphysis and just beyond skin margins laterally.

Dorsoventral
- Place patient in sternal recumbency
- Tie forelegs cranially
- Tie hind legs caudally
- Centre on first lumbar vertebra
- Collimate to tenth thoracic vertebra and cranial wing of ilium and just beyond skin edges laterally.

PROCESSING CHEMICALS

Chemicals can be supplied as powders, liquid concentrates or ready to use liquids. All chemicals should be handled with care, in a well-ventilated room. Gloves, goggles and face mask should be worn. Spilt chemicals should be wiped away immediately.

To dispose of waste chemicals, they should be placed in the original container and collected by an authorised person. Local hospitals and commercial laboratories may provide this service.

Further reading and resources
- Association of British Pharmaceutical Industry, Whitehall, London.
- HMSO Guidance notes. HMSO, London.
- HSE Publications, Health and Safety Executive Books, Sudbury, Suffolk.
- Institute of Environmental Health Officers, London.
- Lavin, L.M. (1994) Radiography in Veterinary Technology. W.B. Saunders, Office of Public Sector Information.
- The Small Animal Veterinary Formulary (2005) BSAVA, Cheltenham.
- Veterinary Medicines Directorate, Addlestone, Surrey.

Exotics

Care of small mammals

Beverly Shingleton

INTRODUCTION

The popularity of rodents and lagomorphs as pets is rapidly increasing, and veterinary practices are not only being required to provide prophylactic and medical treatment for these animals, but also information on their husbandry, nutrition and breeding needs.

ANATOMICAL DIFFERENCES IN SMALL MAMMALS

To help the nurse understand the husbandry requirements of this group of animals it is important to highlight some of the outstanding anatomical and physiological differences between lagomorphs, rodents and the more familiar dog and cat.

Dentition and dental confirmation

Rodents and lagomorphs have open-rooted teeth, which means they continually grow throughout life; they are very sharp, chisel-shaped and ideal for gnawing. Rodents have two upper and two lower incisors, lagomorphs have two pairs of upper incisors positioned one behind the other and one pair of lower incisors. Enamel is only found on the front surface of the incisor teeth, which allows constant wear and re-sharpening.

In all herbivores the canines are absent and a gap called the diastema is present. The premolars and molars are called cheek teeth and are used to grind vegetable material.

See Table 13.1 for dental formula.

Digestive system (Figures 13.1 and 13.2)

All the animals covered in this section are either herbivores or omnivores and modifications to their digestive system can be seen. These anatomical and physiological adaptations allow complex foodstuff eaten to be efficiently digested and assimilated.

Some of the main anatomical and physiological differences are highlighted below and summarised in Table 13.1:

- Rabbits and cavies have a long intestinal tract and large caecum. The caecum contains bacteria that aid in the breakdown of cellulose.
- All species covered in the text carry out coprophagia, which is the re-ingestion of faeces. This process results in ingested food being passed through the digestive system twice, enabling the animal to absorb vital nutrients that would be otherwise lost. This process is best illustrated in the rabbit.
- Rabbits produce two types of faeces: the familiar hard fibrous dropping and a softer caecotroph. Caecotrophs are strong smelling clusters of small green ovoid droppings covered in a layer of mucus. Caecotrophs are ingested directly from the anus and the function of the mucus is to protect the living organisms in the caecotrophs from being destroyed by the acid in the stomach.
- Rabbits tend to produce hard faeces for approximately 4 hours after a meal followed by caecotrophs which are produced for a further 4 hours.

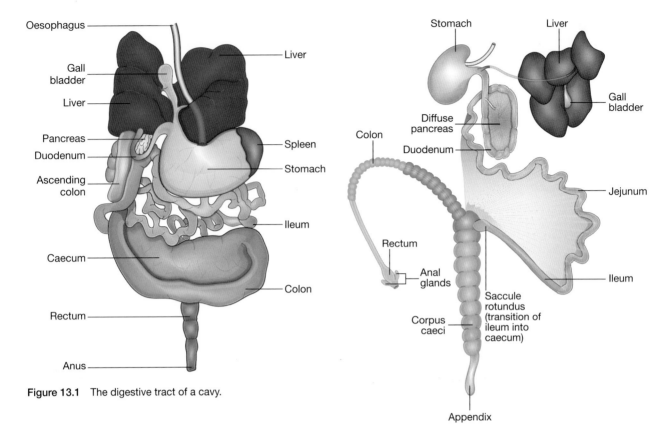

Figure 13.1 The digestive tract of a cavy.

Figure 13.2 Digestive tract of a rabbit.

Table 13.1	Summary of anatomical differences						
	Rabbit	**Cavy**	**Rat**	**Mouse**	**Hamster (Syrian)**	**Gerbil**	**Chinchilla**
Characteristics							
Teeth	Chisel-shaped Open rooted	Chisel-shaped	Chisel-shaped	Chisel-shaped	Chisel-shaped	Chisel-shaped	Chisel-shaped, open rooted
*Dentition	2033 1023	1013 1013	1003 1003	1003 1003	1003 1003	1003 1003	1013 1013
Digestive system	Long Large caecum	Long Large caecum	Long No appendix	Long	Long	Long	Long
Coprophagia	Yes	Yes	Yes	Yes Lesser extent than others	Yes	Only in nutritional deficiency	No evidence found
Oral pouches	No	No	No	No	Yes	No	No
Sebaceous (scent) glands	Anal gland opening into rectum	Grease gland sited base of spine more prominent in males	No	No	Darker patches on flanks	Mid-ventral abdomen May become more pronounced in older animals	No

*NOTE dentition = I/C/PM/M
The wild diet of most of the species above includes abrasive foods that wear down both incisor and molar teeth. If a captive diet is not supplemented with the correct gnawing materials then malocclusion will result. This includes elongation of crowns and roots of teeth, overgrown crowns can result in enamel spurs on the molars and malocclusion of the incisors and/or molars. Overgrown roots can press on the lacrimal gland causing epiphora and if progress into the maxilla or mandible dental abscesses.

The rat digestive system has developed to digest both plant and animal derived nutrients. Their stomach is divided into two sections: a non-glandular forestomach and a distal glandular body and to facilitate digestion of cellulose (plant material) a large caecum. Rats do not have a gall bladder.

Respiratory system

Small mammals share a similar respiratory system to that studied in the cat and dog. Rabbits are nose-breathers (mouth-breathing is indicative of serious illness). The nose moves up and down in a normal rabbit ('twitching') 20–120 times a minute, but this will stop when the rabbit is very relaxed or anaesthetised. The glottis is small and is not easily visualised as it is obscured by the tongue. The thoracic cavity is small, and breathing is mainly diaphragmatic. The lungs have three lobes, and the cranial lung lobes are small (left smaller than right).

Urinary tract (Figure 13.3)

Cavies produce opaque creamy urine; this is perfectly normal. Both rabbits and cavies produce calcium carbonate crystals in their urine and this can account for the build-up of scale in hutches. Food can also influence the colour of the urine; rabbits can produce red-coloured urine if certain plant and vegetable matter is ingested.

Table 13.2 shows normal parameters and species-specific information.

RABBITS (LAGOMORPHS)

Introduction

Nowadays the domestic rabbit is one of the most widely kept small pets and many rabbits have left their cosy hutch to become 'house rabbits' enjoying the same comforts bestowed on our much-cherished dog and cat. Some owners even go to the lengths of teaching them to walk on a harness.

Today indoor rabbits are provided with a strategically placed litter tray, central heating and a nice cosy bed to sleep in, and if in the presence of novice owners, the odd bit of comfort cable nibbling.

History

The domestic rabbit belongs to the order Lagomorpha, but can mistakenly be classified to the order Rodentia. Although rabbits and rodents share many anatomical and behavioural similarities they are classified differently

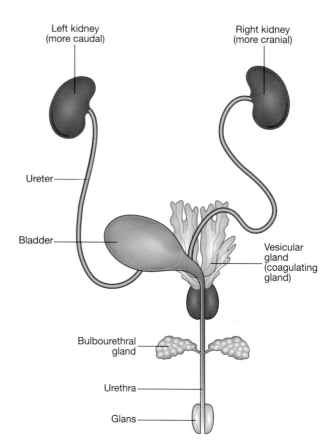

Figure 13.3   Urinary tract of a rabbit.

because rabbits have four upper incisor teeth arranged one pair behind the other, whilst rodents only have the one pair.

The domestic rabbit originated from its wild cousin the European rabbit (*Oryctolagus cuniculus*) and was discovered in Spain. The Romans were the first people to keep rabbits in captivity and were also responsible for their introduction into many parts of Europe including Britain and France. In the Middle Ages French Monks bred rabbits for food and fur. The Monks' interest in breeding these animals played an important part in furthering the domestication of the rabbit and they are probably responsible for many of the different breeds seen today.

Housing

Rabbits can make good and stimulating pets, but when advising on the selection of a rabbit, especially if for a child, the prospective owners need to consider various factors. One of the most important considerations is the eventual size the rabbit will grow to. A common problem and one that leads to the abandonment of many pet rabbits is that the tiny bundle of fluff purchased as a 'dwarf' has grown into a grumpy difficult to handle giant.

Table 13.2 Normal parameters and species-specific information

Parameter	Rabbits	Guinea pigs	Gerbils	Mice	Rats	Hamsters	Chinchillas
Weight (M)	Varies according to species	900–1200 g	46–131 g	20–40 g	267–500 g	87–130 g	400–500 g
Weight (F)	Varies according to species	700–900 g	50–55 g	22–63 g	225–325 g	95–130 g	400–600 g
Life span	7 years (average)	5–6 years	24–39 months	12–36 months	26–40 months	18–36 months	10 years (average)
Body temperature	38.3°C rectal. 37–39.4°C range	37.2–39.5°C	38.2°C	37.1°C	37.7°C	37.6°C	35.4–38.0°C
Heart rate Beats/minute	198–330	240–310	85–160	427–697	313–493	310–471	100
Respiration Breaths/min	30–60	42–150	85–160	91–216	71–146	38–110	45–65
Species gender terminology	Male – buck Female – doe	Male – boar Female – sow	–	–	–	–	–
Classification mammalian order	Lagomorphs	Rodentia	Rodentia	Rodentia	Rodentia	Rodentia	Rodentia
Latin name	*Oryctolagus cuniculus*	*Cauvia porcellus*	*Merione unguiculatus*	*Mus musculus*	*Rattus norvegicus*	(Common hamster) *Cricetus cricetus*	*Chinchilla lanigera*

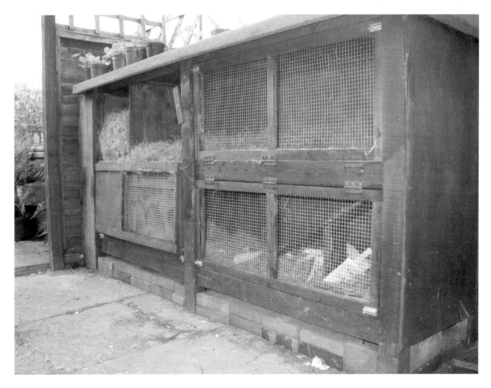

Figure 13.4 Traditional hutch rabbit housing.

The wild rabbit is a sociable creature living in mixed colonies; they enjoy digging producing a network of warrens under the ground. Wild rabbits spend most of their time in these burrows generally only leaving at dawn and dusk to feed.

Obviously it would be difficult and impractical to keep domestic rabbits in such a way but it is essential for the wellbeing of the creature housed that the accommodation provided gives the animal the freedom to move, privacy, safety and is environmentally enriched.

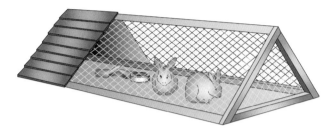

Figure 13.5   A suitable run should include a sheltered area.

As rabbits are sociable animals they are best kept in pairs (minimum). When selecting a companion some caution is advised; two males (bucks) may fight, whereas not all females (does) living together have an amicable relationship and fighting may take place during the breeding season (February to August) or if one is in false pregnancy.

It is worth considering keeping spayed females or neutered males together.

Guinea-pigs can be used as an alternative companion, but extreme care should be taken as a large rabbit has the potential to kick its smaller companion. Some rabbits will mount guinea pigs, whilst some guinea-pigs will chew or barber a rabbit's coat.

The most common methods of keeping a rabbit are either in an outside hutch with run, or indoors giving the rabbit free range of the home and access to a litter tray.

When electing to keep rabbits outdoors in a hutch with access to a run the following points must be considered:

- **Size** – Remember young rabbits grow into larger ones so it is advisable to purchase the largest hutch available; for a medium-sized rabbit, i.e. 3–5 kg, suggested dimensions are 150 cm long × 60 cm wide × 50 cm high. The hutch must allow the rabbits to sit up on its hind legs and stretch out.
- **Siting** – Although rabbits are hardy creatures and can stand fairly low temperatures the hutch should be positioned away from draughts and extremes of temperature and positioned near to the house. In the winter the rabbit hutch can be placed in a well-ventilated airy shed.
- **Construction and materials** – The hutch needs to be constructed in such a way that the occupants are provided with a safe and secure environment with sufficient space to move around and ideally access to a sleeping area. The materials used should be durable and able to withstand the extremes of the British climate (see Figure 13.4). The run must be escape and predator proof with access

to shelter which will act as hiding places. Ideally the run should have two opaque sides, as four open sides will make the rabbit feel very vulnerable. If the rabbit is allowed to roam freely during the day it must be in a securely fenced garden with access to food, water and shelter. The garden must also be safe from visiting predators and owners must be prepared for some warren construction. To prevent tunnelling and escape the base of the wire in a run or perimeter fence must be dug 0.5 m into the ground. The addition of a hide box in the hutch and run will allow the rabbit the security it would gain from being in a burrow.
- **Substrates, bedding and furnishings** (see Tables 13.3 and 13.4) – To ensure the rabbit is comfortable in its surroundings it needs to be provided with adequate bedding and substrate materials, furnished with a food bowl, water bottle, and environmental enrichment. See Table 13.3 for further information on the importance of environmental enrichment.

Hygiene (see Box on next page)

Rabbits are very clean animals, depositing their droppings and urine in the same place each time; this makes it very easy to house-train the indoor rabbit. The hutch should be thoroughly cleaned once a week and depending on the number of rabbits housed spot-cleaned daily.

Nutritional requirements (Table 13.5)

There is a plethora of commercial rabbit foods available on the market ranging from pellets to brightly coloured mixes.

Important points to remember when feeding rabbits include:

- The rabbit is a grazing animal and in the wild spends most of its time eating, therefore it is important that the pet rabbit has access to good quality hay and if possible pasture. This will ensure the diet provides the cellulose (roughage) the rabbit needs.
- Feed diets formulated for the rabbit and not other species.
- Rabbits benefit from small helpings of fresh fruits and vegetables daily (Table 13.5 gives examples of fresh foods that can be offered).
- Do not overfeed as this leads to obesity and prevents the rabbit from performing coprophagia; soiling around the anus can then occur.

Food hygiene storage and feeding tips

- **Rabbit and rodent diets** consist mainly of a course mix or a mono-component diet (complete extrusion diet), supplemented with fresh fruits and vegetables and for those requiring it ad lib hay.
- **Storage of dry foods,** e.g. course mix and mono-component diets, see Figure 13.6.
- **Storage of unopened bags of food:**
  - Unopened bags must be stored off the ground (wooden pallets are good for this) in a dry and rodent-proof room or cupboard.
  - **The room must be kept cool** as increased temperature and humidity cause rapid oxidation of nutrients.
  - **Stock rotation must be adhered to,** with new deliveries placed at the back, bring existing stock forward. When large quantities of food are kept expiry dates must be checked; this will ensure foods are used before 'use by date' and avoids the costly process of having to dispose of out of date food.
- **Opened bags of food** must be stored in airtight containers that will keep the food fresh, dry and free from contamination; bins with lock and seal action lids are ideal for this. Mouldy foods should never be fed as they can contain aflatoxins which if consumed can be fatal.
- **Hay should be kept as for unopened dry food;** it is best stored in cool dry conditions. Increased humidity readily leads to hay going mouldy which must be avoided (see above).
- **Fresh foods**
  - These must be fit for human consumption and stored in a refrigerator at 58°C.
  - Any mouldy, or rotten foods must be immediately disposed of and never offered to the animal.
  - Fresh foods must be washed, free from soil and pollutants; this is especially important when foods are being picked from the garden or hedgerow.
  - Fresh food must be stored so that it does not contaminate that ready for human consumption.
- **Hygiene**
  - Any food preparation must be carried out hygienically with the wellbeing of the animal and the operator considered.
  - Preparation areas must be cleaned before and after food preparation.
  - Hands must be washed before and after food preparation.
  - Food preparation must take place away from human foods.
- As food and water bowls are often used as latrines, daily cleaning is essential.
- The previous day's uneaten food and water must be discarded and fresh provided. Before fresh foods are offered bowls must be washed in mild detergent, rinsed, dried and checks made for cracks, breaks and sharp edges.
- New food must be weighed to stated amount, placed in bowl and positioned in cage where animal can reach it.
- **Care of a gravity fed water bottle**
  - Bottle is cleaned using mild detergent and bottle brush, the spout flushed with water to check ball-bearing is working. Bottle and top rinsed to remove ALL traces of detergent.
  - Water bottle refilled with fresh water and checked for leaks and cracks. Water should flow from the spout when ball mechanism moved but not drip constantly.
  - Bottle should be securely positioned on the cage at a height and angle animal can reach.
- Fresh hay needs to be given daily; hay should be placed in racks as this prevents soiling and being used as bedding.
- Musty smelling hay should not be used as this can be a sign of contamination.
- Observations of animals' feeding and drinking habits are very important as any change can indicate illness, stress or simply excessive or inadequate amounts of food being offered.

■ Adult rabbits eat approximately 90–120 g per day but this can increase 3-fold during lactation and growth. It is advisable to support this by feeding breeders' pellets or the specially formulated diets available on the market.

■ Dietary changes should gradually take place over 4–5 days allowing intestinal microflora to adjust to the new diet.

■ Fresh water should be provided daily. Rabbits consume 5–10 mL of water per 100 g bodyweight

Table 13.3 Substrates, bedding and furnishings

	Substrates	Bedding	Furnishings
Rabbit outside hutch	Thick layer of newspaper, wood shavings, sawdust, straw, hay	Shredded paper Hay	Heavy ceramic or similar food bowl* Water bottle** Hay rack Environmental enrichment (Table 13.4)
Cavy	Thick layer of newspaper, wood shavings, sawdust, straw, hay	Shredded paper Hay	Heavy ceramic or similar food bowl* Water bottle** Hay rack Environmental enrichment (Table 13.4)
Mice and rats	Sawdust, ← wood shavings, ↑ cat litter (made from recycled paper)	Shredded printed paper, tissue paper or kitchen towel Hay	Heavy ceramic or similar food bowl* Water bottle** Environmental enrichment (Table 13.4)
Hamsters	Sawdust, ← wood shavings	Tissue paper or kitchen towel, White shredded paper‡, hay	Heavy ceramic or similar food bowl* Water bottle** Environmental enrichment (Table 13.4)
Gerbils	Mixture of moss peat, wood shavings↑ and chopped straw/hay or just wood shavings↑	White shredded paper, tissue paper or kitchen towel	Heavy ceramic or similar food bowl* Water bottle** Environmental enrichment (Table 13.4)
Chinchillas	Not necessary. Wood shavings, cat litter (made from recycled paper)	Not necessary	Heavy ceramic or similar food bowl* Water bottle** Large, sturdy cat litter tray Environmental enrichment (Table 13.4)

NOTES:

*Nearly all rodents and lagomorphs will overturn and chew food and water bowls so best provide a sturdy food bowl and water via a water bottle that can be attached to the cage.

**Water bottles should be checked to ensure that the drip mechanism is not blocked or leaking. Daily cleaning with a bottlebrush can prevent growth of algae on the inside of the bottle.

←Sawdust must be purchased in prepacked bales; floor sweepings from sawmills are not suitable as these may be contaminated with wild rodent excretions.

↑Care when using wood shavings, especially Red Cedar shavings. As these contain oils and produce much dust both can irritate the respiratory tract and predispose to respiratory disease. If shavings are to be used select those produced, from pine and spruce woods.

‡Newspaper used as bedding must have non-toxic ink and is especially toxic to hamsters. Artificial materials and cotton wool are not suitable bedding materials as they can cause gut impaction and constipation and fibres can get entwined around limbs causing serious injury. In hamsters fibres can impact the pouches.

When cleaning out small rodent accommodation try to replace a small amount of the old bedding and substrate as this will keep the environment familiar to the rodent and lessen stress.

rising to 90 mL/100g bodyweight during lactation and hot weather.

■ Gravity fed (sipper bottles) are recommended over water bowls as they are more hygienic and water consumption is easier to monitor. A cautionary note: the water spout must be checked daily for obstructions, especially the ball bearings as these can get stuck and prevent water flow. Bottles must be cleaned daily using a bottle brush and all signs of green discoloration removed. In winter bottles need to be checked regularly; a frozen water bottle will prevent access to water and as the ice expands the bottle may split.

■ All dry food must be kept in an airtight container in a cool, damp and rodent-free room.

■ Fresh foods must be fit for human consumption and kept in a refrigerator until needed. Mouldy food or those contaminated by vermin should not be offered to any animal as this is a serious health hazard.

Handling and restraint (Figure 13.7)

The more confident the handler is in employing the various handling and restraining techniques the better the experience is for the animal.

Although the majority of pet rabbits enjoy being handled, poor handling can easily stress rabbits causing them to struggle. A frightened rabbit will often wriggle violently kicking out its hind limbs; the result can be fatal causing damage to the rabbit's vertebrae and

Table 13.4	Environmental enrichment	
As we elect to keep more and more animals in captivity it is important that we provide these animals with a stimulating environment, as a stark square cage is not acceptable. The provision of a stimulating environment does not have to cost the pet owner vast amounts of money. Below is a table that demonstrates the types of materials that can be used to enrich a cage.		
Animal	**Materials**	**Benefits**
Cavy, rabbits, mice and rats, gerbils, hamsters, chinchillas	Washed branches from edible fruit trees, hazel, and willow	Stimulates gnawing, helps to grind teeth, play climbing
Cavy, rabbits, mice and rats, gerbils, hamsters	Cardboard cereal boxes/toilet roll tubes	Chewing, nest making, hiding
Mice and rats, gerbils, hamsters	Peat boxes	Stimulate digging and tunnel building, hide food and encourage foraging behaviour
Mice and rats and chinchillas	Ropes, hammocks	Exercise, climbing, chewing
Mice and rats	Balls, dog and cat toys (excludes proprietary hamster balls)	Play, exercise, can place food inside balls
Mice and rats, gerbils, hamsters	Clay pots, jam jars	Hides, toilet areas
Mice and rats, hamsters	DIY wooden maize	Exercise, stimulate brain, chewing
Rabbits, cavies, mice and rats, chinchillas	Plastic drain pipes, ledges	Hides, shelter, security, exercise, ledges to climb on increase surface area and exercise
Mice and rats, gerbils, chinchillas	Rocks, breeze blocks	Different textures wear down nails, look out points
Rabbits	Football	Play and chase games
Rats	Litter tray or heavy dog bowl	*With water great swimming pool
Mice and rats gerbils	Wooden cotton reels	Gnawing
Remember rodents are very destructive and plastic objects are likely to be chewed. *Rats love water and additional exercise can be offered by the occasional dip. Proprietary wheels, ladders and exercise balls should be used with some caution as animals can get their feet caught in the bars and gaps resulting in serious injuries. **Note from the author:** It is quite alarming the amount of toys and gimmicks marketed for small pets, many being expensive to buy. With a little imagination, stimulating toys can be made from cardboard tubes and boxes, cereal packets, glass jars, branches and twigs from fruit trees, ropes and clay pots. Have fun and save money!		

nasty gouges to the handler's arms. Rabbits must be held safely and securely and if being transported any distance even within the surgery it is always best to place them in a secure basket.

Handling rabbits
Two methods can be used:

1. **Method ONE (see Figure 13.7)**
   - Grasp the scruff of the rabbit with one hand.
   - Then place the other hand under the rump bringing the rabbit close into your body.
   - Nervous rabbits benefit from having their head placed under the handler's arm. (This also leaves the handler with a free hand to open cages or doors.)
2. **Method TWO.** Smaller friendlier rabbits may react better to the following method:
   - Place one hand under the thorax gripping each foreleg separately between the thumb and two fingers.
   - With the free hand support the hindquarters.
   - Bring the animal close into the body.

Tips when handling rabbits
- Remember rabbits are preyed upon by silent predators so to reassure them that they are not on the menu, always talk and stroke them.
- Always be confident, animals can sense a nervous handler.
- Never carry a rabbit if it can be placed in a basket and transported in that way.
- Always make sure you restrain the rabbit on a solid non-slip surface.
- Once the rabbit is on the handling table restrain it by placing a hand gently on the scuff and never leave the rabbit unattended.
- If the rabbit panics and starts to struggle during the handling or restraint then hold the rabbit firmly into your body and try to reassure it as described above.
- If having to administer intravenous drugs or carry out nail clipping and the rabbit is objecting to being

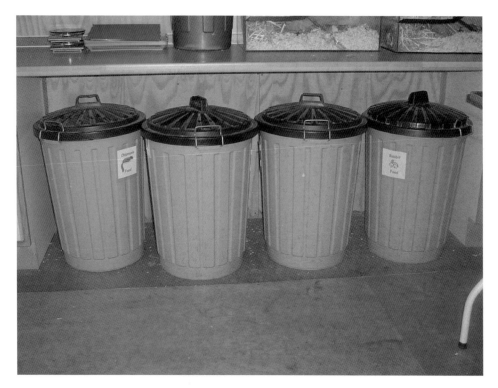

Figure 13.6   Food bins suitable for storing large amounts of dry food.

restrained, it can be useful to place the rabbit in a towel method very similar to that used in cats. Remember to always support the hind limbs.

- If the rabbit is become very distressed chemical restraint may have to be considered.

Sexing and breeding

Sexing rabbits (see Figure 13.8a and b)
To prevent unwanted litters it is important rabbits are correctly sexed; this is not always an easy task as sexing young rabbits under the age of two months can be difficult and even the most experienced breeder can make mistakes. The testicles in the male do not descend until the rabbit is approximately three months old and then rabbits have the ability to retract the testicles into the abdominal cavity. So if in any doubt try and get a second opinion or ask the clients to return to the surgery when the rabbit is a little older.

Breeding rabbits
If rabbits are to be bred it is best to take the doe to the buck – there will be little if any courtship – and once mating has taken place separate the pair returning the doe to her own cage.

The young are born hairless, blind and deaf and will remain in the nest for approximately three weeks. Many novice breeders are alarmed by the lack of parental care displayed by the doe as she spends relatively small amounts of time with her young only returning to feed them once or twice a day. It must be stressed that this is quite normal behaviour and there is no need for the owner to intervene; in fact it is best to give the doe as much privacy as possible as too much attention can cause her to abandon the litter. The young will be ready for re-homing between 8–12 weeks.

For more details on reproductive parameters see Table 13.6.

CAVY (*CAVIA PORCELLUS*) GUINEA PIGS

Introduction

The guinea pig is a gregarious and amiable little creature, with relatively easy husbandry needs. Its short stocky body and little legs make it easy to handle and all of these facts contribute to making the guinea pig a favoured small pet.

History

The guinea pig or cavy (the term cavy originating from its scientific name *Cavia porcellus* meaning 'pig-like

Table 13.5 Fresh foods and supplements

Most rodents and lagomorphs benefit from having fresh foods added to their diet. All fresh foods offered should be fit for human consumption, washed to remove soil and free from toxic chemicals. Fresh foods that are wilted or rotten have no nutritional value and could be detrimental to the health of the animal. Any uneaten food should be removed from the cage and NOT left to rot. Fresh foods are best introduced during weaning, this will prevent digestive upsets later in life. Any new foodstuffs added to the diet should always be introduced slowly.

Rabbit	Cavy	Rats	Mice	Hamsters	Gerbils	Chinchillas
*Cabbage green leaves	*Cabbage green leaves	Dog biscuit	Dog biscuit	Dog biscuit	Dog biscuit	Raisins, no more than 2 daily
Carrots	Carrots	Lean meat	Apple	Apple	Apple	Apple weekly
*Broccoli	*Broccoli	Mealworms	Pear	Pear	Pear	Carrot
*Spinach	*Spinach	Cooked meat bone	Banana	Banana	Banana	Small quantities of dandelion
Swede	Swede	Apple	Tomato	Tomato	Tomato	Small quantities of shepherd's purse
Turnip	Turnip	Pear	Carrot	Carrot	Carrot	Small quantities of dried fruits
Parsnip	Parsnip	Banana	Cherries	Swede	Lettuce	Milk powder
*Brussels sprout leaves	*Brussels sprout leaves	Tomato	Grapes	Grapes	**Sunflower seeds	
Apple	Apple	Cherries	***Nuts	Dandelions	***Nuts	
Pear	Pear	Grapes	Stale toasted bread	Chickweed	Stale bread	
Dandelions	Dandelions	Peas		Groundsel	Dandelions	
Chickweed	Chickweed	Carrots		Stale toasted bread	Chickweed	
Cow parsnip	Cow parsnip	Broccoli		**Sunflower seeds	Groundsel	
Clover	Clover	Potatoes		***Nuts	Shepherds purse	
Comfrey	Comfrey	**Sunflower seeds		Hardboiled egg	Hardboiled egg	
Colts foot	Colts foot	***Nuts		Milk powder	Milk powder	
Hedge parsley	Hedge parsley	Pasta		Cooked meat		
	Vitamin C tablets 1000 mg dissolved in 8 litres of water	Brown rice (cooked)				

Rats, mice, gerbils and chinchillas' food can also be used as an enrichment tool, rather than offering food in a bowl, treats or the normal ration can be hidden in the cage and the rodent can then track it down. Never feed chocolate to rodents as contains a toxic substance alkaloid theobromine.
*GOOD Vitamin C content when fed FRESH.
**Sunflower seeds are particularly addictive and have a low calcium content and high fat content and if eaten in excess can lead to nutritional diseases.
***Peanuts must be stored correctly and not allowed to go mouldy as can contain aflatoxins, which if consumed by the animal can be fatal.
Dog biscuit and toast are good for gnawing and wearing down of teeth. Egg and milk powder are good supplements for lactating females.

cavy') belongs to the order Rodentia and originated from Colombia, Venezuela and Peru in South America. Cavies were probably first kept in captivity centuries ago by the Incas who utilised them as a sacrificial food source. By the end of the sixteenth century, sailors had introduced cavies into Europe and given their endearing characters soon cavies became popular pets.

Cavies are not only favoured children's pets but are enjoyed by many enthusiasts who breed and show them.

There are three principal breed lines distinguished by their coat type: short coated smooth-haired English; the more course haired rosette Abyssinians; and the long-haired Peruvians. From the breeds listed above many more variations can be seen ranging from the spiky rough coated Rex to the elegant long-haired Shelti.

The choice of coat type obviously depends on how much time and effort the owner wants to spend caring for the cavy.

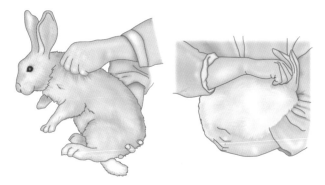

Figure 13.7 Handling and restraining a rabbit.

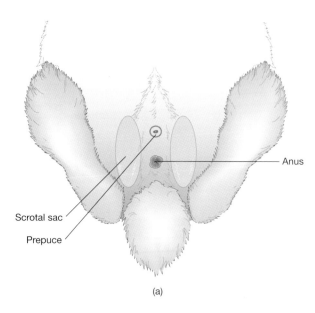

Anus

Scrotal sac

Prepuce

(a)

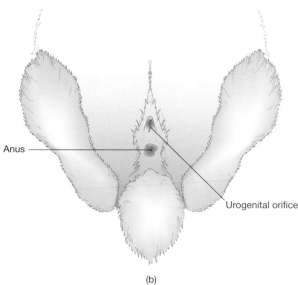

Anus

Urogenital orifice

(b)

Figure 13.8 (a) The male rabbit; (b) the female rabbit.

Housing (Figure 13.9)

The wild cavy (*Cavia aperea*) can be found living in the rocky regions and savannahs of South America; they live in small groups ranging from five to ten comprising of an adult male, two or three females and their offspring of varying ages. In captivity it is advisable to keep cavies in pairs or small same sex groups. Keeping females (sows) together rarely poses a problem, but care should be advised if housing males (boars) together, especially if females are close by as fighting might occur.

The best type of housing to provide for the cavy is similar to that described for the rabbit. Cavies are not as hardy as rabbits and the hutch will need to be well-insulated and placed in a draught-free airy shed or outbuilding. Cavies prefer to be housed at temperatures ranging from 12–20°C (55–70°F) as temperatures in excess of 27–30°C (80–85°F) can cause hyperthermia. The cage needs to be about 30 cm high and allow approximately $0.2 \, m^2$ for each cavy housed. A run or ark is also an essential, as this will provide exercise and a chance for the cavy to graze. Much can be carried out to enrich the run and make it a safe and stimulating environment for the cavies to play. One of the most essential items is a hide box, as it will give the pigs an area to hide and shelter in.

As for the rabbit, the cavy will need to be provided with a sturdy food bowl, gravity drip feed water bottle and a hayrack.

Substrates, bedding and furnishings (see Tables 13.3 and 13.4)

Information on the importance of environmental enrichment is referenced in Table 13.4.

Hygiene (Figure 13.6)

Most cavies are not as discreet in their toilet habits as rabbits and they tend to soil the whole of the cage rather than concentrating on just one area. This obviously makes more work for the owner and daily removal of soiled areas is essential. Hygiene routines are similar to those suggested for the rabbit.

Nutritional requirements

Cavies are herbivores and in the wild would eat a selection of grasses, seeds, weeds and fruit.

The captive cavy should be offered a good quality proprietary dry diet with daily supplementation of fresh fruit and vegetables.

The main dietary considerations are:

Cavies are unable to synthesise their own vitamin C (ascorbic acid) and they are also unable to store vitamin C

Table 13.6 Reproductive parameters of small mammals

Species	Sexual maturity	Oestrous cycle	Gestation	Size of litter	Weaning Age	General
Rabbit Male – buck Female – doe	16–24 weeks Heavier breeds mature later	Seasonally polyoestrous and induced ovulators	30–33 days	4–12 (average 7)	6–8 weeks	Pregnancy diagnosis at 12–14 days by careful abdomen palpation. Altricial young eyes open around 10th day ready for re-homing from 8–12 weeks
Guinea pig (cavy) Male – boar Female – sow	Male: 3–5 weeks Female: 4–6 weeks Recommended breeding age: Male: 3–5 months Female: 4–5 months	15–17 days (polyoestrous) Oestrus lasts 24–48 h Spontaneous ovulation occurs approx. 10 h from onset of oestrus. Sows' external genitalia swell	59–72 days	1–6 (average 3–4)	3 weeks	During oestrus, sows' behaviour changes; she may mount other female occupants, and make purring sounds especially if stroked along back and rump. She will slope her back. Gives birth to precocial young
Rats Male – buck Female – doe	8–10 weeks Recommended breeding age: 4–4 months	Oestrous cycles all year round. 4–5 days (polyoestrous) in oestrus for approx. 14 h	20–22 days	6–16 (average 10)	4 weeks By 10 days have eyes and ears open and hair	In the last third of gestation pregnancy may be detected by gentle abdomen palpation Post-partum oestrus can occur within 24 hours of parturition
Mice	6–7 weeks Recommended breeding age: 11–12 weeks	Oestrous cycles all year round 4–5 days (polyoestrous) in oestrus for approx. 12 h	19–21 days	8–12 (average 10)	3–4 weeks Eyes, ears etc. open as above	Post-partum oestrus can occur within 12 hours of parturition
Gerbils	Males 10–12 weeks Females 12–14 weeks Recommended breeding age: Males 5 months Females 3–4 months	All year round Oestrus every 6 days Oestrus last 12–18 h Mating usually takes place at night	24–26 days	4–6 7 days have covering of hair; 10 days eyes open	21–28 days	Post-partum oestrus lasts 5 h and if mated implantation can be delayed for 2 weeks Gerbils do not mate when lactating. Young start eating solids at 16–21 days

Golden Hamster Syrian	6-weeks Recommended breeding age: Males 10–14 weeks Females 12–14weeks	Oestrus every 4 days Mating usually takes place at night	16–18 days	6–8 5 days young are furred; eyes open 10 days	21–25 days	Parturition normally occurs at night Post-partum oestrus infertile Next fertile oestrus 21–18 days post weaning Females should not be disturbed for 10 days as can abandon or cannibalise young Female will carry neonates in cheek pouches
Hamster Russian	14 weeks	Oestrus every 4 days Mating usually takes place at night	18–21 days	3–7	20–22 days	Russian and Chinese colonies the dominant female most likely to breed and will suppress submissive females
Hamster Chinese	14 weeks	Oestrus every 4 days Mating usually takes place at night	21 days	3–7	20–22 days	Albinos tend to be infertile
Chinchilla	4–8 months Recommended breeding age: 8 months	24–45 days seasonally polyoestrous northern hemisphere matings take place late autumn	111 days By day 90 female should have abdominal enlargement and nipples reddened	1–5 (average 2)	6–8 weeks	At beginning of oestrus female may produce a waxy plug After mating males penis should be checked for presence of hair that can encircle penis and cause much discomfort Parturition normally occurs early morning duration of approx. 4h

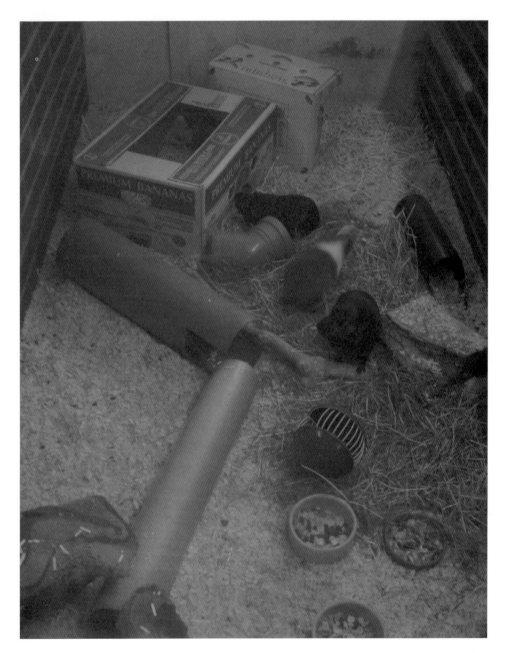

Figure 13.9 Indoor run for cavies. Observe variety of enrichment.

in their bodies for any length of time. Therefore, it is essential that this vitamin be supplemented on a daily basis through the diet. The normal daily requirement for vitamin C is 10 mg/kg, but this increases to 30 mg/kg during pregnancy. Vitamin C plays an important role in the cavies' metabolism and a deficiency can cause degeneration of connective tissues, which can lead to structural abnormalities in bone, teeth, cartilage and muscles. Clinical signs of vitamin C deficiency or scurvy are bleeding gums, weight loss, pain and poor movement.

There are good proprietary diets on the market that are already supplemented with vitamin C and combined with daily fresh green vegetables can provide a good diet for the cavy. (Table 13.5 gives examples of fresh foods that can be offered to cavies.)

Other methods of introducing vitamin C into the diet include adding it to the drinking water in the form of effervescent tablets. Some care should be taken as organic matter easily inactivates vitamin C and drinking bottles should have stainless steel spouts as

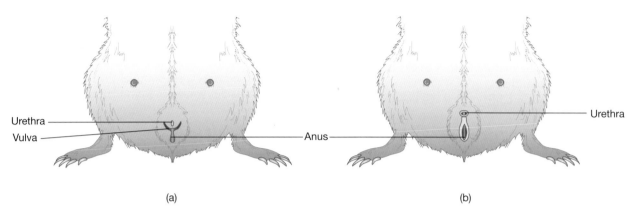

Figure 13.10   Sexing guinea pigs: (a) female and (b) male.

other metals can cause the breakdown of the ascorbic acid.

Roughage (cellulose) is another main consideration in the cavies' diet. Roughage especially in the form of fresh hay is essential in maintaining the health of the gastrointestinal tract and will aid in the prevention of diarrhoea and caecal impaction. Roughage also helps to prevent boredom and helps in the wearing down of the teeth. A bored cavy will often look to its companions for extra stimulation and this attention is usually in the form of barbering (nibbling of the hair).

Vitamin A has been proven to be required in greater amounts compared to that required by the rabbit and other rodents.

Do not give cavies rabbit food as it may contain a coccidiostat which could harm the cavy, also some rabbits foods are high in vitamin D and can cause hyper-vitaminosis D.

Similar to the rabbit, cavies carry out coprophagia; this is a normal process and aids in the re-absorption of the B group vitamins.

Cavies require access to clean fresh water (see discussion under rabbits).

Handling and restraint

Cavies are gentle creatures that rarely bite, but incorrect handling can lead to a very distressed creature that will protest by emitting a high pitched squeak, struggle and possibly bite.

Cavies are best transported in small pet carriers as this limits the amount of space they have available to start a 'chase me game'.

When handling a cavy be calm, confident and exact.

Method
- Making a 'V' shape with your thumb and fourth finger place one hand across the cavy's shoulders.
- The thumb should rest behind the front leg with the 'V' of the hand extending over the shoulders.

- The fourth and middle finger will support the other foreleg and the rest of the fingers will curl just underneath the ribcage.
- The free hand should be placed under the cavy's rump.
- The cavy can now be safely and securely handled.

Tips
- Always talk to the cavy; remember predators are silent.
- If the cavy struggles, hold it into your body and reassure it.
- Cavies have sharp chiselled incisors, which can inflict much pain when they bite so endeavour to make handling and restraint as stress free as possible.

Sexing and breeding

Sexing (see Figure 13.10)
To prevent indiscriminate breeding and unwanted piglets' knowledge on how to sex cavies is essential.

Sexing cavies is a relatively straightforward process and can be carried out soon after birth. In both males and females the anus is closely associated to the urogenital openings.

In males by applying gentle pressure either side of the genital opening the penis can be protruded. In females there is a hairless area of skin and in the centre a 'Y' shape can be seen this 'Y' represents the vaginal groove which sits between the urethral opening and the anus.

Breeding
Main points to consider when breeding cavies include:

- Females can be bred from as early as 4–5 weeks but to give the cavy the opportunity to develop wait until 12 weeks.
- By the age of 10 months the sow's pelvis fuses therefore to prevent problems during parturition

it is necessary to be breed sows before they reach this age.

■ Take the female to the male.

■ Males are sexually mature from 4 weeks but best to breed from 4 months.

■ If a boar by the time he is a year old has not been used for mating then his libido and fertility is compromised.

■ The sow has a relatively long gestation period and she gives birth to precocial young. The young are born with their eyes open, normal body hair and will take solid food within 24–48 hours.

■ Remove boar before parturition as sow returns to oestrus 6–48 hours post partum.

For further details on reproductive parameters see Table 13.6.

RATS AND MICE (*RATTUS NORVEGICUS*) AND (*MUS MUSCULUS*)

Introduction

Rats and mice are often thought of as vermin and disease carriers. Fortunately for rats and mice this is not a view shared by all and the domestic rat or fancy rat (*Rattus norvegicus*) and mouse (*Mus musculus*) are frequently kept as children's pets and by enthusiasts for breeding and showing.

There are many coat and colour variations seen in both species ranging from the solid self-colours, i.e. white, agouti, brown, silver and chocolate to the hooded varieties in rats and tan mice where they have a tan underside and contrasting solid colour on the upper body. Coat variations can also be seen ranging from short to long coats, curly rex coats and silky satin coats.

History

Rats and mice belong to the order of mammals called the Rodentia.

Two species of rat the Black rat (*Rattus rattus*) and the Brown rat (*Rattus norvegicus*) have been domesticated, but it is the brown rat that has been bred to produce the fancy rat. The brown rat originated from Eastern Asia and Northern China; it was established in Europe in the 1800s and has been bred in captivity and domesticated for over 150 years.

Mice originated from Asia and given their reproductive behaviour and ability to adapt to nearly any condition they have spread rapidly throughout the world. History tells us of mice being regarded as sacred animals and having temples constructed for their worship. The Romans used mice in the formulation of medicine to treat a variety of ills. In more recent times mice have been bred to aid in medical research and kept as pets.

Housing (Figures 13.11, 13.12, 13.13)

Rats and mice share similar housing requirements albeit on a varying scale. There is a wide variety of rodent housing on the market, but some of the most important aspects to consider when accommodating rats and mice include:

■ Both species need to be kept indoors.

■ Good ventilation is important as both can suffer from respiratory disease.

■ Room temperature should be between 15–27°C; temperatures above 30°C can cause heat stroke.

■ Rats and mice both gnaw so any accommodation provided should be gnaw and escape proof.

■ The materials used in the construction of the cage must be safe and easy to clean as both can produce pungent urine.

■ Rats and mice are both active creatures and require space to climb and explore so the larger the accommodation the better. The recommended minimum cage size to house a single rat or two mice is 45 cm × 30 cm × 25 cm.

■ Cages with vertical bars provide extra exercise as do those with ledges and platforms.

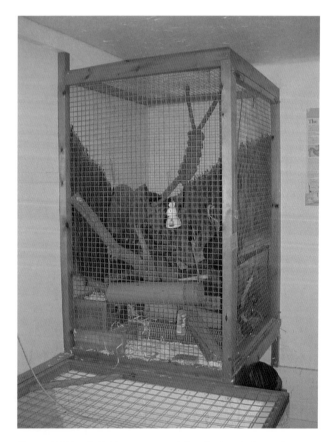

Figure 13.11 Suitable accommodation for two to four rats.

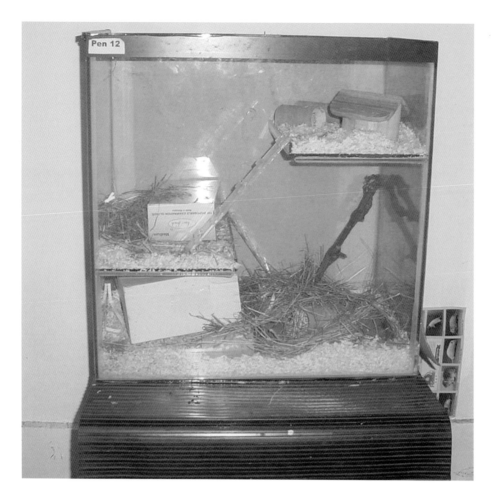

Figure 13.12   Mouse emporium.

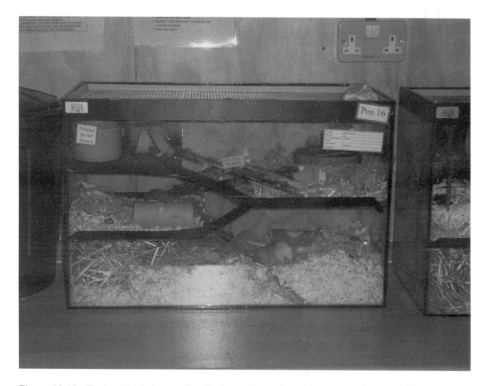

Figure 13.13   Tank suitable for small rodent species such as hamsters, mice or gerbils.

- Rats and mice are inquisitive creatures and benefit from much environmental enrichment. It must be highlighted the more space provided the greater the scope for enrichment activities and therefore the happier the occupants (see Table 13.4).
- Mice and rats are social animals and enjoy the company of their own species. They are best kept in single sex pairs or small colonies and when selecting pairs it is advisable to keep litter mates together. If males are to be kept together some caution is advised especially if females are near by as fighting may take place.

Furnishings, substrates and bedding

See Tables 13.3 and 13.4.

Hygiene (Figure 13.6)

Good hygiene procedures are essential in maintaining the health of the rodents housed. As mentioned earlier, rats and mice produce quite pungent urine and if left the ammonia from the urine will accumulate in the cage causing respiratory problems.

A recommended routine is to spot-clean soiled areas daily (this is especially important if animals are kept in large colonies) and a total clean can be carried out once a week.

Nutritional requirements

Rats and mice have similar nutritional requirements; they are both omnivores and benefit from a wide variety of foodstuffs being offered in their diet.

There are some excellent commercial diets available on the market especially those formulated as complete diets for rats and mice.

The main dietary considerations when providing food for rats and mice are:

- Rats need to be provided with an animal source of protein in their diet; this can be achieved either by feeding one of the proprietary mixes that include dog biscuits in the ration or by daily supplementation of animal protein, i.e. cooked chicken.
- The diet of a rat should contain 14% protein for maintenance increasing to 24% for optimum reproductive ability. Premium puppy foods are a useful supplement for reproducing and growing rats; these foods can be fed up to 10–12 weeks of age.
- Both rats and mice can be selective in their feeding habits, rejecting foodstuffs they do not like; this is especially true when feeding formulated rations. The best way to overcome this is to feed small amounts of food at a time, ensuring all except the grain husks and alfalfa pellets are eaten before offering more food.
- Rats and mice diet should be regularly supplemented with fresh fruits and vegetables (see Table 13.5).
- Rats and to some extend mice will eat almost any type of food offered, so special care should be taken on the types of treats given. Do not feed foods high in fat and sugar as these can cause obesity.
- Rats can synthesise their own vitamin C.
- Rats carry out coprophagia, which aids digestion and supplies the B vitamins, which are produced by the gut flora.
- Clean fresh water should be provided daily and available at all times; it can either be provided in a heavy bowl or gravity feed bottle.
- Rats water intake 10 mL/100 g body weight/day. Adult mice require 4 mL/day.

Handling and restraint of rats and mice

Rats

A well-handled rat rarely bites unless it is in pain or stressed.

To pick up a rat, place one hand around the shoulders and use the free hand to support the rest of the body (see Figure 13.14).

When restraining a rat, try to avoid grasping the animal too tightly around the chest, as this will cause it to struggle and bite.

Mice

Young or nervous mice are very lively and may panic and bite when being handled. Therefore, to ensure a good grip, mice need to be grasped at the base of the tail and

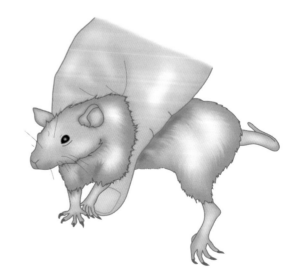

Figure 13.14 Handling a tame rat.

then placed either onto a rough surface where they can then be scruffed or onto the palm of the hand.

Always keep hold of the base of the tail and do not allow the animal to run freely.

If having to transport rats or mice always place them in a small, secure and well-ventilated container.

Sexing and breeding rats and mice

Sexing rats (see Figure 13.15)

Sexing rats is possible from a young age, although in the very young animal more skill is required. Males have a longer anogenital gap, approximately twice that of the females. In juvenile rats the testicles are already descended and when the rat is held in an upright position the testicles are visible in the scrotal sac.

Sexing mice (see Figure 13.16)

Males have a longer anogenital gap, approximately twice that of the females. Younger mice are more difficult to sex, but if animals of both sexes are available then comparisons can be made.

Rats and mice are prolific breeders and to prevent a population explosion of unwanted animals careful consideration MUST be taken before breeding.

Breeding

Main points to consider when breeding rats and mice include:

- Rats and mice can be kept in breeding pairs or in a polygamous system, which can consist of one male to two–six females.
- If a male and female are to be paired for the purpose of mating the female must be taken to the male's cage and not vice versa or alternatively both can be introduced on neutral territory.

- Signs of oestrus in rats include lordosis, a willingness to be mounted by the male and the vulva appears open and purple in colour.
- After mating a waxy plug forms in the vagina; this plug is produced from the male ejaculate and its function is to prevent leakage of semen from the vagina. In rats the plug soon shrinks and drops out in approximately 24 hours; in mice it can remain for up to 24–48 hours.
- Female rats should be separated from the male or colony by the 16–20th day of pregnancy. This is a safeguard against post-partum mating and cannibalism.
- Both rats and mice display nesting behaviour a few days pre-partum.
- Rats and mice give birth to altricial young, i.e. they are blind, deaf and hairless.

For more details on reproductive parameters see Table 13.6.

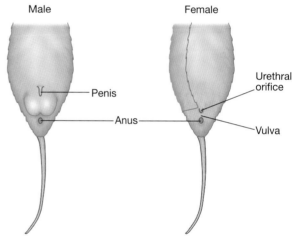

Figure 13.16   Sexing mice.

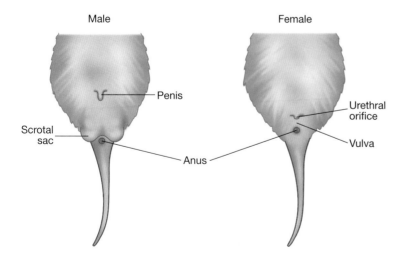

Figure 13.15   Sexing rats.

HAMSTERS

Introduction

Hamsters are one of the most popular rodents and a favoured small pet with many children. But their crepuscular lifestyle, i.e. being active at dawn and dusk, does not always make the hamster the amenable small pet we would imagine them to be, and interaction with them during the day, especially when the hamster is trying to sleep, can prove somewhat hazardous to the handler.

History

Hamsters belong to the order Rodentia; the most common species kept in captivity is the Golden or Syrian hamster (*Mesocricetus auratus*). Other species of hamster that are available include the Russian hamster (*Phodopus sungorus*), Chinese hamster (*Cricetulus cricetus*) and the Roborovski hamster (*Phodopus roborovskii*).

Golden hamsters are native to Bulgaria, Romania, and the Middle East and have been bred to produce a variety of coat types and colours.

Russian hamsters are native to Russia, Mongolia and China; there are two species: Campbells and the Djungarian. Russian hamsters range in colour from the original grey with dark dorsal strip to black with various colours in between.

Chinese hamsters are native to many parts of Eurasia ranging from Siberia to Tibet. They are mouse-like in their appearance with a short tail, and are usually brown with a black dorsal stripe or greyish brown with white patches.

Roborovski hamster is the smallest of the dwarf hamsters and is golden brown in colour with distinctive white eyebrows.

The first Golden hamsters were discovered in 1930 in Aleppo Syria by an archaeologist and it is considered that the majority of the golden hamsters kept as pets today are the descendants of those found in Aleppo.

Housing

In the wild hamsters live in underground tunnels and spend the day sleeping and night foraging for food.

As mentioned earlier Golden hamsters are solitary animals and should be housed on their own. Russian and Chinese hamsters are more sociable animals and can live together either as single or mixed sexed pairs or in small colonies. The Roborovski hamster is better kept in pairs. It is not advisable to mix the different dwarf species.

Main housing considerations include:

- Like the other rodents covered, hamsters love to gnaw and are best kept in metal or plastic containers. Converted aquariums can be used as long as good ventilation is provided and enrichment is carried out. Tanks are especially suitable for small colonies of Russian, Chinese or Roborovski hamsters.
- If a barred cage is used the bars should run vertically, not horizontally as this will give the hamster extra climbing area.
- Some of the more elaborate rodent accommodation made up of a network of tubes can look impressive but is not very practical. Apart from the cost, this type of housing provides poor ventilation, and inside condensation soon builds up. The accommodation is not easy to clean and animals can get their feet caught in the ventilation slits.
- If wooden accommodation is to be used the owner must be advised to use hardwood of at least 1 cm thickness and ensure no raw edges are exposed as these will be chewed.
- Hamsters are excellent escape artists and all steps must be taken to ensure the accommodation is secure. Hamsters can flatten their bodies and squeeze through very small gaps so check sizes of mesh and bars.
- Minimum cage size is 60 cm long × 30 cm wide × 23 cm high.

Siting of accommodation

As for all rodents, accommodation must not be sited by a heat source or window and extremes of temperature must be avoided. Ideal temperature should be between 18°C and 21°C with a relative humidity of 40–60%.

Providing ample bedding is given, hamsters are better adapted to coping with cold rather than heat. Dwarf hamsters are especially susceptible to heat stroke and Golden hamsters can go into a state of immobility called *sleeper's disease* if the temperature reaches 22–25°C.

For further information on environmental enrichment see Table 13.4.

Substrates, bedding and furnishings

See Tables 13.3 and 13.4. Hamsters require a sleeping box and plenty of bedding material.

Hygiene (Figure 13.6)

The animal's accommodation should be cleaned weekly if colonies are kept then more frequent cleaning may be necessary.

When cleaning hamster's accommodation always check the food store and remove any mouldy or stale food. Try not to remove their entire store, as this will cause the hamster much stress. When replenishing the bedding material include a small amount of the old bedding in with the new. Hamsters will generally adopt an area within the cage in which to urinate and defecate; this area can be cleaned daily and if a jam jar or shallow tray is placed in the toilet area, then the hamster will soon adopt this as its latrine.

Nutritional requirements

Hamsters are omnivores and their natural diet would include a mixture of seeds, grains and grasses with the additional supplement of grubs and insects.

In captivity hamsters should be offered a proprietary dry mixture of cereals, seeds and nuts supplemented with a small amount of fresh foods daily (see Table 13.5).

Hamsters should be fed once a day ideally early evening (an adult hamster will consume approximately 5–7 g dry food/day).

Other important points to remember when feeding hamsters are:

- As hamsters are natural hoarders and place food in their large expandable pouches it is NOT advisable to offer sharp foods that could puncture the lining of the pouches or sticky foods that can cause impaction.
- Excess water on fresh foods can cause diarrhoea.
- High fat seeds such as sunflower seeds and peanuts are extremely palatable and can lead to obesity. Sunflower seeds if eaten in excess can exacerbate the onset of osteoporosis.
- If invertebrates are going to be included in the diet then these should be introduced early in the animal's life as the intestinal microflora has to adapt to this food source. Late introduction can lead to diarrhoea and other intestinal disorders.
- Like rats hamsters also carry out coprophagia; this aids the digestion and supplies vitamins B and K produced by the gut flora.
- Hamsters should always have access to fresh clean water, preferably offered in a gravity feed bottle with a stainless steel spout. Water intake for adults is 15–20 mL/day.

Handling and restraint

Hamsters have a reputation for inflicting painful bites and should always be handled with care. If startled or frightened a hamster may role onto its back, raising its front feet and showing its teeth; at this stage it is best to let the hamster calm down before attempting to handle it again.

General procedure and precautions
- Never handle or scruff a hamster with full pouches.
- As hamsters are usually asleep during the day the handler must ensure the sleeping hamster is slowly and gently roused from its slumber.
- Prior to handling a little substrate from the animal's cage can be rubbed into the handler's hands, this will then give the strange hand a familiar smell.
- Hamsters are short-sighted and if approached too hurriedly or if the hand smells of food the hamster may bite.
- A friendly hamster can be cupped in both hands and if further examination required the hamster could be scruffed by grasping the large amounts of loose skin at the back of the neck and down the back.

Sexing and breeding

Sexing (see Figure 13.17)
Males have a longer anogenital gap compared to that of the females. The scrotal sacs of the male are also visible. Females have a rounder rump than the males and seven pairs of nipples whereas the male usually has a more pointed rump and no nipples.

Hamsters possess bilateral sebaceous glands on their flanks; they are more pronounced in the male and appear as dark circular areas.

Breeding
Main points to remember when breeding hamsters include:

- **Golden hamsters**
  - To prevent fighting the female must be taken to the male's cage and not vice versa or alternatively both can be introduced on neutral territory.
  - Hamsters should be mated late evening.
  - Even when in oestrus the female hamster is often aggressive toward the male and they should be separated immediately after mating.
  - When in oestrus the female will exhibit lordosis crouching and holding her tail in the air.
  - During oestrus the female produces a slightly stringy, clear, mucoid vaginal discharge which post oestrus appears cloudy.
  - Male will repeatedly mount the female and mating may last for 10 minutes; once mating

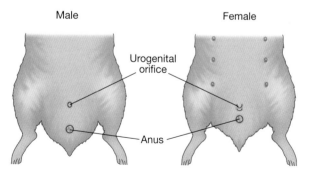

Figure 13.17   Sexing hamsters.

is complete the pair should be separated and returned to their accommodation.

– Pregnant females must have access to plenty of nesting materials.

■ **Russian and Roborovski hamsters**

– These can be kept in breeding pairs or colonies and both male and female will play a part in rearing the young.

■ **Chinese hamsters**

– As for Russian hamsters but the pregnant female may display signs of aggression toward the male banishing him from the nest until the young are born.

For more details on reproductive parameters see Table 13.6.

GERBILS (*MERIONES UNGUICULATUS*)

Introduction

Gerbils are one of the few diurnal rodents, and being active during the day makes them very interesting and lively animals to keep as pets.

History

The species of gerbil commonly kept as a pet is called the Mongolian gerbil (*Meriones unguiculatus*). The Mongolian gerbil is closely related to the hamster and its Latin name means clawed warrior. Like rats and mice, gerbils belong to the order Rodentia.

Mongolian gerbils are a desert species originating from Mongolia and North-eastern China. Other species of gerbil kept as pets include the larger Shaw's jird (*Meriones shawii*); this species originates from the arid areas of North Africa and the Middle East.

The domestication of the Mongolian gerbil began in 1935 in Tokyo when Japanese scientists used 40 wild caught animals for breeding, however, the Mongolian gerbil did not reach Britain until 1964 and over the years, its popularity as a small pet and show animal has slowly developed. The most common coat colours seen include the original agouti, white, black and blue.

Housing (see Figure 13.18)

Gerbils are natural diggers and in their native habitat they live in colonies and produce a complex network of underground tunnels, which consist of storage rooms, sleeping quarters and adjoining tunnels with two exits providing adequate escape routes if danger looms.

Mongolian gerbils are social animals and are best kept in groups within a gerbilarium.

Females will live quite happily together; males can live together but it is advisable to introduce them at

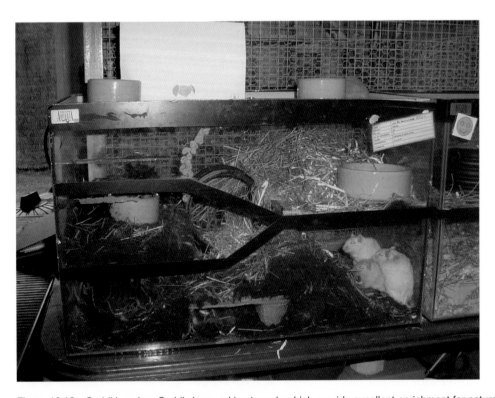

Figure 13.18 Gerbil housing. Gerbils love making tunnels which provide excellent enrichment for natural behaviour. Bowls contain chinchilla sand for bathing.

an early age or select littermates, but fighting may still occur.

Making a gerbilarium

Converting a glass or plastic aquarium and covering it with a well-fitting fine mesh lid can produce a gerbilarium. The best substrate to include in the gerbilarium is a mixture of moss peat, wood shavings (not cedar), chopped straw or hay. The mixture needs to be at least 10cm deep; shredded white paper or tissue can be offered as a suitable bedding material.

Other types of accommodation that can be used include:

- A wire or plastic cage, but as gerbils love to gnaw wood is not a suitable medium. A hide box must be provided as this gives the gerbils privacy and somewhere to sleep.
- The minimum cage size for two Mongolian gerbils is 60cm × 25cm × 25cm but the more space that can be offered the greater the opportunity for exercise.
- Ideal environmental temperature for gerbils is 15–20°C.

Other considerations when housing gerbils include:

- Gerbils are very active and can jump so ensure lids are well fitting and check for signs of chewing especially to plastic containers.
- If barred cages are used the animal must be observed for bar gnawing as this can lead to stereotypical behaviour and can also cause injuries to the gerbil's nose. Good environmental enrichment and a good-sized cage with deep litter can overcome much of this behaviour. (For further information on environmental enrichment, see Table 13.4.)
- Another disadvantage of using a barred cage is that the substrate can be kicked out as the gerbils dig.
- Sand is not recommended as a substrate, but a small bowl placed in the cage can act as a good sand bath.
- Remember – *Gerbils are very destructive and will chew anything placed in their cage or if in a gerbilarium will most likely bury it, so plastic items, especially food and water bowls, are not recommended.*

Furnishings, substrates and bedding

See Tables 13.3 and 13.4.

Hygiene (Figure 13.6)

Gerbils are relatively odourless animals and coming from a harsh arid environment produce very little urine and faecal matter.

If a peat mix gerbilarium is used then the animals only require cleaning approximately every three months. If other types of accommodation are used, then weekly cleaning and replenishing of substrates and bedding materials is necessary.

With both types of accommodation daily checks should be undertaken to remove any stale or mouldy foods.

Shaw's jirds

Shaw's jirds can be kept very much as stated for the Mongolian gerbil, but the accommodation must be larger. Males can be kept in pairs especially if litter mates or introduced at an early age. Female however are very aggressive and territorial and are best kept singly.

Nutritional requirements

Gerbils are omnivores and in the wild they eat a wide selection of grasses, grains seeds, stalks, roots supplemented with insects and grubs. Offering gerbils one of the proprietary gerbil rations can simulate this natural diet. Gerbils should be fed once a day (an adult gerbil will consume approximately 10–15g/day) and any uneaten food removed; scatter feeding is a very good way to enhance natural foraging behaviour. Like other rodents, gerbils can be selective feeders and if allowed will exclusively eat sunflower seeds, which are high in fat and low in calcium. This selective diet can lead to calcium deficiencies and obesity.

Gerbils benefit from having fresh foods included in their diet (see Table 13.5).

Gerbils are desert animals and although their water requirement is relatively low (50mL/kg/day), they should always have access to fresh clean water preferable offered in a gravity feed bottle.

Shaw's jirds

Shaw's jird diet is very similar to that for the Mongolian gerbil. Their diet can be supplemented with fruits and vegetables and also offered meat proteins in the form of cat or dog food or mealworms.

Handling and restraint

Gerbils are generally easy to handle and rarely bite, but some caution must be taken as they have no perception of height and will readily jump off a hand or table.

Method

Grasp the gerbil at the base of the tail and place onto the palm of the hand. Slightly cup the hand to prevent the gerbil jumping. Always keep hold of the base of the tail and do not allow the animal to run freely. NEVER grasp a gerbil at the tip of the tail as the skin may shed.

For jirds, it is best to handle them using the method suggested for rats.

If having to transport gerbils or jirds, always place them in a small, secure and well-ventilated container.

Sexing and breeding

Sexing (see Figure 13.19)

Males have a longer anogenital gap, approximately twice that of the females. Sexing is possible from an early age; by 4 weeks the scrotal sacs of the male become visible.

Males have a more pronounced ventral scent gland, which is a hairless area found on the mid-ventral abdomen.

Breeding

Main points to consider when breeding gerbils include:

- Gerbils can be kept in monogamous breeding pairs or in a polygamous system.
- If electing to breed using the polygamous system it is best to establish colonies when the animals are between 8–10 weeks old as this will help to prevent fighting.
- If a male and female are to be paired for the purpose of mating the female must be taken to the male's cage and not vice versa or alternatively both can be introduced on neutral territory.
- The female produces no vaginal plug, but because the mating process continues over several hours' sores can be seen in both sexes around the perineal area. This usually heals in 2–3 days.
- Gerbils if disturbed or stressed and those that have small litters have been known to kill and cannibalise their young.
- Gerbils and jirds give birth to altricial young, i.e. they are blind, deaf and hairless.
- Female jirds will only accept the male when in oestrus and then he will only be tolerated for up to 2 hours.

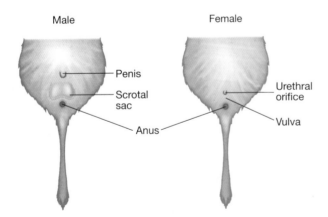

Male   Female

— Penis
— Scrotal sac
— Anus
— Urethral orifice
— Vulva

Figure 13.19 Sexing gerbils.

For more details on reproductive parameters see Table 13.6.

CHINCHILLAS (*CHINCHILLA LANIGERA*)

Introduction

Chinchillas are agile, cheeky animals with squirrel-like characteristics; they are closely related to the cavy and porcupine. Chinchillas make excellent and interesting pets for adults and older children.

History

The chinchilla (*Chinchilla lanigera*) originates from the Andes in South America; they inhabit very barren areas and survive at altitudes up to 4500 m (15 000 feet). They shelter in holes and crevices amongst the rocks and are thought to be nocturnal.

The Incas were one of the first groups to identify the value of chinchilla fur. In the 1920s fur farms were established and in the 1960s chinchillas were eventually recognised as being suitable pets. The wild chinchilla is a blue-grey colour, but many variations have now been bred ranging from white, silver, beige, and black.

Housing (Figures 13.20 and 13.21)

Chinchillas love to gnaw, so they are best kept in metal cages. If a wooden frame is constructed then no raw edges must be accessible, and all exposed wood must be covered with fine wire mesh. Wood must be treated using a non-toxic chemical.

Chinchillas need plenty of space to exercise and a cage of $2 \text{m} \times 1 \text{m} \times 0.45 \text{m}$ (L × W × H) will happily accommodate two chinchillas, but the more space that can be provided the better for the animal housed.

Good ventilation is essential; chinchillas do not like the heat or high humidity and are best kept at temperatures ranging from 10–15°C.

Chinchillas are social animals and can be kept in pairs, colonies or polygamous units; as with other rodents chinchillas should be introduced to one another while young.

Furnishings and enrichment are essential in the welfare of the chinchilla (see Table 13.3).

Substrates, bedding and furnishings (see Tables 13.3 and 13.4)

The main points to highlight here are:

- The provision of a nest box, which should be one per chinchilla housed.
- A large cat litter tray containing silver sand to act as a dust bath; this should be left in the accommodation daily for 10–15 minutes. Any

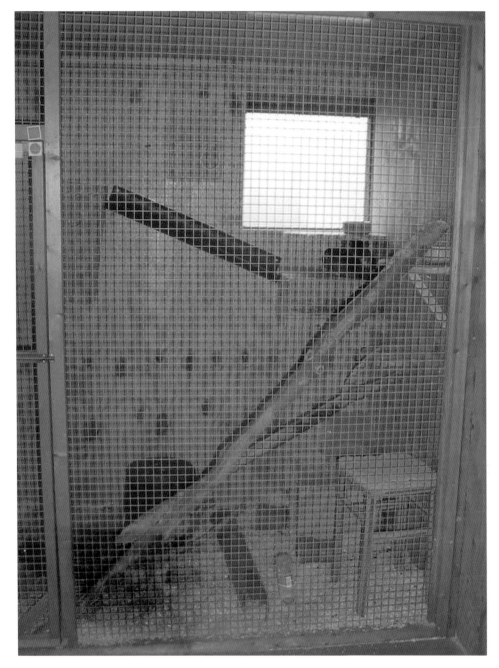

Figure 13.20   Large walk-in chinchilla cage and hide boxes.

longer than this will result in the chinchilla soiling the bath and over-bathing itself.

■ Remember due to the constant gnawing of these creatures any wooden objects placed in the cage will need to be replaced regularly, for example: wooden ledges, hide boxes and branches.

Hygiene (Figure 13.6)

Chinchillas are relatively odourless animals and should have their soiled areas cleaned daily and a total clean each week. It is essential that the sand bath is sieved daily to remove any faeces or urine as a soiled coat will damage fur.

Nutritional requirements

In the wild the chinchilla would enjoy a high fibre diet consisting of grasses, fruits, leaves, bark stems and roots.

In captivity chinchillas can be fed either a complete pelleted ration or a specially formulated course mix.

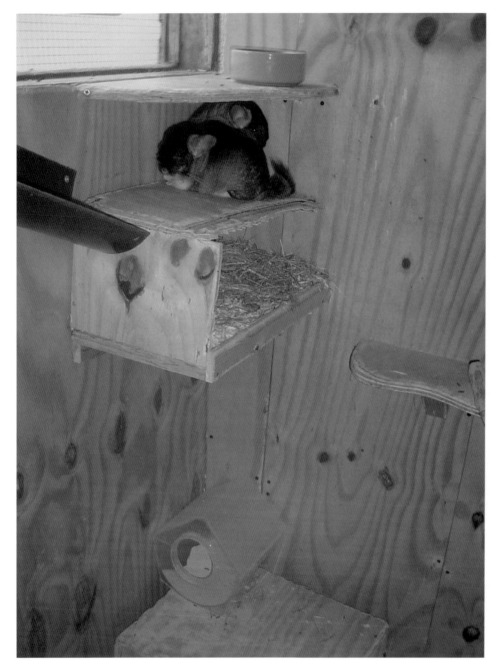

Figure 13.21 Although chinchillas are not climbing animals, they enjoy moving from ledge to ledge and have a choice of hide boxes. They are gnawing animals – see damage done to wooden boxes.

They need access to good quality hay (to prevent soiling it should be placed in a hay rack) and have access to fresh water.

Chinchillas' main nutritional considerations are as follows:

- They need to be fed daily, preferably early evening, just before their main period of activity and again in the morning.

- To prevent gastrointestinal disorders and possibility of boredom, chinchillas require high levels of fibre in their diet.
- Chinchillas are unable to synthesise certain unsaturated fatty acids and so these need to be present in the diet. Deficiencies of fatty acids such as linoleic acid can lead to poor fur condition and growth.

- Chinchillas are unable to synthesise their own vitamin A and any deficiency can cause poor night vision, skin conditions, reproduction and gastrointestinal problems.
- Calcium, phosphorus and vitamin D levels are also important for maintaining good bone and teeth formation. Deficiencies can lead to musculoskeletal weakness, bone deformities and cramping. To prevent deficiency diseases occurring, calcium and phosphorus need to be present in the diet at a ratio of between 1:1 and 2:1 (calcium : phosphorus).
- It should be stressed that as long as a good commercial diet is being fed, owners should not be advised to supplement their chinchilla's diet as this could lead to disease from excess.
- Food must be offered in a heavy earthenware type bowl and fresh water provided via a gravity feed bottle with a stainless steel spout.
- Care should be taken when offering treats to chinchillas, as they are prone to dietary-induced diarrhoea.

See Table 13.5 for suitable fresh foodstuffs.

Handling and restraint of chinchillas

Chinchillas are lively creatures and if used to being handled will rarely bite. However, a chinchilla that has not been handled regularly can be difficult to restrain and will struggle, catapulting itself forward away from the grasp of the handler.

The chinchilla should be restrained by picking it up at the base of the tail close to the body, then the free hand can be placed underneath the chinchilla to support the body. Once restrained the handler should bring the chinchilla in close to his or her own body, or once the tail has been grasped the chinchilla can be placed straight onto the handler's arm.

The chinchilla may be picked up by placing a hand round the shoulders, but grasping or rough handling can lead to shedding of the fur and cause much distress to the chinchilla.

Sexing and breeding

Sexing (see Figure 13.22)
In the male there is a considerable distance between the anus and the penis.

In the female the anus and the genital papilla are closer together. The urethral orifice is at the end of the genital papilla and a slit-like vulva is found at the base of the genital papilla. The vulva is normally closed apart from 3–5 days when the chinchilla is in season.

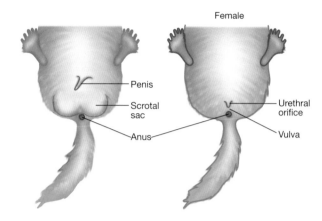

Figure 13.22   Sexing chinchillas.

Breeding
Main points to consider when breeding chinchillas include:

- Like the cavy chinchillas have a long gestation period resulting in precocial young that are fully furred with eyes open.
- Chinchillas can be bred as pairs or in a polygamous unit, which consist of one male to several females.
- New breeding pairs must be introduced slowly; one way this can be achieved is by placing the individual chinchilla cages side by side. Once the breeding pair has become accustomed to one another they can be placed in a neutral cage and allowed to mate; best time to introduce new breeding pairs is during the day when they are less active.
- When ready to mate the male makes cooing and chuckling noises, whereas the female's vagina opens and a mucous discharge can be seen.
- Mating normally takes place at night.
- As explained under the section on rats, the female chinchilla produces a copulatory plug or 'stopper' which is normally passed a few hours after mating; it is approximately 3 cm long and although white at first soon shrivels and appears yellow in colour.
- During the gestation period the breeding pair can be kept together, but approximately 12 hours after parturition the female experiences a fertile post-partum oestrus, which can last 2 days and mating at this time should be discouraged.
- Chinchillas do not build nests but a nest box should be provided, as young born on the cage floor are susceptible to hypothermia. Just before parturition females can become aggressive toward the male and refuse food.

For more details on reproductive parameters see Table 13.6.

References and further reading

- Beynon, P.H., Cooper, J.E. (1991) Manual of Exotic Pets. BSAVA, Cheltenham.
- British Rabbit Council, various leaflets.
- Brown, S.A. (1997) Gastrointestinal Physiology and Disease in the Domestic Rabbit. Waltham/OSU Symposium.
- Hill, L. (1997) Complete Hamster Internet Web Site.
- Hillyer, Quesenberry, K. (1997) Ferrets, Rabbits and Rodents. Clinical Medicine and Surgery. W.B. Saunders, London.
- Laber-Laird, K., Swindle, M.M., Flecknell, P. (1996) Handbook of Rodent and Rabbit Medicine. Pergamon, Oxford.
- National Fancy Rat Society (1998) www.national/fancyrat-society.co.uk
- Okerman, L. Diseases of Domestic Rabbits. Blackwell Science, Oxford.
- Quesenberry, K. (1997) Medical Management of Gerbil, Hamsters and Guinea Pigs. Waltham/OSU Symposium.
- Richardson, V.C.G. Diseases of Domestic Guinea Pigs. Blackwell Science, Oxford.
- Richardson, V.C.G. Diseases of Small Domestic Rodents. Blackwell Science, Oxford.
- Supreme Pet Foods Small Animal Directory (2000) Supreme Pat Foods, Southampton.
- The RSPCA Official Guides (1995) Rabbits, Guinea Pigs and Hamsters. Collins, London.

Care of birds, reptiles and fish

Chapter

14

Caroline Gosden

Chapter objectives

This chapter gives an introduction to:

- Basic comparative anatomy
- Species and breeds
- Housing requirements
- Handling and restraint
- Feeding requirements
- Breeding

PART I – HUSBANDRY

Before keeping any exotic species, thorough research should be undertaken as to its natural habits and habitat. This in itself presents a formidable challenge; if you take any three sources of information the chances are that they will invariably contradict each other, particularly in the case of reptiles. This probably reflects the fact that there is no single right way to care for these species and it is a matter of deciding what is best for each particular set of circumstances.

REPTILES

Suitability as pets

An important point to bear in mind is that they should not be considered a 'children's pet', as adults must be involved with their care.

Very few species are suitable for beginners. For a first time owner I would suggest leopard gecko, corn snake or king snake.

Species such as tortoises and terrapins whilst not too difficult to maintain, do require specialised equipment and set-ups initially to house them adequately.

Green iguanas are not suitable for any but the most experienced keepers.

Most reptiles do not appreciate being handled in the same way that a mammal does and are usually stressed to a greater or lesser degree (depending on the individual) by the experience.

Good husbandry is the key to healthy reptiles, and the majority of illnesses are avoidable. Therefore, it is important to know what is and is not acceptable as this may give you the reasons for the illness of a given animal.

Factors to be taken into consideration when caring for a reptile are:

- **Specific requirements of a given species, e.g.**
  geographical origin
  natural habitat
  wild diet
  biological data
- **Housing:**
  size
  accident-free environment
  temperature
  humidity
  lighting
  ventilation
- **Feeding:**
  correct diet
  supplements if necessary
  variety
- **Stress:**
  overhandling
  lack of stimulation
  overcrowding
  species-specific information.

Before acquiring a reptile it is important to find out as much as possible about how it lives in the wild. Table 14.1 gives basic information on some of the more commonly kept species.

Environmental stimulation is particularly relevant with reptiles, one method of providing this is with companionship. A little research is necessary to establish the best group size and mix of sexes and as a rule,

Table 14.1	Species-specific information for reptiles				
Species	Scientific name	Geographical origin	Natural habitat	Wild diet	Activity time
Spur-thighed tortoise	*Testudo graeca*	Southern Europe, North Africa and South West Asia	Open steppe with scattered rocks and bushes. Hot, dry summers, cool, wet winters. 5–30°C. Terrestrial	Flowers, leaves, fruit, succulents. Opportunistic carnivore	Diurnal
Red-eared terrapin	*Chrysemys scripta elegans*	Northern USA	Ponds, swamps etc. 10–30°C. Semi-aquatic	Water insects and plants, small vertebrates, e.g. fish, frogs, waterfowl chicks	Diurnal
Corn snake	*Elaphe guttata*	South-eastern USA	Pine forests, fields/paddocks, rockpiles, small rodent burrows, abandoned buildings. 5–30°C. Terrestrial	Small lizards, frogs, rodents, birds	Crepuscular/ nocturnal
Leopard gecko	*Eublepharis macularius*	South Central Asia to Iraq to North West India	Steppe and mountain regions up to 2000 m, semi-desert, scrub-land. 10–35°C. Terrestrial, hides under rocks or in burrows	Grasshoppers, small lizards, scorpions, young rodents	Crepuscular/ nocturnal
Green iguana	*Iguana iguana*	Central and South America	Tropical and sub-tropical rain forest below 900 m, high to moderate rainfall, near large bodies of water. 15°C–30°C. Arboreal, good swimmers	Leaves and shoots, flowers, soft fruits, occasional insect (more so as youngsters)	Diurnal

different species should not be housed together. Even if the species has a solitary lifestyle in the wild, I prefer to give my reptiles company, provided of course, that it does not have any contraindications, king snakes are a notable example of this given that they have a tendency to eat each other!

Housing

The following applies to all reptiles *including* tortoises. It is not sufficient to put a tortoise in a part of the garden during the summer and then hibernate it in the winter. There are not many days in the year when it is hot enough to leave a tortoise outside with no supplementary heating etc.

Design
Vivaria can be made as complicated as you wish, there are no hard and fast rules about sizes. Many people keep and breed reptiles using very simple set-ups such as the drawer system (Figure 14.1). However, I prefer to provide as much room and variation as possible (Figures 14.2, 14.6).

For short-term accommodation, e.g. hospitalisation, the very minimum that an animal needs is heat, light, a hide and water and if you are housing an animal for just a few days the set-up could be as simple as a fauna box lined with newspaper, containing a hide and a water bowl and placed on a heat mat (Figure 14.3). However,

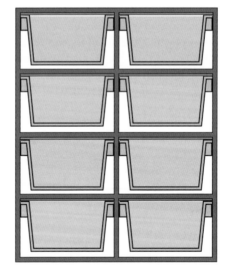

Figure 14.1 Drawer system for keeping reptiles.

for longer term/permanent some basic criteria need to be addressed:

The exact size depends on the size of the species and the number of individuals housed. As a rough guide a pair of adult corn snakes can be comfortably housed in a vivarium measuring 60 cm high × 60 cm deep × 2 m long.

The shape should reflect the reptiles' natural habits, i.e. an arboreal (tree living) species should be provided

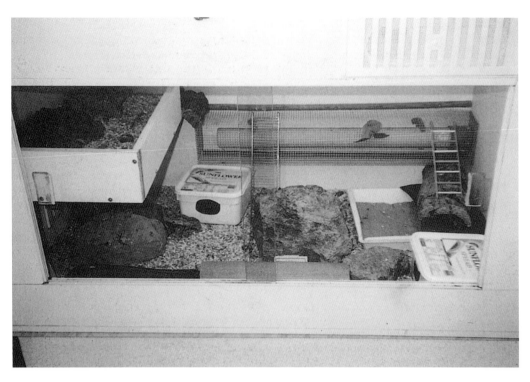

Figure 14.2   Vivarium for leopard geckos.

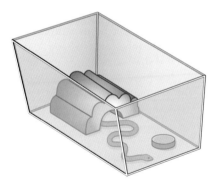

Figure 14.3   Simple or short-term set-up.

with plenty of height, whilst a fossorial (burrowing) species needs a deep layer of substrate (Figure 14.4).

Heating
There are a number of methods available, some are suitable for most vivariums and some have very limited use.

- The background temperature is best maintained by ceramic or tubular greenhouse heaters, etc.
- Hot rocks should not be used as they can result in burns.
- Light bulbs are not suitable for providing background heat.
- Heat mats are not suitable for most set-ups.
- All heaters must be connected to a thermostatic control unit.

- Heaters must be guarded with a wire mesh cage to prevent burns.
- A heat gradient should be provided within the vivarium to allow the reptile to thermoregulate. This is achieved by keeping everything that produces heat at one end.
- If the preferred body temperature (PBT) is not known most species will tolerate a gradient of 25°C at the cool end rising to 30°C at the hot end.
- Spotlights can be used to provide daytime basking areas but these should also have a guard around them.
- The system should take into account day/night and summer/winter variations in temperature that reflect the animals' natural habitat.

Lighting
Full spectrum lighting which includes ultraviolet (to assist with calcium metabolism) is usually required by all chelonia (tortoises, terrapins, turtles) and diurnal lizards, e.g. green iguana. This is usually provided in the form of fluorescent tubes which are available with various levels of UV.

Snakes and most nocturnal lizards, e.g. leopard gecko, do not generally require UV when adult. However, they do need some form of lighting so that they can register the difference between night/day and summer/winter in order to regulate their circadian cycle. Incandescent light bulbs are usually used to provide lighting for these species, they are also useful as a basking spot for all species whether they require UV or not. Ensure this type of bulb is also guarded as even a very low wattage bulb will produce enough heat to cause a burn.

All forms of lighting will produce a certain amount of heat (some more than others) and so should be placed at the hot end of the vivarium. They should not, however, be considered as a primary heat source, as they will need to be turned off at night.

All lighting should be turned off at night otherwise the animals' sense of time will become confused. Lighting cycles should also take into account the differing day length between summer and winter where applicable.

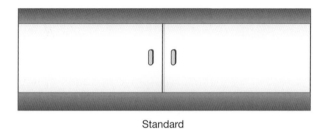

Standard

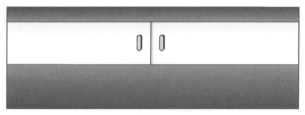

Fossorial

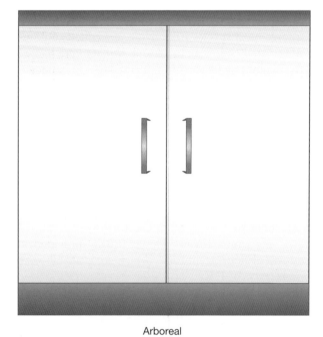

Arboreal

Figure 14.4 Vivarium shapes.

Ventilation

Very important to provide a good through flow of air to prevent air stagnating but must avoid creating a draught (Figure 14.5).

Humidity

It is important to ascertain if a particular species needs high humidity, or not. Too low and it can cause difficulty in sloughing (dydecdysis) and too high and it can result in blisters and respiratory problems.

Most commonly kept species require medium to low humidity, e.g. corn snake, leopard gecko, bearded dragon. The green iguana requires high humidity and the royal python needs a rainy season and a dry season.

The most common method of providing humidity is to use a spray bottle filled with warm water. The vivarium can be sprayed as often as necessary to maintain the correct humidity.

Décor

Use plenty of rocks, branches, cork bark, clay pots etc. to provide environmental stimulation and security. If species is arboreal, e.g. green iguana, ensure there is the means to gain height and clamber about amongst branches (Figure 14.6).

There must be at least one hide per individual (within reason) and these should be at both hot and cold ends so that the reptile does not have to compromise security for thermoregulation. Hides can be as simple as a cardboard box or a more elaborate construction, e.g. a rock pile, but this must be stable and secure.

Some furniture can also provide hotter or cooler areas to aid with thermoregulation, e.g. inside a clay pipe is cooler than outside, a large rock placed under the basking lamp etc.

One essential item is a container, e.g. a margarine tub, lined with damp moss or peat with a hole cut into the side. This provides three important functions:

- A damp area to aid sloughing. Most lizards (not geckos) usually shed their skin in bits and pieces and may take several days. Snakes should shed in one piece within a few hours.

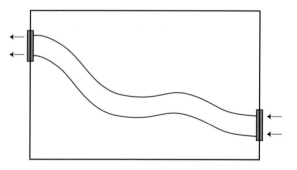

Figure 14.5 A good 'through flow' of air is essential.

■ A cooler area for thermoregulation.

■ A place for females to lay their eggs, as if she cannot find a suitable place she may retain them which may lead to egg binding. (It is worth noting that a female does not need to be with a male in order to produce eggs.)

All furniture should be secured or, if moveable, will not harm the animal if it falls on it. Heavy items such as rocks or drainpipes that rest on the floor must be in full contact with the vivarium floor so that the animal cannot burrow underneath it and get squashed!

Various forms of substrate are available. Ensure the type used is suitable for the environment and the depth suits the animal's habits, i.e. deep enough to allow

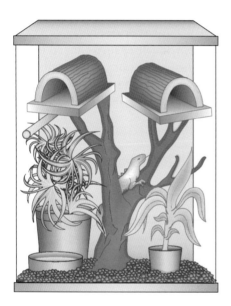

Figure 14.6   Natural set-up vivarium.

burrowing/digging in if appropriate, e.g. blue tongue skink. Consideration needs to be given to the size of granules, especially with insectivores, as they may ingest quantities with the food.

Feeding

What to feed and how often? Another area where there is no one right way but there are several wrong ways. It would be possible to write an entire chapter on the principles of feeding and nutrition for reptiles (indeed, I have). However, I will attempt to offer some general guidelines, which should, hopefully, give some idea as to the basic principles.

Obviously it is most important to ascertain what the animal eats in the wild. If this cannot be replicated there are a number of acceptable alternatives available (Table 14.2).

However, many species do not fall conveniently into one category, they may be predominantly herbivorous but also take insects occasionally.

One of the most important points is to provide as great a variety as possible (see Table 14.3). This prevents monotony and nutritional imbalances (see Table 14.4). This is easy for herbivores and omnivores, but a little more difficult for insectivores as there is not the range available. Snakes are the exception as they tend to have the same food item all the time.

Especially prepared pelleted food is also available for some species, e.g. iguana, bearded dragon, tortoise, terrapin. Pellets should not be used as a complete diet, rather one constituent of a varied diet.

Species classified as herbivores should be given fresh food daily but it is not necessary or indeed desirable to feed all species every day. Most adult snakes are fed no more than once a week, e.g. corn snake, or even once a

Table 14.2   Food alternatives

Feeder type	Alternative	Supplements	Example species
Carnivore	Pinkies, fluffs, rat pups, mice, gerbils, rats, cavies, rabbits, chicken, 'snake sausages'	Not normally necessary	Most snakes e.g. Corn snakes Burmese python
Herbivore	Fruit, vegetables, herbs, garden flowers, weeds	Multivitamin/mineral	Mediterranean tortoise Iguanas (also occasional insects) Bearded dragons (also insects)
Insectivore	Crickets, locusts, waxmoth larvae, mealworms	Multivitamin/mineral	Leopard geckos (may also take occasional pinkie) Day geckos (need nectar substitute occasionally e.g. honey)
Omnivore	All of the above but may also take: prawns, fish, snails, worms and eggs	Multivitamin/mineral	Red eared terrapin Blue tongued skink (not sea food)

month depending on their size and therefore the size of the food item. Those classified as insectivores or omnivores tend to muddy the waters a bit. Certainly it is not essential to feed on a daily basis but the environmental enrichment provided by feeding should not be underestimated. The primary consideration in this case should be how much to feed on say, a weekly basis, then divide this into the number of feeds to be given.

So, for example if a leopard gecko eats 21 crickets a week, it could be given three every day OR seven three times a week.

See sample diet sheets in Tables 14.5, 14.6, 14.7, 14.8 and 14.9.

General points to bear in mind:

- Fruit should be used carefully as it can promote diarrhoea and fussy eaters.
- Temperature needs to be at the PBT for digestion to occur properly.
- Some foods should not be fed too regularly as they can become 'addictive', e.g. bananas and prawns.
- Do not be tempted to use cat or dog food as these can also become addictive and can cause problems with obesity and fatty liver disease.
- Remember that live prey items such as crickets need to be fed as well. If you do not feed these then all the reptile will eat is an empty husk. Proprietary diets are available or I have found that apple (for moisture) and fish flakes works well.
- Most species need supplements added to their diet. A specific reptile multivitamin/mineral should be

Table 14.3 Examples of herbivorous foods

Vegetables	Fruit	Weeds/flowers	Herbs
Broccoli	Apple	Clover flowers and leaves	Basil
Cabbage	Banana	Dandelion leaves and flowers	Coriander
Carrot (grated)	Blackberries and leaves		Parsley
Cauliflower	Grapes	Groundsel	Rocket
Chard	Kiwi	Nasturtiums	
Chinese leaves	Melon		
Cress	Peach		
Cucumber	Pear		
Curly kale	Plum		
Mange tout	Strawberry		
Mushroom			
Pak choi			
Runner beans and leaves			
Spinach			
Tomato			
Watercress			

Table 14.5 Corn snake

Day	Food/s	Amount	Supplement
Monday	Adult mice	2	Not necessary
Tuesday			
Wednesday			
Thursday			
Friday			
Saturday			
Sunday			

Table 14.4 Common nutritional problems in reptiles

Problem	Cause	Symptoms	Comments
Hypovitaminosis D/Calcium deficiency In chelonia is often known as soft shell	Usually insufficient supplements or UV provision Particularly common in growing animals as a result of too high a quality diet (too much protein)	Weakening and deformities of the limbs Initially the plates just above the tail are soft and bend easily, this area extends until the whole shell is affected and the animal is extremely debilitated	These two conditions are usually associated as vitamin D assists the uptake of calcium
Hypovitaminosis A	Insufficient supplementation	Swollen eyelids, anorexia, lethargy	
Hypovitaminosis B	Most often due to thiamine deficiency in animals fed a high fish diet	Weak limbs, blindness, paralysis, convulsions	Frozen fish contains thiaminase which destroys vitamin B1 (thiamine) The best way to avoid this is to provide a varied diet

used. The correct dose rate will be written on the label. The exception is again snakes because they eat the entire carcass. This provides a complete diet and is often not too dissimilar to their natural diet.

When feeding snakes there are a number of factors to be considered:

■ The size and frequency of food depends on the size of the animal, e.g. a hatchling corn snake

Table 14.6	Green Iguana		
Day	Food/s	Amount	Supplement
Monday	Fruit and vegetable mix plus crickets or waxworms once a month	3 large handfuls 4/5	Yes
Tuesday	Garden weeds and flowers when in season, otherwise herbs	3 large handfuls	
Wednesday	Soaked iguana pellets	1 heaped tablespoon	Yes
Thursday	Different selection of fruit and vegetable mix	3 large handfuls	
Friday	Garden flowers and weeds when in season, otherwise herbs	3 large handfuls	Yes
Saturday	Different selection of fruit and vegetable mix	3 large handfuls	
Sunday	Different selection of fruit and vegetable mix	3 large handfuls	

Table 14.7	Spur Thighed Tortoise		
Day	Food/s	Amount	Supplement
Monday	Garden weeds and flowers when in season otherwise mixed herbs	A handful per tortoise	Nutrobal
Tuesday	Selection from the fruit and vegetable mix	As above	
Wednesday	Soaked herbivore pellets	A dessertspoon (when dry) per tortoise	Yes
Thursday	Different selection from the fruit and vegetable mix	A handful per tortoise	
Friday	As for Monday	As above	Yes
Saturday	Different selection from fruit and vegetable mix	As above	
Sunday	As for Wednesday	A dessert spoon (when dry) per tortoise	Yes

Table 14.8	Red Eared Terrapin – Week 1		
Day	Food/s	Amount	Supplement
Monday	Fish	2 small (2″ long) each	Yes
Tuesday	Floating sticks (pelleted food)	5 each	
Wednesday	Crickets	4 each	
Thursday	Floating sticks	5 each	
Friday	Pinkies	1 each	Yes
Saturday	Cabbage/ lettuce leaf	1 leaf	
Sunday	Worms/snails	3 each	

Table 14.9	Red Eared Terrapin – Week 2		
Day	Food/s	Amount	Supplement
Monday	Floating sticks	5 each	
Tuesday	Prawns	2 each	Yes
Wednesday	Cabbage leaf		
Thursday	Crickets	4 each	
Friday	Floating sticks	5 each	
Saturday	Banana	2 slices each (approx. 1 cm wide)	Yes
Sunday	Floating sticks	5 each	

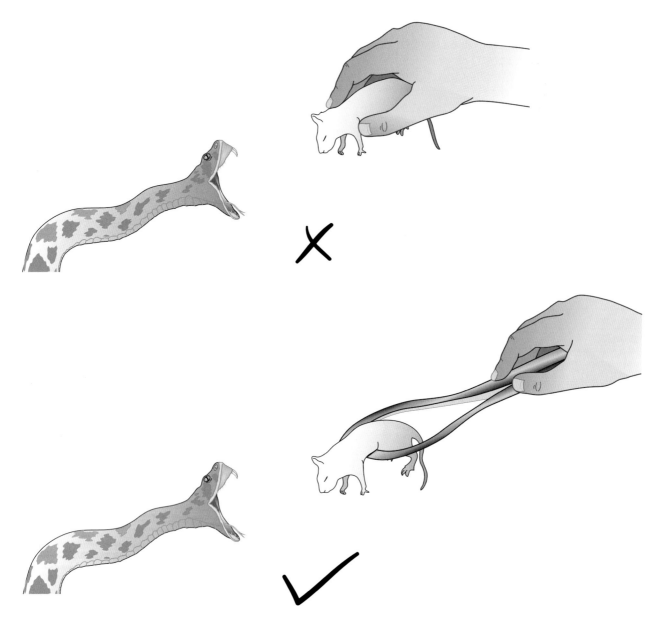

Figure 14.7 Diagram showing incorrect and correct feeding methods.

may take one pinkie 2–3 times a week, whereas an adult might take 1–2 adult mice once a week, and a large Burmese python a rabbit every three weeks.
- Snakes should not be unduly stressed (e.g. handled) on the day of feeding and for the day afterwards, as they may then either refuse to feed or regurgitate their meal.
- As a general rule, if there is more than one snake kept in the same vivarium, they should be separated for feeding.
- ALWAYS use feeding tongs to offer the food NEVER your hands (Figure 14.7).

Hibernation

To hibernate or not to hibernate?
- Only hibernate a species if it does so in the wild.
- Do not hibernate underweight or sick individuals.
- The smaller/younger an individual the shorter the hibernation length.
- Very young tortoises should only be hibernated by experienced keepers.

Preparation
Ensure adequate bodyweight. Figure 14.8 shows a graph that can be used to ascertain if a tortoise is within

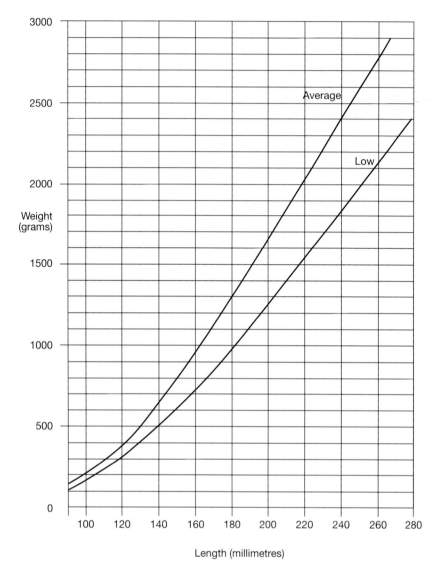

Figure 14.8 The Jackson ratio. Reproduced by kind permission of the British Chelonia Group.

an acceptable range. **This graph is only for use with Mediterranean species, e.g. Spur Thighed.**

Stop feeding approximately four to six weeks prior to hibernation (it takes that long for the digestive tract to empty). Any food left in the tract will ferment causing gas which constricts the lungs and may also cause bacterial infection.

Continue to allow to drink as adequate hydration during hibernation is very important.

Health check and worming
Prepare accommodation:

▨ Ideally in a fridge which is set to run between 4–6°C. Put tortoise in a sturdy box with ventilation holes in sides and lid and pack tortoise snugly with shredded paper; this is preferable to hay or straw as these may contain fungal spores which can take advantage of the depressed immune system during hibernation. NB. Ensure fridge is not airtight.

OR

▨ Put tortoise in box as above, then put that in a slightly larger, rodent proof box and again pack between the boxes with shredded paper. Place whole thing somewhere between 2–8°C (not a garage where carbon monoxide may build up) (Figure 14.9).

During hibernation
▨ Monitor temperature regularly. This should preferably be maintained at between 4–6°C. Above 10°C the tortoise may wake up, below freezing it may suffer frost damage or even die.
▨ Check weight regularly. An adult Hermans/Spur Thighed tortoise loses approximately 1% body-weight per month. If it loses too much, wake it up.
▨ There is some discussion as to whether a tortoise should be allowed to go back into hibernation if it wakes up prematurely. There have been instances

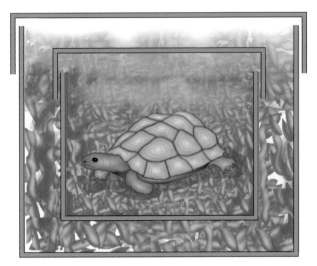

Figure 14.9 Hibernation accommodation for a tortoise.

when an individual that re-hibernated did not have sufficient energy stores to 'kick start' its metabolism for a second time and consequently died. However, many keepers report that their tortoise often wakes during its hibernation with no ill effects at all. I would suggest that the former was the result of an individual being or becoming underweight prior to or during its hibernation.
- Healthy adults should be allowed to hibernate for about 16 weeks.

Post-hibernation
- Once awake bring box into a warm room for a few hours.
- When sufficiently warmed, remove from box into a warm, bright environment.
- When fully awake put in a warmish bath just deep enough for it to drink properly, i.e. about half way up its shell. This is very important as it allows it to re-hydrate; bathing also stimulates urination thus eliminating the toxic by-products of metabolism that have built up during hibernation.
- Should start to feed within 48 hours. If not seek veterinary attention.

Over-wintering
If not allowing to go into hibernation, the day length and temperature must be kept up. Therefore in August, when both start to decline, artificial light and heat must be provided.

Once a tortoise has decided it is going to hibernate it can be extremely difficult to reverse the process; in this instance a very short hibernation may have to be allowed.

Table 14.10	Chelonians
Males:	
A. Slightly concave plastron.	
B. Longer, thicker tail.	
C. Wider rear plastral lobe.	

Table 14.11	Lizards
Males:	
A. Hemipenal bulges at base of tail	
B. Larger/more robust	
C. Larger crests/dewlaps etc	
D. More pronounced femoral and preanal pores	

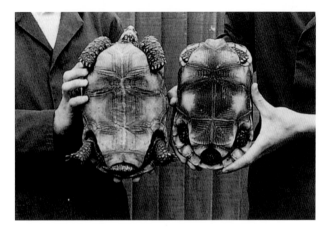

Figure 14.10 Sexing tortoises showing rear plastral lobes. The male is on the left, with the wider lobes.

Breeding

Sex determination
Individual species vary, but in very general terms please see Tables 14.10 and 14.11, Figures 14.10 and 14.11.

Snakes: The only reliable way to sex most snakes is to get an expert to probe them.

Mating
Many of the most commonly kept species can be left together all year round and will probably mate without any special care (although why anyone would wish to breed red eared terrapins or iguanas is beyond me when rescue centres have so many they can not house them all). However, if problems are being experienced consider the following:

- Are they a true pair?
- Many species require a winter cooling to stimulate mating activity in the spring.
- Housing the species separately and introducing them after the cooling down for mating.

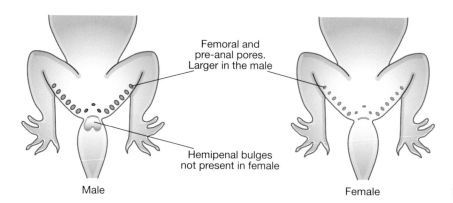

Male   Female   **Figure 14.11**   Male and female lizards.

Femoral and
pre-anal pores.
Larger in the male

Hemipenal bulges
not present in female

Incubation

Some species do not lay eggs, rather give birth to live young. This is not quite the same as mammalian live bearing process A basic distinction between these three forms is as follows:

- **Oviparous** – Animals which lay eggs.
  Reptilian examples are: all chelonia, most snakes, geckos, iguanas, bearded dragon.
- **Ovoviviparous** – These species produce eggs but instead of being laid they are retained within the female for the duration of incubation. The embryo is still nourished by the egg yolk (in some species there is also some degree of placental nourishment to a greater or lesser extent, depending on the species) but there is no shell surrounding the egg. At the end of the incubation period the self sufficient young emerge in a similar manner to that of mammals.
  Reptilian examples are: boas, blue tongued skink, monkey tailed skink.
- **Viviparous** – species in which the eggs are retained within the female and are entirely dependent upon her to nourish them via a fully developed placenta, e.g. most mammals. True viviparity is not known amongst reptiles.

In captivity it is usual to remove the eggs of oviparous species once they have been laid and incubate them artificially. As most reptiles do not have any further parental input there is a better success rate this way. Some keepers, however, prefer to leave the eggs with those species that do incubate them, e.g. pythons.

If artificial incubation is to be attempted the following should be considered:

- A suitable egg laying receptacle must be provided in the vivarium, e.g. an area/container filled with damp peat or moss, otherwise the female may be disinclined to lay her eggs, resulting in egg binding.

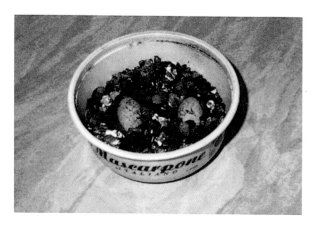

Figure 14.12   Incubating eggs.

- Once laid, in most cases, the eggs should be removed to the incubator as soon as possible. Care must be taken when moving/unearthing the eggs not to rotate them from the laying position as this will kill them.

In order to incubate the eggs successfully, you should find out the specific requirements of the species in question, however, as a basic guideline I have had success using the following techniques:

- Place the eggs in a container $\frac{3}{4}$ filled with damp vermiculite (1 mL water per 1 g vermiculite) so that they lie snugly but are not completed covered.
- If possible place the eggs so that they do not touch each other in order to prevent contamination (this is no always possible as many species' eggs will be connected or stuck to each other) (Figure 14.12).
- Put ventilation holes in the lid of the container.
- Place in the incubator (this could be a spare vivarium) and monitor regularly throughout the incubation replacing water as necessary.
- Only remove individual eggs if they smell bad, collapse or are badly affected by mould (Table 14.12).

In many species the sex of the young can be determined by the temperature they were incubated at; this is known as temperature dependent sex determination (Table 14.13).

Care of hatchlings
■ Hatching can last 24 hours or more. This is not a problem provided it can poke its head clear in order to breath and the urge to intervene should be resisted.
■ As each hatchling emerges remove it to its own separate, small, container which has a hide and water (Figure 14.13).
■ Terrapins will need shallow water with a ramp to a land area.
■ Snakes need high humidity to aid their first slough, so container should be lined with moist tissue paper.

■ The yolk may still be attached. Leave it alone; it will shrivel up within a few days.
■ Maintain a constant temperature of about 30°C for the first few days.
■ Lizards and chelonia may eat straight away or may take a few days.
■ Snakes probably will not eat until after their first slough.
■ Offer food of suitable size.

BIRDS

Bird keeping has been a very popular pasttime for many years. Consequently, it is possible to obtain captive bred individuals for all of the commonly kept species, along with sound advice on their husbandry. Therefore, there are very few justifiable reasons why wild caught specimens should be in captivity as household pets.

As with any exotic animal, some homework is required to establish species-specific information. Table 14.14 gives an example of the basic information on some of the more commonly kept species.

Table 14.12	Incubation lengths
Species	**Incubation length**
Corn snake	55–72 days at 25–30°C
Green iguana	3–4 months at 28–30°C
Spur thighed tortoise	2–3 months at 26–30°C
Red eared terrapin	8–12 weeks at 26–30°C
Leopard gecko	55–65 days at 26–30°C

Table 14.13	Temperature dependent sex determination	
	Predominant sex of hatchlings if incubated at:	
	High end of range	**Low end of range**
Lizards	Male	Female
Chelonia	Female	Male
Snakes	N/A	N/A

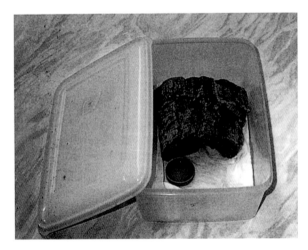

Figure 14.13 Hatchling container.

Table 14.14	Species-specific information for birds				
Species	**Scientific name**	**Geographical origin**	**Natural habitat**	**Wild diet**	**Activity time**
Budgerigar	*Melopsittacus undulatas*	Australian interior	Semi-arid grassland with trees, near water holes. Very hot	Fruit, seeds, fungi, occasional insect	Diurnal
Canary	*Serinus canaria*	Canary Islands, Azores, Madeira	Scrublands, fields, pastures	Seeds, grasses	Diurnal
Cockatiel	*Nymphicus hollandicus*	Australian interior – the west coast	Dry savannah, grassland trees	Grasses, plants, seeds, fruit, berries	Diurnal
African grey parrot	*Psittacus erithacus*	West and Central Africa	Lowland forests, wooded savannah	Seeds, fruit, nuts	Diurnal

Housing

There are very few absolute dos and don'ts, and mostly it is a matter of common sense; however, listed below are a few guidelines/recommendations.

Aviaries – basic design

- Size – This is a tricky one, I hesitate to state X dimensions for X many individuals for X species, as anyone you talk to will tell you something different. The best advice is as large as possible taking into account the size of the bird and its flight requirements.
- Height needs to be enough for ease of cleaning but not so high that the birds can sit up in the rafters laughing down at you when you try to catch them.
- A double entry door is a very good idea to prevent accidental escapes.
- A concrete base is a good idea for ease of cleaning and keeping rodents out.
- A low brick wall on which the wood and wire sides sit is again a good idea for cleaning and discouraging rodents.
- Larger parrots will demolish wood and small gauge netting. Many like to climb the wire, e.g. cockatiels.
- Welded wire is useful for destructive birds, but does not 'give' as much as chicken wire if the bird should fly into it.
- Ideally adjoining aviaries should be separated by a double layer of wire to prevent malicious injury.
- Water birds will need a pond area.
- The aviary should be south facing preferably.

Shelter

- Ideally a large shed or bird room connected to the aviary. Most cage/aviary species are from warmer climates and therefore heat and light may be required but definitely a good weather proof area where they can escape the wind, rain etc.
- Nest boxes are just that, birds will not normally utilise them for shelter etc.
- Nest boxes should be provided both inside and out. The size and shape varies between species, e.g. in the wild, parrots tend to use rotten tree trunks or logs and dig them out, whereas finches will weave their nests from grasses.
- Provide more nest boxes than required. This helps to prevent squabbling over the least desired ones.
- Wooden boxes may need reinforcement with wire as some species will destroy them with exasperating frequency.
- It is a good idea to cover a portion of the roof and maybe one or two sides (depending on prevailing weather conditions) with something like corrugated plastic sheets as additional weather protection.

Perching

- Ensure perching is arranged to allow an uninterrupted flight path.
- Natural perches, i.e. branches, are best as they provide variable width and surface which helps to prevent foot problems. It also provides environmental stimulation by way of seeing how quickly they can destroy them.
- Ropes should be used with care as they may cause damage especially during mating.
- Ground dwelling species, e.g. pheasants, quail may appreciate low level perches.
- Bushes and shrubs in pots provide natural greenery/cover but careful thought needs to be given as to which plants are suitable. They should be non-toxic, have branches that will bear the weight of the bird and not be too densely foliated. They will also need watering etc.

Indoor cages

- I am not an advocate of keeping birds in cages, however, if there is no choice, considerable effort should be expended to meet species' needs and provide them with sufficient stimulation.
- Size should again be as large as possible, but legally, must be at least big enough to allow the bird to stretch its wings fully in every direction.
- Position the cage away from draughts, windows, gas cookers/heaters etc.
- Should be considered as the shelter and the bird allowed to fly free frequently.
- Do not chain birds to cages or perches as injury can occur if the bird takes fright at something.
- Rather than clipping wings to allow easy retrieval when the bird is free, concentrate on training the bird to come to you.
- Vitamin D must be provided if they do not have access to direct sunshine.
- Baths and showers should be provided regularly.
- Perches should be of natural material, i.e. branches.

Feeding

Birds are divided into two basic categories as far as deciding what sort of food forms the basis of their diet:

- **Hard bills** – seed eaters, e.g. parrot, dove, canary, finch.
- **Soft bills** – fruit/nectar eaters, e.g. mynah, lorie.

However, having said that, it does not mean that hard bills eat seed exclusively. All birds need fruit/vegetables to a greater or lesser extent.

Table 14.15	Food for different species of bird								
Species	Basic mix	Fruit/veg.	Grasses, herbs, weeds	Mineral block	Cuttlefish	Grit	Dried mix	Comments	
Budgie	Budgie	✓		✓	✓	✓		Feeding guide is approx. 2 × level teaspoons of mix a day	
Canary	Canary	✓		✓	✓	✓		As above	
Cockatiel	Cockatiel	✓	✓	✓	✓	✓			
African Gray	Parrot	✓	✓	✓	✓	✓	✓	Feeding guide is approx. 60–125 mL of mix a day. Sunflower seeds and peanuts are a favourite but should only be a treat. Fruit and veg. should form approx. 20–25% of the diet	

Basic principles

Obviously the first step is to find out what they eat in the wild (Table 14.15), e.g. whilst most parrots are hard bills, rainforest species will eat a large amount of fruit.

For many species there is a proprietary food mix which can form the basis of most diets, e.g. budgie mix, canary mix etc. Cheap mixes should be avoided.

In addition to the base mix the following are important in the diet, although not all are relevant for all species (see Table 14.15).

- Water: obviously
- Cuttlefish: calcium and beak trimming
- Grit: calcium and food breakdown
- Grasses: long grass with the seed heads intact
- Herbs/weeds: variety and interest
- Fruit/veg: wide a variety as possible (see below). Some experimentation may be needed to find out individual preference:

Apple	Peas (in pod)	Corn on	Tomato
Kiwi	Banana	the cob	Grapes
Papaya	Mango	Spinach	Orange
Pomegranate	Pear	Melon	Raspberry
Asparagus	Strawberry	Peach	Carrot and tops
Cucumber	Broccoli	Plum	Kale

NB. Mynahs should not be given foods that are high in iron, e.g. grapes, banana, spinach or foods that enhance iron absorption, e.g. kiwi, papaya, orange, sour apples, tomato.

- Dried mix: consists of dried fruits and nuts, e.g. sultanas, nuts (of appropriate size), coconut, banana, dates, pineapple, etc.

- Live food: crickets, mealworms, flies, spiders, woodlice, moths etc.
- Spray millet: interest and novelty.

Many species when eating fruit will take a bite then drop it. This does not necessarily mean they do not like it as in the wild they will often go from branch to branch taking a bite out of each fruit.

To prevent 'picky feeding' give only the daily requirement of the basic mix and offer it before preferred items, e.g. fruit.

Vitamin/mineral supplements can be provided in a number of different forms and different species' needs vary so some research is required. However, calcium is always required, especially during breeding.

Most species are diurnal and will therefore only eat during daylight hours.

The husks of eaten seeds will need to be blown away regularly to allow the bird to get to the seed underneath.

VARIETY IS THE KEY TO A BALANCED DIET.

Containers

There are many different types of food and water containers available and common sense should tell you which are the most appropriate for any given situation but the following points should be considered:

- Bear in mind the destructive force of the bird, i.e. plastic containers will not last long with larger parrots.
- Do not put citrus fruit into galvanised metal containers as the citric acid may react with the metal with fatal results.
- Feeding stations should be easy for the birds to get to, e.g. doves and quails are ground

Table 14.16 Common avian nutritional problems

Disorder	Cause	Symptoms	Notes
Avitaminosis A (retinol)	Common in birds maintained on a seed only diet	Respiratory signs, poor eye sight, dead-in-shell, loss of muscle control	
Avitaminosis B (riboflavin)		Mouth and skin lesions, poor feather quality	Supplementation is best given with all the B complex group. Macaws are particularly susceptible
Avitaminosis C		Susceptibility to infections, slow healing of wounds, swellings, general debilitation	Vitamin C is used particularly during illness and stress. African Greys are particularly susceptible
Iodine deficiency	Usually seen in birds maintained on cheaper seed mixes	Elevation of neck, change/loss of voice, enlarged thyroid, breathing difficulties	Budgies are particularly susceptible
Calcium deficiency		Shifting lameness, droopy wings, soft shells	African Greys again very susceptible
Haemochromatosis	Too much iron in the diet causes excess iron to accumulate in the liver resulting in liver failure	Anorexia, ascites, dyspnoea, weight loss, sudden death	Mynah birds are particularly susceptible therefore foods rich in iron should be avoided, e.g. All tinned fruit All dried fruit Apricot; blackberry; mango Blackcurrant; water melon; olive Passion fruit; raspberry Also avoid foods that are high in ascorbic acid (citrus) as this enhances iron absorption, e.g. sour apple; pineapple; orange; tomato
Sour crop	Fungal infection Nutritional deficiency (? Vit. A)	Vomiting foul smelling fluid	
Soft shelled eggs	Infection Overlaying Nutritional deficiency (Vit. D and/or calcium)	Either fragile shells or no shells at all	
Infertile eggs/poor hatching rate	Parents too old Not a true pair Hereditary Infection Excessive breeding Infertile parents (?Vit. E) Poor nutrition (esp. B complex)		

feeders, whereas cockatiels prefer them off the ground.

- Food and water containers should not be positioned underneath perches, in direct sunlight or where they can get wet.
- Gravity fed water containers are more hygienic than open bowls.

Table 14.16 contains problems that are not necessarily nutritional but might be. I have given several possible causes as well as nutritional.

Sex determination

Many species are sexually monomorphic (both sexes have the same outward appearance) and therefore the only reliable way of sexing them is either surgically or DNA testing.

- **Budgerigar:** The normal colour of the cere in a healthy male is blue and in the female pink/brown.
- **Canary:** Monomorphic, but the male tends to be more vocal.

■ **Cockatiel:** Several factors can be considered but none of them are guaranteed, e.g. the male has a more colourful crest and is more vocal and the female has grey extending into her crest and horizontal tail bars on the underside. However, with the various colour phases these may not apply.

■ **African Grey:** Monomorphic.

Breeding

Some species of bird will breed readily without any special care or attention, budgies are a good example; very often all that is needed is an aviary with a group of birds and several nesting boxes and nature will then take its course. However, if you want to maintain any sort of control over the breeding it has to be a little more structured. The following are guidelines for breeding budgies but could equally apply to other species.

Conditioning

■ **Age:** Hens particularly should not be bred from before they're a year old, as they are not fully grown or mature until then. The maximum age is rather less specific and ultimately depends on the individual, as an average, hens may start to produce small young after about 5 years,

cocks generally go on for longer and in extreme circumstances have still been breeding into their late teens.

■ **Health:** Obviously only fit birds should be bred from.

■ **Day length:** Budgies tend to breed in the summer when the temperature and day length are conducive.

■ **Food:** A good breeding/rearing mix should be given. This is higher in protein. Calcium supplementation should also be given.

■ **Sociability:** In the wild budgies breed in flocks, so in order to encourage breeding activity in captivity they should also be in the company of several other budgies.

Breeding cages

Having decided on which individuals to pair up they should be brought into the bird room and placed in the prepared breeding cages.

These should be as large as possible bearing in mind they will be spending several months in them (e.g. one meter in length).

Each cage needs a nest box, perching, food/water containers. There should be several within sight and sound of each other (Figure 14.14).

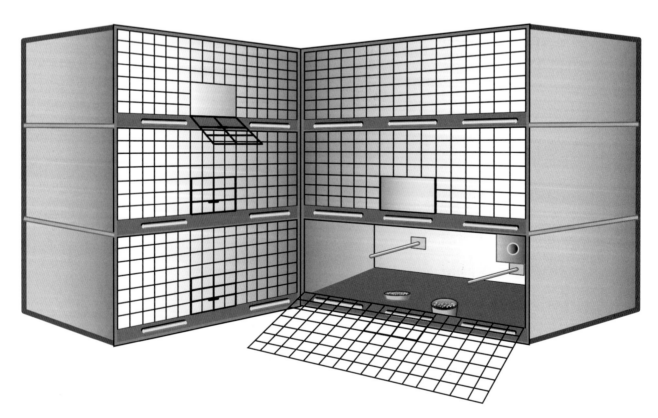

Figure 14.14 Breeding cages for budgies.

Nest boxes

The exact measurements vary between different breeders, however, an example is given in Figures 14.15–14.17.

At one end there should be a sliding flap to allow for inspection and a sliding glass panel behind this.

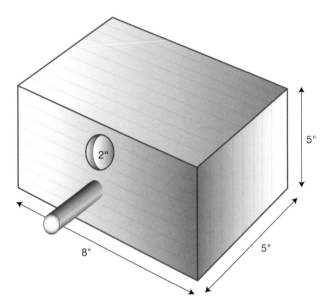

Figure 14.15   Nest box.

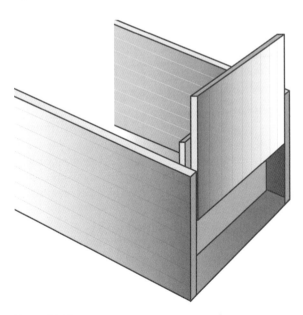

Figure 14.16

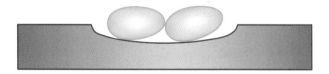

Figure 14.17

This prevents eggs/chicks accidentally falling out (Figure 14.16).

As budgies do not make nests the base of the box should have a concave area in it – this prevents eggs rolling away into the corners and keeps the chicks together (Figure 14.17).

The base should be removable as it will become heavily soiled during rearing. It is best to have at least two interchangeable bases for each box, this allows the base to be thoroughly cleaned and dried.

As an alternative or in addition to this some breeders like to provide a layer of sawdust in the bottom of the box.

If breeding in an aviary plenty of nest boxes should be available to allow choice and prevent fighting.

Egg laying and incubation

- Eggs are laid every other day. Clutch size is usually 3–5, although can be up to 8.
- Only the hen incubates.
- Incubation is about 18 days.
- Humidity may need to be provided in hot/dry summers.
- Heating may need to be provided if there is a cold snap.

Should you need to artificially incubate the eggs, suitable incubators can be purchased specifically for bird eggs. Some designs will have automatic turning which is preferable to manual turning. The incubator should be set to the following:

Temperature: 37.5°C
Humidity: 45–55% (wet bulb thermometer – 80–84°F)
Turnings: 24 side over side a day; 3/5 end over end a day.

Rearing

- Initially the hen does all the feeding.
- Strict hygiene and regular cleaning of the base of the nest box is essential during rearing.
- The claws and beaks of the young birds are liable to become clogged with excreta, if this happens it should be cleaned off GENTLY by dipping/bathing with warm water to soften caked on material then removed with a cotton bud.
- After about 4–5 weeks the chicks begin to emerge. The cock then takes over the feeding.
- Seed should be made readily available for the youngsters.
- The young should be removed when fully independent (approx. 6 weeks) as by then the hen will be looking after the second clutch.
- Pairs should not be allowed to rear more than two clutches per season.

FISH

Keeping fish is a very popular and relaxing pastime. Set-ups can be simple or complicated. Provided that the individual requirements of the fish have been researched the whole process can be very enjoyable. It is a sad fact, however, that people are still to be found keeping goldfish in a small bowl/tank with no company whatsoever. Beginners should not attempt marine fish keeping until they have become experienced with freshwater set-ups.

There are many books available that give a step by step account of how to set up an aquarium; the following notes are brief but will hopefully point you in the right direction to get started.

Accommodation

Size

This will dictate the number and size of the inhabitants, so as usual, the bigger the better. The calculation is usually based on volume and size of fish (when measuring the length of fish exclude the tail fin):

Cold freshwater – 2.6 litres of water per cm of fish
Tropical freshwater – 0.9 litres of water per cm
of fish.

Remember that some fish are territorial and that may limit the number of individuals in the tank.

If a community aquarium is desired then obviously compatible species must be selected.

Siting

Avoid draughts, heaters and direct sunlight and ensure that whatever the tank is put on can hold the not inconsiderable weight.

Tanks should always be placed on a layer of polystyrene as this will provide even support.

Tank cover

Most aquaria come complete with a hood, this will reduce heat loss and evaporation and also provide protection from 'Tiddles'.

Lighting

Most fish and plants need an average of 12 hours of light a day and this is best provided artificially. Most aquarium lids have a space in them for the fluorescent tubes specifically designed for such a purpose. An important point to remember is that too much light will cause algal blooms.

Filtration

Waste occurs from excess food, faeces, urine and plant material build up in the tank. As they decompose they become toxic. A filter will remove and convert harmful chemicals.

There are three basic types; all employ both biological (bacterial) and mechanical filtration; under gravel (which is least effective and not generally recommended), internal or external. These latter two work in a similar manner and the deciding factor is usually the amount of water that they have to cope with (i.e. the size of the tank).

Water quality is the key to good fish husbandry, so seek proper advice as to which would be most appropriate for a given set-up.

Heating

Different species have different temperature requirements. As a basic guideline most community tropical aquariums should run between 23 and 27°C.

Always use a thermostat with a heater in order to maintain the temperature accurately and ensure the heater is able to heat the whole tank.

Cold water aquariums, e.g. those for goldfish, do not require heating. If sited indoors the ambient temperature of most houses is sufficient. If in an outside pond ensure the pond is deep enough for them to hibernate in winter.

Aeration

This ensures sufficient oxygen in the aquarium and can be provided through air pumps and/or air stones but is most often part of the function of the filter.

As the air drawn into the pump comes from the room, it is important to remember that fumes from smoke, paint, aerosols etc. will also be drawn into the tank and may harm the fish.

Décor

Gravel is the usual substrate. A variety of decorative items can be acquired from specialist aquarist shops e.g. castles, rock-like formations.

Slate, bogwood, clay pipes and rocks can also be used; ensure the rocks are appropriate to use in an aquarium and always thoroughly clean everything before putting it in.

Real/plastic plants: If real plants are to be used research the best type to use and how to get them established.

Maturation

Once the set-up is complete it must be allowed to run for several days before adding the fish. This is to allow the bacteria necessary for bacterial filtration to develop.

Special additives can be acquired which speed up the maturation process, or adding a quantity of water from an established, disease free aquarium is an alternative.

Fish can only be added when the water quality has settled down to normal levels.

Water quality

Maintaining correct water quality is crucial. If the tank set-up is in balance the following should occur:

- Decaying food and the waste products of respiration and digestion result in the production of ammonia.
- As ammonia oxidises it produces toxic nitrites.
- Nitrites are converted to less harmful nitrates by bacterial filtration.
- Nitrates feed the plants (Figure 14.18).

If this cycle get out of balance it can cause serious problems for the fish which may result in death.

The aquarium water should be tested weekly for all three substances plus pH levels as this affects the toxicity of ammonia. There are a number of test kits available from aquarist shops for this purpose. The kits will give instructions on how to use them and what the respective levels should be.

Partial water changes, i.e. up to $\frac{1}{3}$ of the total volume, should be carried out every 2–3 weeks.

Feeding

There are a number of points to be considered:

There is a bewildering variety of foods available. Initially it is probably easiest to use one of the complete diets for whatever the species of fish, e.g. goldfish flakes, tropical community, koi pellets and take advice as to what other form of food might be appropriate, e.g. freeze dried, live.

Most fish can be classified into one of three groups: top, middle or bottom feeders; as the names imply this describes where, within the aquarium, they prefer to take their food. Some can adapt to various positions but others, like the catfish have no choice as their mouths face downward, therefore, they should be feed pellets that sink to the bottom of the aquarium.

Establishing the correct amount of food required is very important as too much will result in poor water quality. Two methods available are commonly used:

1. Add a few (flakes) at a time and keep going until the fish no longer take any; that will indicate how much needs to be given at one time.

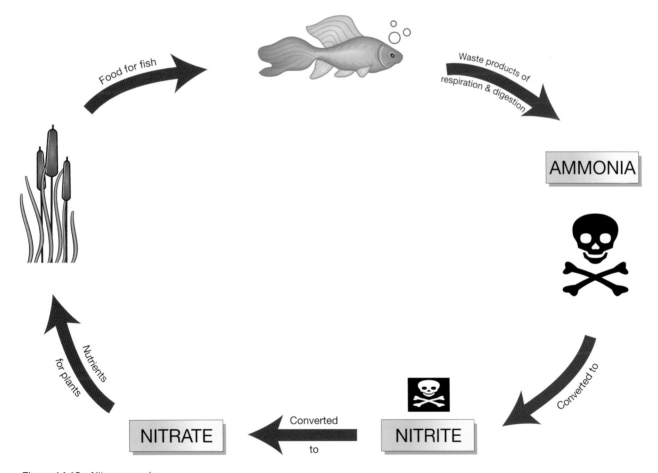

Figure 14.18   Nitrogen cycle.

2. Any food that is left after 2 or 3 minutes should be removed and the amount adjusted accordingly next time.

Small feeds throughout the day is preferable, however, not practical for most people but twice a day is fine.

If you go on holiday the fish can be left for up to two weeks without being fed. Do not be tempted to 'feed them up' prior to leaving or to 'make up for it' on your return. If you ask a neighbour to feed them, prepare each feed in a little parcel before you go so that they will not over feed.

PART 2 – ANATOMY

For most vertebrate classes of animal it is not difficult to relate the internal anatomy to that of the dog/cat. Obviously there are differences but most of the organs are readily identifiable and in a similar position, snakes however, take a few liberties owing to their long, slender shape (Figures 14.19–14.24).

SKELETAL SYSTEMS

Again, the skeletal systems of the different classes are all variations on a theme. The differences are as a result of the animals' lifestyles and the most variation is seen in the limbs, which, of course, reflects the animals' locomotive adaptations (Figures 14.25–14.29).

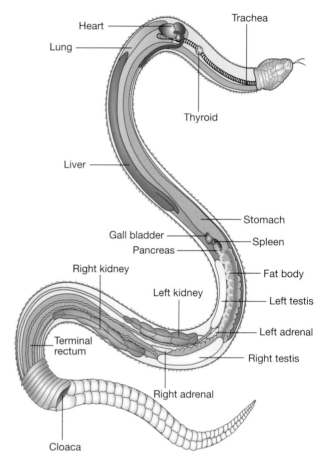

Figure 14.19 Internal anatomy of a typical male snake.

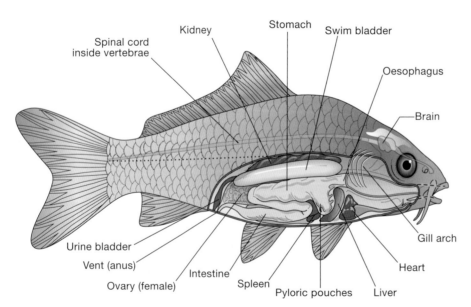

Figure 14.20 Internal anatomy of a typical bony fish.

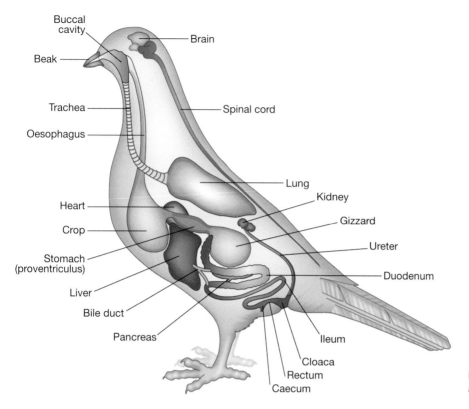

Figure 14.21 Internal anatomy of a pigeon.

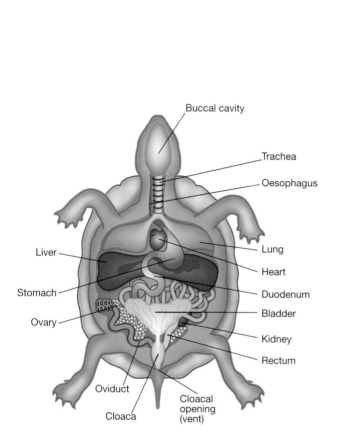

Figure 14.22 Internal anatomy of a female tortoise.

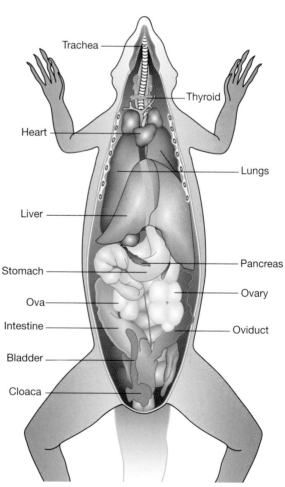

Figure 14.23 Internal anatomy of a typical female lizard.

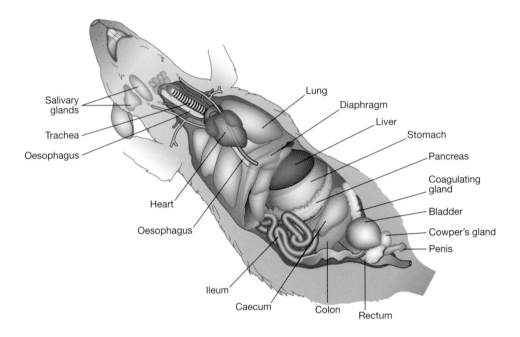

Figure 14.24 Internal anatomy of the rat.

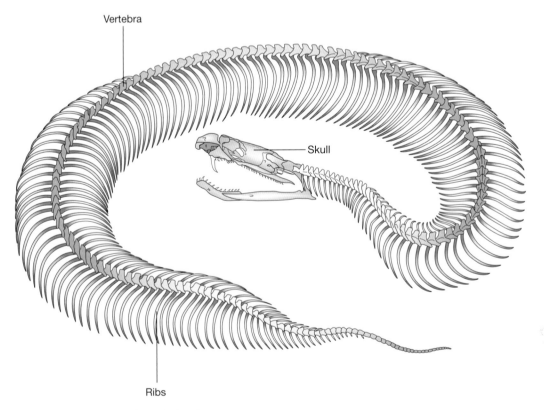

Figure 14.25 Skeleton of a typical snake.

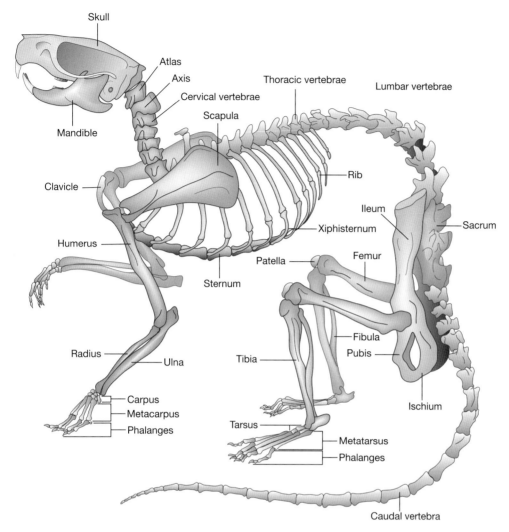

Figure 14.26 Skeleton of a rat.

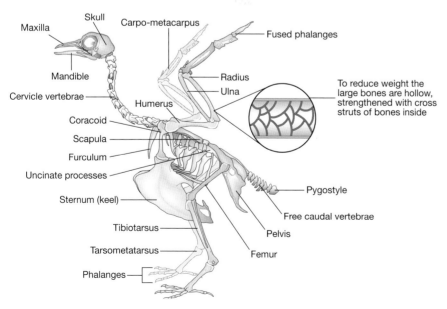

Figure 14.27 Skeleton of a typical bird.

A few of the key variations are outlined below:

Birds

- Cervical vertebrae vary in number from 13–25.
- Many of the vertebrae along the trunk have fused to form a single bone (like the sacrum in mammals).

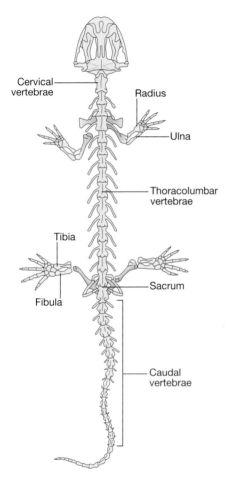

Figure 14.28   Skeleton of a typical lizard.

- The last few tail vertebrae have fused to form the pygostyle.
- The sternum has become greatly enlarged in many of the flying birds to form the keel. This provides anchorage for the large muscles that power the wings.
- The ribs are often jointed in the middle and many have a projection called the uncinate process. This overlaps one or more adjacent ribs and provides extra rigidity for the rib cage. This is particularly important in diving birds.
- The clavicles are fused together to form the furcula (wishbone), which acts as a brace to keep the wings apart. The furcula is absent in some parrots and owls.
- The scapula is long and flattened and attached to the ribs.
- The corocoid is an extra bone which helps to brace the wings.
- Many of the bones of the 'hand' are lost or fused.
- There are only two carpus bones; the rest are absent or fused with the metacarpus to form the carpometacarpus.
- Similarly, some of the bones of the leg have become lost or fused, i.e. some of the tarsus have fused with the tibia to form the tibiotarsus. The remaining tarsus have fused with some of the metatarsus to become the tarsometatarsus.
- Many bones, especially the long bones, are air filled (pneumatic) (Figure 14.30). This aids both flying and respiration. Flying birds have far more extensively pneumatised bones than those that dive.

Reptiles

Ophidia (snakes)

- Extremely flexible jaws. The two halves of the lower mandible are not fused and can be moved independently when gripping prey. In addition there are four other jaw joints (Figure 14.31).

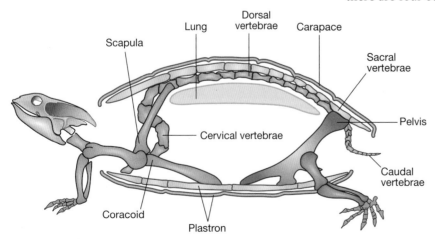

Figure 14.29   Skeleton of a typical tortoise.

■ No sternum or pectoral girdle, therefore no obstruction to swallowing large prey items. However, some pythons and boas retain spurs which are what remain of the claws of the vestigial hind limbs.

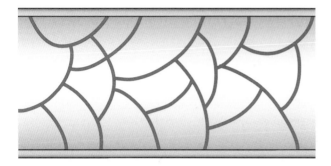

Figure 14.30 Pneumatic bone.

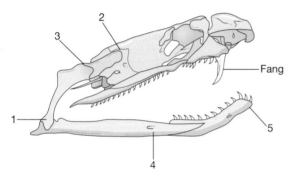

Figure 14.31 Diagram showing the five joints in a jaw of a snake.

■ Between 130–500 vertebrae.
■ Between 100–435 pairs of ribs which are very flexible and will flex outwards to accommodate large food items.

All of the above mean that a snake is able to swallow prey that is much wider than itself.

Chelonia (tortoises, terrapins and turtles)

First and most obvious difference is the shell. It is living tissue and consists of an outer layer of horny plates called scutes and an inner layer of bone. The upper shell called the carapace and the lower shell the plastron. They are joined together at the sides.

The ribs and many of the vertebrae are fused to the carapace (the cervical and caudal (tail) vertebrae are free moving). Therefore they cannot be used to ventilate the lungs, instead various muscles, especially those of the abdomen and limbs, expand and contract to alter the amount of space in the shell.

The acromion is a hook-like projection from the scapula. It is the articulation point for the clavicle.

Fish (Figure 14.32)

Fins are supported by fin rays and fin supports.
Each of the fins has a specific function:

■ Caudal – Forward propulsion
■ Dorsal – Stops side to side rolling

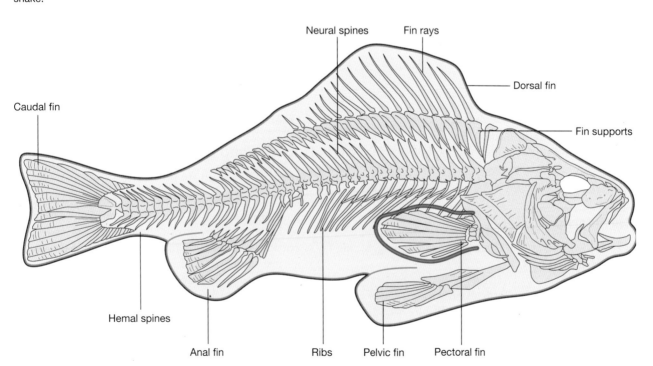

Figure 14.32 Generalised skeleton of a fish.

Table 14.17   Mammals and reptiles

Species	Fore foot	Hind foot
Rabbit N.B. The rabbit has no foot pads	4 + dew	4
Cavy	4 + dew	4
Chinchilla	5	4
Mouse and rat	4	5
Gerbil, hamster, etc.	4	5
Most lizards e.g. Green iguana	5	5
Chameleon (zygodactyl)	4	4

Table 14.18   Birds

Species	Forward pointing	Backward pointing
Psittacines (zygodactyl)	2	2
Most others	3	1

- Anal – Stops side to side rolling
- Pelvic – Stops side to side rolling and used for braking
- Pectoral – Braking slow manoeuvring and display.

Neural and hemal spines provide large areas for muscle attachment.

Digit numbers

See Tables 14.17 and 14.18.

DENTITION

By looking at an animal's dentition it is usually possible to tell whether it is a carnivore or herbivore. However, within each of these groups there is considerable variation, especially amongst the herbivores.

Carnivores

The carnivore dentition is adapted for catching, killing and slicing their prey.

- Carnassials are present in all carnivores. These are specialised, enlarged molars (Figure 14.33) or pre-molars that act like scissors, slicing the meat. Usually there is one carnassial in each quadrant.
- The dental pattern will vary between species, particularly if the diet is very specialised.

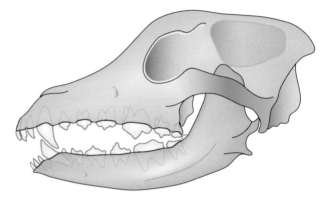

Figure 14.33   Dentition of a carnivore (dog).

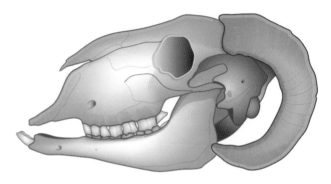

Figure 14.34   Sheep dentition.

Herbivores

These show marked variation:

- The incisors are generally used for cropping and sometimes only present in one jaw, e.g. most ruminants
- Canines are absent
- Molars and pre-molars have multiple cutting edges used for ruminant dentition for cutting up the cropped vegetation (Figure 14.34).

Rodents and lagomorphs (Figure 14.35)

Three types of teeth are present:

- **Incisors** – These have sharp edges designed for gnawing. There is an open/persistant pulp cavity which means they grow continuously. The sharp cutting edge is maintained by the wear of the top against the bottom and they are chisel-shaped because only the anterior surface is covered with enamel which therefore wears down more slowly. If the incisors are not worn down, usually due to malocclusion or insufficient material to gnaw, they will overgrow (Figure 14.36).
- **Pre-molars** – As for molars (absent in some species, e.g. rat).

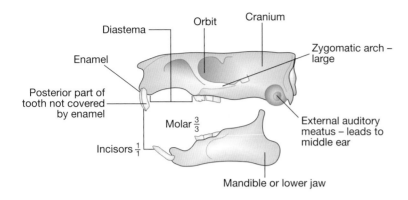

Figure 14.35   Rat dentition.

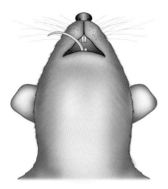

Figure 14.36   Overgrown tooth of a rat.

■ **Molars** – These show limited growth, enamal does not form on the tips and as they wear down they expose widening areas of dentine surrounded by enamel, this improves the chewing efficiency.

The diastema is the gap between the incisors and pre-molars/molars. Whilst gnawing at food it can be prevented from moving to the back of the mouth by folding the skin of the cheeks across the diastema.

Lagomorphs can be distinguished by the presence of the 'peg teeth', a smaller set of incisors behind the front ones on the top jaw only (Figure 14.37).

Rodent incisors are often coloured brown/orange; this is due to an iron pigment. If this colouration is not present it may be due to a diet deficient in iron.

In Rodentia the molars of the upper jaw bite inside those of the lower, whilst in Lagomorpha the upper molars bite outside the lower (Table 14.19).

Birds

The lack of teeth is thought to be a weight saving device. As with mammals the shape of the beak is largely related to the diet, e.g.

■ **Parrots** – Seeds, nuts and fruit. Short and stout, upper bill strongly downward curved and overlapping the lower. For cracking nuts.

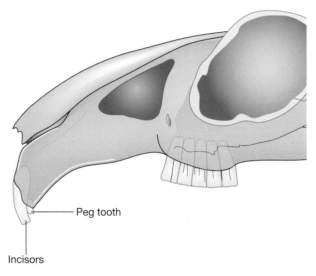

Figure 14.37   Lagomorph dentition.

Table 14.19	Dental formulae			
Species	I	C	PM	M
Rabbit	2/1	0/0	3/2	3/3
Cavy	1/1	0/0	1/1	3/3
Rat	1/1	0/0	0/0	3/3

■ **Finches** – Seeds. Short, stout and strong. For cracking seeds.
■ **Mynah bird** – Insects, fruit. Straight, moderately strong. To bite off pieces of food.
■ **Parakeets** – Seeds. Similar to macaw but smaller and less strong.

Reptiles

■ Snakes and lizards typically have a row of conical teeth of varying size which undergo continuous succession (polyphyodont) (Figure 14.38).
■ Some have more complex dentitions for piercing, cutting and/or crushing.

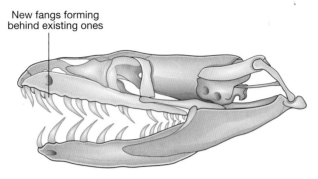

Figure 14.38 Fang succession in the snake.

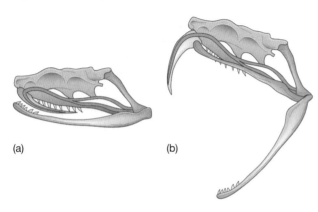

(a)   (b)

Figure 14.39 Skull of a poisonous snake with (a) its mouth closed and the fangs folded up along the roof of the mouth; (b) the jaw opened with the fangs in position.

■ In some species of snake certain teeth are adapted as venom fangs. These may be immovable or fold backwards against the roof of the mouth when it is closed and automatically drop down when the mouth opens (Figure 14.39).

■ Teeth are found in all species except chelonia, instead they have jaws that are covered with a horny substance that forms a beak-like structure.

DIGESTIVE SYSTEMS

Methods of obtaining energy from food (digestion) vary enormously. Amongst the higher animals a basic difference is found between those of carnivores and those of herbivores. Carnivores generally have a shorter digestive tract than herbivores as the cellulose of plant material takes a longer time to break down than animal protein.

In many of the lower vertebrates, i.e. some fish, amphibians, reptiles, birds and monotremes there is a common exit for the digestive, urinary and reproductive systems; this is called the cloaca.

Mammals

Amongst the herbivores the greatest variety occurs. They need to overcome the problem of breaking down

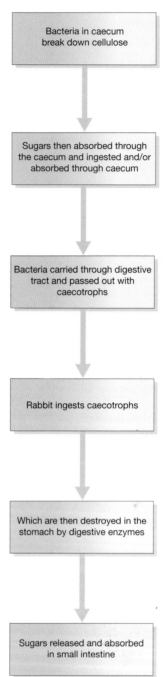

Figure 14.40 Flow chart of symbiosis.

the tough cellulose of plant material. This is achieved by having special bacteria in the gut that do this for them. The bacteria do this because after they have broken the cellulose down (fermentation), they will then feed off the end product, simple sugars.

The host benefits because the bacteria break down the cellulose, and the bacteria benefit because they get food. This relationship is known as a symbiosis (Figure 14.40). However, often the bacteria themselves are

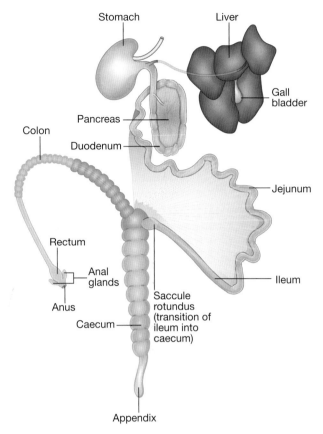

Figure 14.41 The digestive system of the rabbit.

then broken down (digested) by the host, thus releasing the sugars and making them available to the host.

The fermentation site varies with species, usually it is either in the stomach – ruminants, e.g. cow, goat, sheep – or in the caecum and/or colon – hind guts, e.g. horse, rabbit, cavy.

Rabbit (Figure 14.41)
Along the first part of the tract, food is dealt with in a similar manner to that of the dog. However, when it reaches the caecum it spends several hours there where it is subject to bacterial fermentation.

Eventually it is passed through the rest of the large intestine where it is formed into faecal pellets called caecotrophs. These are large, soft and covered in mucus.

Caecotrophs contain partially digested cellulose, bacteria and vitamins. When the caecotrophs are passed the rabbit will eat them directly from the anus.

The pellets are then subject to a second trip through the digestive tract. They spend several hours in the stomach, protected from the gastric juice by the mucus that covers them.

Whilst in the stomach the bacteria continue to ferment. Eventually though, the mucus becomes eroded and the pellets are broken down by the gastric juice in the normal way.

Digestion of the pellets then continues in the normal way, absorption occurring in the small intestine etc. The remaining pellet material passes relatively quickly through the caecum and when the pellets are passed this time they are smaller and harder than the caecotrophs and left as normal excreta.

The process of passing food through the system twice is called caecotrophy.

Baby rabbits will often eat their mother's caecotrophs in order to populate their own tract with the correct bacteria.

Many rodents including cavies and rats will also indulge in caecotrophy. Their digestive system is very similar to that of the rabbit. However one variation of note is that rats do not have a gall bladder.

Birds (Figures 14.42 and 14.43)

Again, enormous variation dependent on diet, including mechanisms such as the gizzard and enlarged caeca.

The first and most obvious difference is that birds have a beak rather than a mouth and they do not possess teeth. Food is therefore swallowed whole or broken off into chunks.

Some species have a dilation of the oesophagus called the crop, e.g. pigeon, dove, parrots, ducks, and raptors (except owls). This functions as a storage area.

The size and shape of the crop varies between species and whilst diet is the obvious reason it does not fully explain the differences (Figure 14.43).

In pigeons and doves the crop has another function, the production of 'crop milk'. This consists of fluid filled cells sloughed from the crop lining rich in protein, fat and vitamins. Both sexes produce it.

The crop leads to the stomach, which in most birds is divided into two parts:

1. The first part is called the proventriculus. This is the glandular part and it acts in a similar manner to the stomach of mammals. Food is mixed with gastric juice and chemical digestion occurs here. Budgies produce a similar nutritive secretion to pigeons for their chicks, but it is 'proventriculus milk.'
2. From the proventriculus food is passed into the gizzard (ventriculus). This is the muscular part where mechanical breakdown occurs.

The type of gizzard is again dependent on diet. Insectivores, seed eaters and herbivores have well developed gizzard musculature which when it contracts exerts pressure on its contents. In addition, glands lining the gizzard secrete a substance that forms grinding plates called cuticles which mill the food between them. Species which eat very hard nuts etc. have hard, pointed,

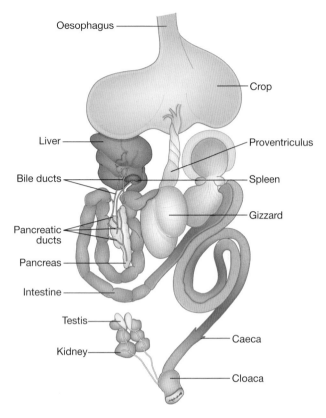

Figure 14.42 The digestive system of a pigeon.

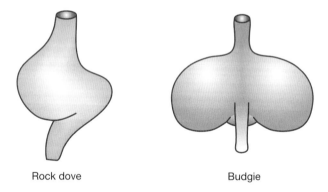

Rock dove   Budgie

Figure 14.43 Crop types – rock dove and budgie.

conical processes on the surface of the cuticles; these interlock with each other in a cog-like fashion and grind the nuts.

The effect of the gizzard is further aided by the presence of stones/grit which the bird ingests.

Fish and meat eaters have a thin walled sac which is more for storage than mechanical breakdown.

The digestive tract executes a reverse peristalsis action. Food is shunted backwards and forwards between proventriculus and gizzard in a complex cycle of contractions which assists digestion. In raptors, e.g. owls, falcons, hawks etc, the gizzard filters out indigestible items like bones, feathers and fur which are then regurgitated as pellets.

The small intestine follows much the same pattern as in mammals. Generally, the meat and fish eaters have a shorter tract than the others.

Some species lack a gall bladder, e.g. pigeons. In these species bile goes directly into the small intestine.

Most birds have two caeca; in some species, e.g. chickens, these may be very large and even divided into sacs. This is because, as in some herbivorous mammals, the caeca are a fermenting chamber for cellulose. A few species, e.g. kestrel, have one caecum and in some they are rudimentary/completely absent, e.g. parrots, pigeons, budgie (Figure 14.44).

There is no colon and a short rectum joins the caeca to the cloaca, which is also where the urogenital tract opens.

In the absence of a urinary bladder, the rectum resorbs water which has been excreted by the kidneys and retrogressively enters the rectum via the cloaca. An especially important adaption in desert dwelling birds.

The 'bursa of Fabricus' is a sac-like structure located in the cloaca (Figure 14.45). This aids in the production of lymphocytes and is particularly prominent in young birds.

Overall, absorption is efficient and food passes through the system rapidly, e.g. a warbler may pass berries through in a matter of minutes, and a chicken (Figure 14.46) takes only 12–24 hours to digest hard grains.

Reptiles

Ophidia (Figure 14.47)

The garter snake is a typical example of most snakes.

The tongue is forked and is also a major sense organ. It is often seen flicking in and out gathering scent particles.

Extremely flexible jaws enable them to swallow prey several times wider than themselves (see skeletal section).

As with most of the internal organs, those of the digestive have become narrow and elongated, especially the stomach which is not always differentiated from the oesophagus. It contains pepsin and HCl.

The intestine is short and terminates at the cloaca.

Chelonia (Figure 14.48)

Most tortoises are herbivores whilst most terrapins and turtles are omnivores. They do not possess teeth and the jaws are covered with a horny substance that forms a beak. Therefore, they are unable to chew their food so break off chunks and gulp it down. The system terminates at the cloaca.

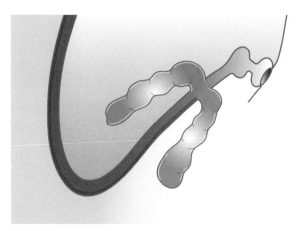

(a) Chicken

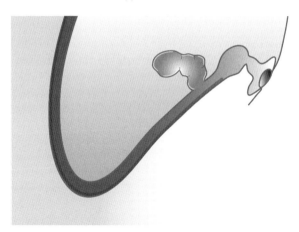

(b) Kestrel

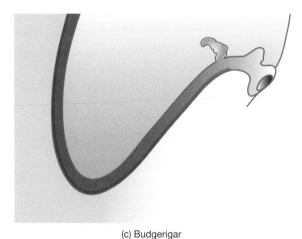

(c) Budgerigar

Figure 14.44   Caeca variations.

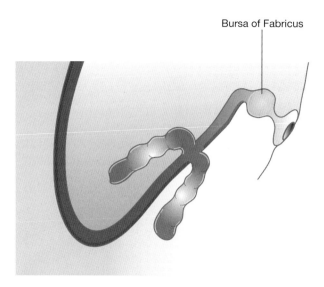

Figure 14.45   Diagram of bursa of Fabricus.

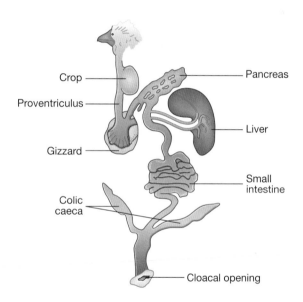

Figure 14.46   The digestive system of a chicken.

Fish (Figure 14.49)

There is a huge variation amongst the different fish species.

Generally herbivores have a longer tract than carnivorous species.

Most have teeth, some have teeth that extend into the pharynx (pharyngeal teeth), and some, like the goldfish, have only pharyngeal teeth which roughly grind the food against a bony pad on top of the pharynx.

Those species that do not possess teeth either swallow chunks of food whole or use a method called filter feeding which filters incoming water for food particles.

The oesophagus is usually highly distensible.

Some fish (e.g. Koi) do not have a stomach as such rather, an expanded section of the intestines (similar to the crop of birds). Because there is no stomach, food cannot be broken down by gastric enzymes, however,

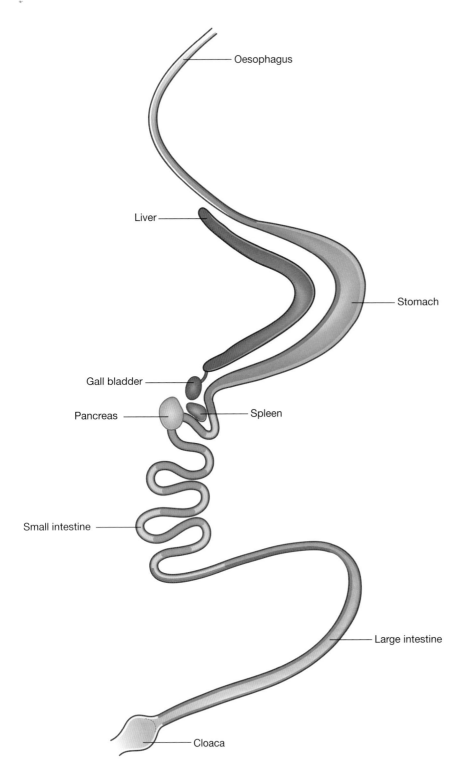

Figure 14.47 Digestive system of a snake.

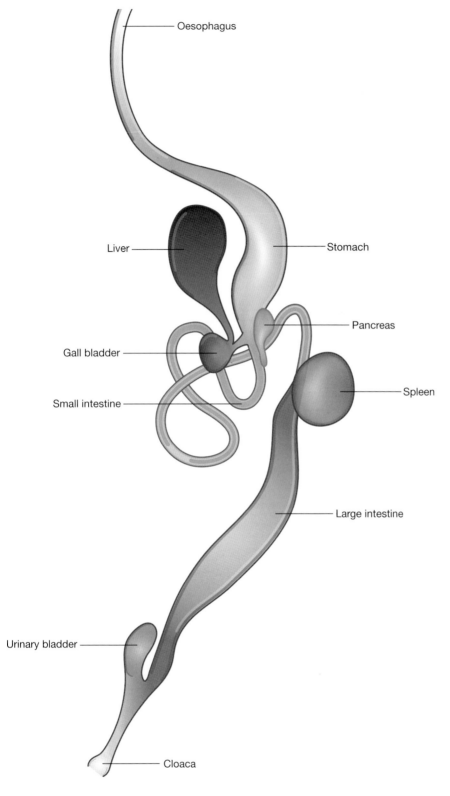

Oesophagus

Liver

Stomach

Pancreas

Gall bladder

Spleen

Small intestine

Large intestine

Urinary bladder

Cloaca

Figure 14.48 Digestive system of a tortoise.

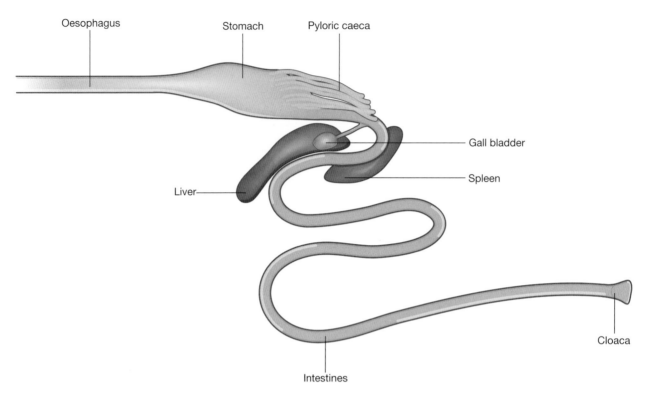

Figure 14.49 Digestive system of a fish.

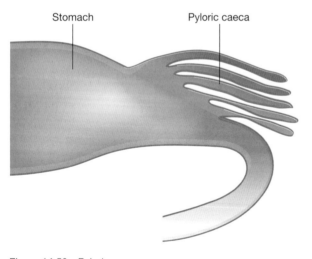

Figure 14.50 Pyloric caeca.

pancreatic and bile enzymes which enter the intestines at a point before the stomach seem to perform the function sufficiently.

Pyloric caeca (Figure 14.50) are finger-like projections located near the junction between the 'stomach' and intestines. They secrete enzymes that aid digestion and/or absorb digested food. Intestines are not divided into small and large.

Some species have separate exits from the body for digestive waste (anus) and urogenital (urogenital opening) functions. Others have a cloaca, e.g. goldfish.

RESPIRATORY SYSTEM

In birds and reptiles, pulmonary gaseous exchange occurs in the same manner as mammals. Most fish do not have lungs (although some species can breathe air through simplified lung structures) and obtain their oxygen from the water via the gills.

Birds

The upper part of the respiratory tract is similar to that of mammals, however, some birds, usually those that plunge from a height into water, do not have external nares and breathe through their mouths. The syrinx is the equivalent to the mammalian larynx (Figure 14.51).

- There is no diaphragm.
- Birds have not only lungs but air sacs as well. These are situated throughout the body and connect to the lungs.
- The lungs are small compared to a mammal of similar size but in conjunction with the air sacs the avian respiratory system is approximately double that of mammals of comparable size.
- The trachea divides into two bronchi which then divide into smaller and smaller bronchi which then spread throughout the lungs in decreasing diameter until eventually they are fine capillaries, which terminate in structures rather like alveoli.

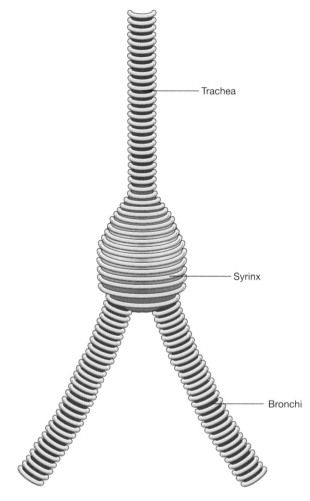

Figure 14.51 Avian syrinx.

- The lungs are rigid and do not expand as they fill with air.
- There are nine air sacs in most species, although some have eleven.
- Some of the air sacs extend into the pneumatic bones, e.g. the interclavicular air sac extends into the humerus.
- Respiration involves pumping the air through both the air sacs and lungs in a continuous one way system. To achieve this, the air sacs are inflated and deflated in sequence like a series of interconnected bellows (Figure 14.52).

It requires two inspirations and two expirations for the air to travel through the whole system:

1. On the first inhalation air goes into the posterior air sacs.
2. On the 1st exhalation the air is pumped into the lungs. This is where gaseous exchange occurs.

3. On the second inhalation the air is passed into the anterior air sacs.
4. On the 2nd exhalation the air exits the body.

This system results in much better O_2 uptake than mammals, mainly because there is no residual air left in the system.

Reptiles

The basic physiology of the system is the same as mammals. All species possess a trachea and lungs (Figure 14.53a, b).

In snakes the lungs are very elongated; some species have two, e.g. royal python; some have one functional lung (right) and one vestigial, e.g. corn snake; and some only one, e.g. most vipers.

A tracheal lung is found in some snake species (usually aquatic). This is a membrane with a limited blood supply that is wrapped around the trachea. It means that if the snake is eating a large prey item and the lung is compressed, gaseous exchange can still occur.

In snakes the trachea will move sideways whilst a large prey item is being swallowed.

Most species do not possess a diaphragm.

Ventilation is achieved by moving the ribs and/or muscles in the surrounding area. However, this is not possible in chelonia (as the ribs are fused to the carapace) so they utilise the muscles of the limb pockets to expand and contract the lungs. Abdominal muscles are also used.

Many aquatic species also respire through the skin, the lining of the throat and/or cloacal bursae (thin walled sacs in the cloaca). Gaseous exchange is limited in these areas but is sufficient for example to maintain a terrapin hibernating at the bottom of a pond.

Reptiles' lungs are sac-like and have faveoli, instead of alveoli, which are small divisions of the lung lining which open into the lung cavity.

In snakes gaseous exchange only occurs in the proximal region of the lung/s as this is the area where vascular tissue is most dense, distally there is none at all (Figure 14.54).

Fish

The gills are the respiratory apparatus of fish. They are located on either side of the pharynx at the back of the mouth in an area called the opercular cavity.

Most bony fish have one large gill pouch, with a single opening to the exterior. This is covered by the mobile, bony operculum.

Gills consist of four pairs of gill arches. Each gill arch has two rows of gill filaments called primary lamellae.

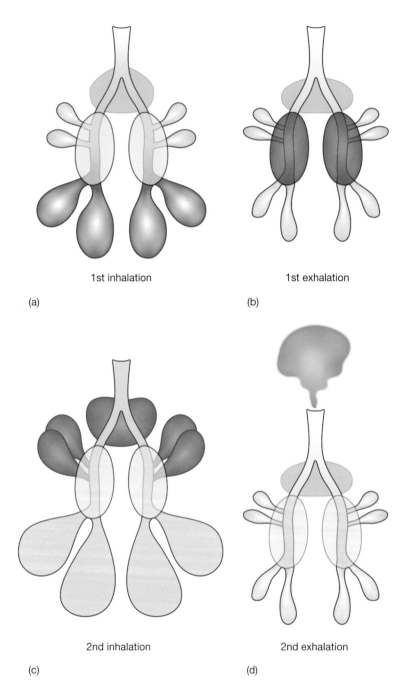

1st inhalation

(a)

1st exhalation

(b)

2nd inhalation

(c)

2nd exhalation

(d)

Figure 14.52 Avian respiratory cycle.

Each primary lamella has two rows of folded, vascular membranes called secondary lamellae. This is where gaseous exchange occurs. Gill rakers, located on the opposite side of the gill arch, help to trap debris in the water and prevent the gills becoming clogged.

Two arteries run through the gill arches:

- **afferent artery** – which carries oxygen-depleted blood from the heart to the gills
- **efferent artery** – which carries oxygen-enriched blood from the gills to the rest of the body.

Mechanics of fish respiration (Figure 14.55)

1. The mouth is opened and water is drawn in. At the same time the operculum (flexible edge of each gill) is closed, thus preventing water entry.
2. The mouth is then closed and the buccal floor brought upwards. This forces the gill slits open and the water over the gills.
3. As the water passes over the secondary lamellae gaseous exchange occurs.

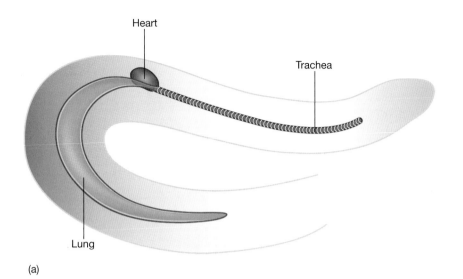

(a)

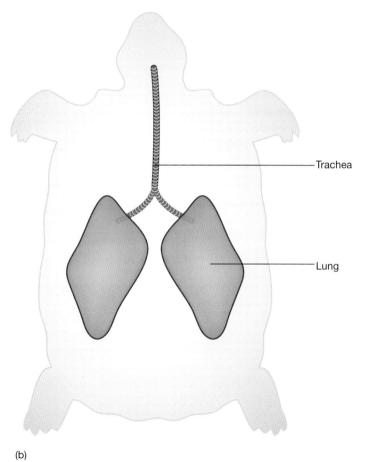

(b)

Figure 14.53   (a) Snake respiratory system, (b) tortoise respiratory system.

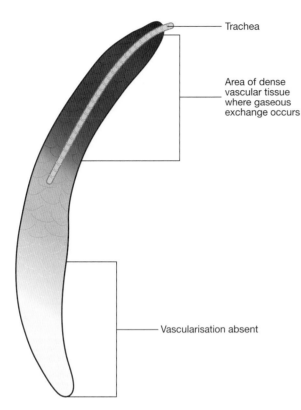

Trachea

Area of dense vascular tissue where gaseous exchange occurs

Vascularisation absent

Figure 14.54   Snake lung.

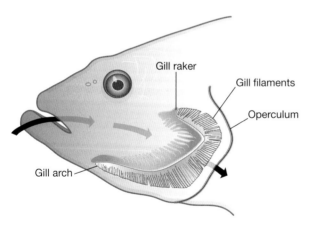

Gill raker

Gill filaments

Operculum

Gill arch

Figure 14.55   Gills and respiration.

UROGENITAL SYSTEM

Birds

There is no urinary bladder (except in the ostrich).

The system terminates at the cloaca which is a common chamber for digestive, urinary and reproductive systems.

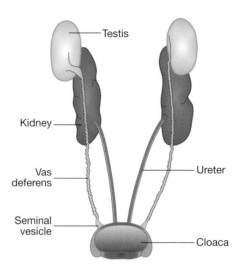

Testis

Kidney

Vas deferens

Seminal vesicle

Ureter

Cloaca

Figure 14.56   Urogenital system of a typical male bird.

Birds do not produce urea, instead they produce uric acid. This is white in colour and much less toxic than urea and therefore requires less water to dilute it.

Sex determination is opposite that of mammals. Males carry ZZ chromosomes and females WZ. Therefore it is the female who determines the sex of the embryo.

Male

The testes are internal and located cranial to the kidneys (Figure 14.56).

Outside the breeding season they are very much reduced in size, however, during the breeding season they may increase up to 1000 times.

Sperm travels down the vas deferens to an expansion called the seminal vesicle.

During mating the cloaca of the male is brought into close apposition with that of the female and the sperm is transferred. This is sometimes referred to as a 'cloacal kiss'.

In some species, e.g. ducks and geese, there is a rudimentary penis (papilla) at the base of the cloaca. During mating the papilla is everted and comes into close contact with the female's cloaca; sperm then flows down a groove on its surface.

Birds have none of the accessory glands of mammals, but vascular bodies at the end of the vas deferens dilute the sperm.

Female

There are two ovaries but only the left is fully developed in most species. This is another weight saving device (Figure 14.57).

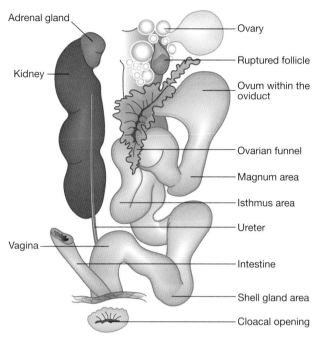
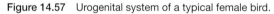

Figure 14.57   Urogenital system of a typical female bird.

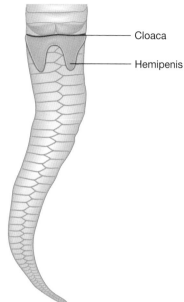

Figure 14.58   Snake hemipenis.

If the left ovary becomes damaged the vestigial right ovary will usually develop but into an ovotestis that secretes testerone and causes the development of male characteristics. Like the male, the ovaries are greatly enlarged during the breeding season.

Yolk material (produced in the liver) is gathered from the blood supply by the follicle containing the oocyte.

During the breeding season the ovary contains several oocytes in various stages of development. The one with the most yolk is the first to be ovulated. The others follow at regular intervals depending on the species, e.g. every 24h.

At ovulation the oocyte passes into the ovarian funnel (infundibulum). As it moves along the oviduct various layers are laid down around the yolk: albumin, shell membranes, water, calcium, shell markings.

Finally the egg passes into the cloaca and is laid.

The female can store viable sperm in sperm storage tubules at the junction of the shell gland and vagina for between 1 week and 1 year.

The amount of calcium needed for a hen's egg is approximately 2 grams. As no more than 25 milligrams are contained within the blood of a hen the rest must be mobilised from her reserves, i.e. the bones.

Females tend to lay down calcium in the marrow cavity of their bones in the weeks prior to laying.

Reptiles

The reptilian system is very similar to that of birds. All reptiles produce uric acid. The main differences are outlined below.

Ophidia

The most unusual feature of snakes (and lizards) is the possession by the male of two penises. They are referred to as hemipenes (Figure 14.58). Unlike the mammalian penis the hemipenis is an intromittent organ used purely to deliver sperm and has no urinary function. The sperm runs down a groove on the surface. They are located at the base of the tail and when at rest they are everted (turned inside out) and lie inside the body (like the finger of a rubber glove that has been pushed in).

They do not possess a urinary bladder; however, chelonia and most lizards do.

In some species of snake the female can store viable sperm for several months (same as birds) enabling several batches of eggs to be fertilised following one mating.

Females of very slender species, e.g. thread snakes, have lost one oviduct.

Most species lay eggs and some will show a degree of parental protection, e.g. most pythons will incubate but generally they will not return to the eggs once they are laid. Some species are live bearing, e.g. most boas.

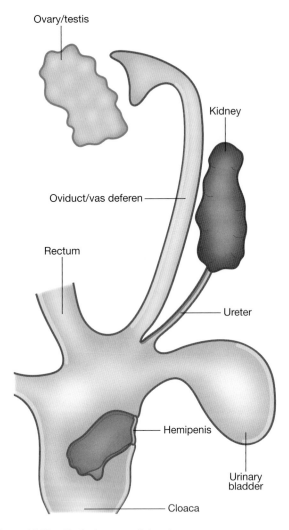

Figure 14.59 Chelonia urogenital system.

Chelonia (Figure 14.59)

All species lay eggs on land; however, the shells may be hard shelled, e.g. most tortoises and terrapins or soft shelled, e.g. turtles.

Females may store fertilised sperm for several years in some species and some may retain fertilised eggs for up to one year.

Chelonia do possess a urinary bladder. This is an important site for resorption of water.

Males only have one hemipenis.

Veterinary reception and administration

Veterinary reception and administration skills

Jennifer Seymour

ENGLISH LANGUAGE

The use of correct spelling, grammar and punctuation is important within the veterinary practice environment to ensure effective communication between staff members and also between staff and clients.

Spelling

Not only should students be competent at spelling everyday words in the English language but also they should have a basic knowledge of how to spell and define Veterinary terminology routinely used in practice.

Punctuation

Using correct punctuation ensures that written text is easy to read and understand.

Capital letters

Capital letters are used:

- at the beginning of all sentences
- when using proper nouns such as names of people and places, days and months
- when using the word 'I'
- at the beginning of reported speech

- for words indicating rank or profession
- for each important word in a title.

Examples:
The black dog in the waiting room is called Jake. He belongs to Ms Meredith from Burnley. He must return to the surgery on Wednesday 6th of March.

The nurse was reading The Veterinary Nursing Journal. She asked her friend, 'Have you read this?' Her friend replied, 'No I have not received my copy yet.'

Full stops (.)

- A full stop is written at the end of a sentence. It is used to denote a long pause.
- Question marks (?) and exclamation marks (!) may also be used.

Examples:
Mrs Mason took her dog Wilber to the Veterinary surgery in Wolverhampton.

'What is wrong with my cat?' asked Mr Collins.

'I have passed my ANA examination!' said Rebecca.

Commas (,)

- The comma denotes a short pause. It helps to clarify the meaning of a sentence.

Examples:
In the kennels were three dogs, two cats and one rabbit.

Holly the Border collie, who was very nervous, trembled on the operating table.

It should be noted that in the UK we do not use a serial comma (i.e. before 'and'), but in the US a serial comma is correct.

When writing spoken words, a comma is placed between the spoken words and the unspoken words.

Example:
The head nurse said, 'Please bandage the dog's paw.'

Semicolon (;)

▪ A semi colon is an intermediate pause between a full stop and a comma. It is used to separate two complete but related sentences.

Examples:
Claire was confident as she looked at the examination paper; she knew she had worked hard.

The stray dog was miserable; he was lonely, cold and hungry.

Colon (:)

▪ A colon is used to demonstrate a pause in a sentence longer than a semi colon but less than a full stop. It is commonly used to denote the beginning of a list.

Examples:
The clinical signs of canine distemper virus include:
Coughing
Hyperkeratitis of nose and pads
Lethargy
Convulsions.

The inpatients in the kennel ward were:
An elderly Cocker spaniel with congestive heart failure
A kitten with a fractured jaw
Two Labrador puppies suffering from parvovirus
A rabbit with myxomatosis.

Apostrophe (')

▪ An apostrophe is used

(a) When shortening two words to use them as one.

Examples:
I'd like to go home (I would like to go home).

It's cold today (It is cold today).

You're late for work (You are late for work).

(b) To show possession.

Examples:
The rabbit's ear was bleeding.

The nurse's uniform was torn.

My colleague's dog is in the car.

When the item belongs to more than one person or animal, the apostrophe is placed after the s.

Examples:
The three dogs' tails wagged.

The guinea pigs' food bowls were empty.

My flock of birds' feathers are moulting.

Inverted commas (' ')

▪ These are used to indicate spoken words.

Examples:
'Please restrain this dog,' said the Veterinary Surgeon.

Robert said 'I will clean out the kennel for you.'

'We will return later,' said Stephen 'after lunch.'

Grammar

This refers to the correct use of spoken and written language. Proper use of grammar ensures understanding and maintains a professional image within the practice.

Tenses
▪ The tense of a verb tells **when** the action takes place.

Present tense
▪ This indicates that the action is happening now.

Examples:
I am stroking the dog.

She is going to work.

They are studying for their examinations.

Past tense
▪ This is used to illustrate events that occurred **before** the present time.
Present tense: I am walking the dog.
Past tense: I walked the dog.
Present tense: I hurry to work
Past tense: I hurried to work.

Future tense
▪ This is used to demonstrate events that will occur **after** the present.

Present tense
Joanne goes to college.

The Dalmatian is having his operation.

Future tense
Joanne will go to college.

The Dalmatian will have his operation on Tuesday.

Nouns

A noun is a word that is used to represent an object, a living thing or place.

Examples:
Dog, cat, bone, Veterinary Nurse, ambulance, library.

Proper nouns

These are used when naming people, places days and months.

Examples:
The dog's name is **Archie**.
The nurse lives in **Liverpool**
The cat was born on **Tuesday** 4th **April**.
The locum veterinary surgeon originates from **New Zealand**.

Collective nouns

These are used to name groups of many similar things.

Examples:

Table 15.1 Nouns and collective nouns	
Noun	Collective noun
Dogs	Pack
Kittens	Litter
Students	Class
Insects	Swarm
Books	Library

Abstract nouns

These are the names of things we are unable to see or feel, such as qualities and ideas.

Examples:
The fear of examinations.
The decision was made by the head nurse.
The dog demonstrated great strength.

Abstract nouns can be formed from verbs.

Examples:

Table 15.2 Verbs and nouns	
Verb	Noun
Communicate	Communication
Laugh	Laughter
Know	Knowledge

Pronouns

Pronouns are short words used to take the place of nouns.

Examples:
I, it, you, he, she, we, they, me, her.

Verbs

A verb is a word used to show action.

Examples:
Tilly the cat **wakes** up and **eats** her breakfast.
Max the dog **limped** to the bed, **went** to sleep and started to **snore**.
The terrier **snapped** at the nurse's hand when she tried to **apply** a bandage to his foot.

Adverbs

An adverb is used to describe how actions are performed.

Examples:
The kitten hissed **noisily** at the adult cat.
The nurse **carefully** carried the dog to the operating theatre.
The Animal Nursing Assistant students waited **anxiously** for their examination results.

Adjectives

An adjective is used to **describe** a noun. Numbers are also adjectives, as are words such as some, few, many and all.

Examples:
The stray dog was **frightened**, **hungry** and **exhausted**.
The dog was **loyal** to his owner.
Biddy the mongrel had a **shaggy** coat, **droopy** ears and a **wagging** tail.

Adjectives may be formed from nouns.

Examples:

Table 15.3 Nouns and adjectives	
Noun	Adjectives
Noise	Noisy
Poison	Poisonous
Sense	Sensible

Prepositions

Prepositions are used before a noun. They connect the noun with the rest of the sentence.

Examples:
The chinchilla was placed **on** the consulting room table.
The frightened dog shivered **under** the bed.
The veterinary surgeon looked **at** the cat as she walked **between** the two dogs.

COMMUNICATION SKILLS

Verbal communications – clients in reception

The reception area of a veterinary practice is the first place that clients will see. It is therefore important that it creates a professional and welcoming image to the public. The area should be constantly checked to ensure it is clean, tidy and odour free.

There is nothing worse when entering any establishment than to be ignored. It is important that every visitor to the practice is greeted in a friendly and professional manner.

Even when on the telephone or dealing with another client, an acknowledging gesture such as a smile or eye contact will reassure the client that they have been noticed and will be dealt with presently. All reasonable clients will accept that you are busy and will wait patiently until you are free.

The needs of clients should take precedence over all but the most urgent conversations between staff members.

Whenever possible the client should be greeted by name. Owners also always appreciate a suitable greeting to their animal. Specific or general enquiries regarding the health or well being of their pet promotes a feeling of belonging to the practice and is likely to encourage loyalty from the client.

Inevitably the nurse will at times encounter difficult clients. These clients may cause distress, anger or embarrassment and may prove very difficult to manage.

It is important to remember, however, that ordinary, reasonable people can easily become angry or upset when they are worried about the welfare of their pet or the cost of its treatment. Much can be said in the heat of the moment that will be regretted at a later time.

A calm, sympathetic attitude can assist enormously to diffuse a potentially unpleasant situation. The following are useful guidelines to consider when dealing with difficult clients:

- Remain calm.
- Avoid a scene in the waiting room – invite difficult clients into a consulting room or office so they may be dealt with in private.
- Reassure the client that you understand their feelings.
- Do not attempt to answer questions or justify actions if you are not absolutely sure of the facts.
- If you cannot deal with the situation seek assistance from a senior staff member.
- Do not take sides or place blame in an argument between clients or staff members.
- Allow clients to voice their anger without retaliating.
- Do not take personal offence at anything said.

Confidentiality

In every veterinary practice there will be certain information that must be treated in a confidential manner. The Animal Nursing Assistant should be aware of which information may be disclosed to members of the public and which should be withheld.

The following are examples of information that may be deemed confidential unless told otherwise by a senior member of staff:

- Results of other client's laboratory tests or radiographs.
- The diagnosis or prognosis of another client's animal.
- Any private conversations held in the surgery regarding clients or staff members.
- The home telephone numbers of staff members.

Telephone/electronic communication

The telephone is an important means of communication in the veterinary practice. Without even entering the surgery, clients will form an impression of the practice according to the way they are treated on the telephone and this will form the basis of any further communication. It is therefore vitally important that answering and talking on the telephone is carried out in a professional manner.

There are several general rules regarding the use of the telephone:

- Answer the call promptly.
- Clearly state a greeting in accordance with practice policy.
- Speak in a professional but friendly voice; your voice should be clearly audible.
- Always be polite and courteous – even if the caller is not!
- Establish all the details of the call including client's name, address and reason for call.
- If you must hold the line find out the nature of the call first – it may be something that cannot wait.
- If the client must be left waiting, apologise for the delay and explain the reason.
- It may be better to ask the client to call back later or take a number and call them back at a more convenient time – remember keeping clients holding on costs the caller money and time. It also engages the line maybe preventing urgent calls from getting through.

When discussing patients with their owners, use the animal's name and indicate that you know whether it is male or female. This reassures the client that their pet is a known individual, rather than just another animal.

Writing a letter

Most practices will use prepared headed paper, often with a company logo, when sending written communication to clients or business associates. This creates a professional and readily recognisable image to the correspondent.

There are various acceptable formats for a formal letter, but the following information should be included:

- Name of sender
- Sender's reference
- Address and postcode of sender
- Date
- Name and address of recipient
- An introductory salutation
- Reference of letter
- Complimentary close
- Name, qualifications and position of sender

The following are examples of the correct layout of a formal letter.

The Grove Veterinary Hospital
93 Grove Square, Southampton
SH23 7KD
Telephone 01364 287372

Mr P Thompson
23 Casey Drive
Southampton
SH 12 4KP

11 December 2006

Dear Mr Thompson

Referral appointment for 'Barney'

Please be advised that an appointment has been made for you to attend the orthopaedic referral centre in Portsmouth at 3.30 pm on Wednesday 31st January 2007.

In the meantime, please continue with Barney's medication as directed.

If you have any questions or if Barney's condition should deteriorate please do not hesitate to contact the surgery.

Yours sincerely

Alison Draycott VN
Head Nurse

Figure 15.1   The correct layout of a formal letter: example 1.

Ref: JW/booster

Mr A Kennedy   **R G McCormack MRCVS**
4 St Helens Way   **Copthorne Veterinary Centre**
Liverpool   **21 Hatherton Avenue**
L7 4KP   **Liverpool**
                                                L4 9AN

28th September 2000

Dear Sir

Booster vaccination reminder

According to our records your cat 'Smokey' is due for her booster vaccination and routine worming in November. Please contact the surgery to arrange an appointment.

We look forward to seeing you.

Yours faithfully

Christine Jones
Practice Manager

Figure 15.2   The correct layout of a formal letter: example 2.

Note:
When the salutation of a letter is addressed to a **named** person such as Mr Callaghan, Dr Andrews or Stacey the complimentary close should be 'Yours sincerely'.

When the salutation of a letter is addressed to **Sir**, **Madam** or a **non-specified person** such as veterinary nurse or client, the complimentary close should be 'Yours faithfully'.

Less formal letters may be ended with a closure such as Best wishes, Regards or Kind regards.

It is obviously important that all letters use correct spelling and grammar throughout.

Writing a curriculum vitae (CV)

The term curriculum vitae originates from the Latin expression 'The course of your life'. It is used to give prospective employers information about you in a concise, accessible manner.

There are no rigid rules for compiling a CV. It is, by definition a personal document and as such should have an individual style.

However, the following information should be included:

- Personal details
- Education
- Employment details such as job title, activities, achievements and location
- Interests

■ Other skills
■ References.

STATEMENTS OF EMPLOYMENT

All employees are entitled to a written statement of employment, which must be provided no later than two months after work commences.

The specific contents of the statement may vary between employers but the following details are usually included:

■ Name(s) of employer
■ Name of employee
■ Date of commencement of employment
■ Job title
■ Rate of pay
■ Pay intervals, i.e. weekly, monthly
■ Terms and conditions relating to hours of work
■ Terms and conditions relating to holiday entitlement
■ Terms and conditions relating to sickness
■ Place of work
■ Details of any pension scheme
■ Length of notice required
■ Disciplinary procedures.

PROFESSIONAL ORGANISATIONS
Royal College of Veterinary Surgeons

The RCVS is the regulatory body for the veterinary profession in the United Kingdom. It deals with issues of veterinary professional conduct, monitors standards of veterinary education and maintains a register of veterinary surgeons that are eligible to practise in the UK.

The RCVS VN Council is charged with the regulation of the veterinary nursing profession. The names of all currently Listed Veterinary Nurses (VNs) are also maintained by the RCVS.

British Veterinary Association

The BVA is the national representative body for the veterinary profession. It promotes the interests of its membership and the animals under their care and develops and maintains communication with Government and the media. It has 51 divisions representing the whole spectrum of species and specialities within veterinary science.

British Small Animal Veterinary Association

The BSAVA is a division of BVA and exists to promote high scientific and educational standards of small animal medicine and surgery in practice, teaching and research.

British Veterinary Nursing Association

The BVNA is the only representative body for veterinary nurses, animal nursing assistants and practice staff. One of its primary aims is to promote the standards of veterinary nursing throughout the UK and quality assure and further develop veterinary nurse education as well as seeking and actioning on the opinions of its members.

The Veterinary Defence Society

The VDS supplies insured defence for veterinary practices and their staff in the UK as protection against litigation from the general public.

Administration

Angela North

COMMUNICATION

Basic needs for communication

The varied role of the student nurse does of course involve the application of the key skills we have developed throughout our lives. With the 'office' aspect of our role it is necessary to communicate effectively, both in written form, verbal form and in terms of finding out information.

As 'first line' staff the public will predetermine the service of the surgery by their first impression. Not only are actual communication skills important, but physical appearance, hygiene, body language and facial expression play a role in the customer's opinion of not only the administrator but also the practice.

This first impression plays a valuable marketing tool. A client who feels comfortable and confident will market the organisation using word of mouth – expressing satisfaction!

To this end, of course, the reception area should be perceived as an informative yet calm and organised area until a problem arises. The service given to clients or customers with a grievance can be taken personally by those in the environment. Equally, the ability of the reception staff to diffuse a situation but still deal with the matter fairly is a skilled job.

Dealing with customer complaints

By law, as a business the veterinary practice is a retail outlet, providing a specialised service for keepers of animals. All clients and customers must be treated equally, and without judgment or opinion. It is vitally important that a nurse learns to disguise personal feeling to provide an appropriate service to all clients.

As those in direct contact with members of the public we are also asked frequently for advice or opinion. Employees often forget that when we are working behind reception we are the company representative; any recommendations we put forward are seen to be the opinion of the workplace, rather than a personal one.

For example, by recommending a local boarding kennel or cattery, as an employee of the veterinary practice, you are endorsing the establishment and its actions. Should an incident occur, the client could hold the practice partially responsible. Clients should be advised to select

---

Considerations for pet insurance

- **General cover:** comparison of included aspects. Maximum claim amounts. Monthly outlay
- **Death:** remuneration available
- **Loss:** aid to locate lost pet, remuneration of market value
- **Veterinary fees:** amount available PER CONDITION, exclusion clauses, supportive therapies, initial 'excess' fee etc.
- **Third party:** amount of insurance available in the event that the insured animal causes accident or injury to third parties
- **Optional extras**
  - Boarding during owner hospitalisation
  - Advertising costs to recover lost pets
  - Wider therapy cover

a boarding establishment from a given list and inspect it themselves. Similarly, practice employees are not permitted to recommend specific insurance policies (see Box in previous page).

General advice for clients selecting pet insurance

▪ Always check the small print across a range of policies
▪ Look for hidden costs – large breed loading, age loading etc.
▪ Check that cover is adequate
▪ Check policy does not stipulate TIME LIMITS for claims – this affects degenerative, chronic and recurring conditions
▪ Is MAXIMUM benefit PER YEAR or PER CONDITION?
▪ Check insurance extends to aged animals as time goes on
▪ Double check that congenital, hip, dental, behaviour and diet related treatments are included to some extent!

Owners are responsible to complete and submit claim forms, with veterinary records to be supplied by practice staff. At all times this must be accurate, correct and clear to avoid discrepancies or queries. Claim forms are a legal document and can be used as evidence in case of fraudulent claim.

RECORD SYSTEMS

In today's society, we manage information in a range of ways. Records are kept in veterinary practice to cover a range of management systems: staff information; client details; patient records, diagnostic results, stock control etc.

The way in which records are maintained relates to the facilities available and of course the nature of the information (see Table 16.1).

Clearly not all information can be attached to a patient's records; to amalgamate records, there is usually a cross referencing system to align different storage methods. Here the client central record would contain the cross reference indicator to other storage systems such as laboratory reports, radiographic images etc.

Table 16.1 Methods and examples of filing systems within veterinary practice		
Type of system	Example of records	Method of filing
Filing cabinets	Grouped sets of information – staff files, client records, radiographs, laboratory results etc.	Various Alphabetical Alphabetical or numerical Chronological
Rotary files (circular, revolving card index)	Contact name/telephone numbers Equipment locations/availability	Alphabetical Alphanumerical (e.g. Grouped equipment – S3 could label an item of surgical equipment, stored on shelf 3) or geographical
Postcard filing	Small practice client files Vaccine reminders by month 'Practice Plan' installments	Alphabetical Chronological
Loose leaf	Central system to store specified information – i.e. all radiographic images, laboratory results, ECG tracings, in-patient details of care etc.	By chronological or numerical order, stored in logical sequence – collated in a central file or folder
Computerised systems	Client and patient details, record of consultation by client/pet, stock control, staff details, rotas, staff holidays accounting, appointments, spread sheet analysis of cash flow, database containing client/pet details for general mailing, storing correspondence etc.	IT system dependent. Alphabetical, chronological, numerical, geographical by client address, alphanumerically.
NB: Pre-printed manual card systems can contain detailed descriptors for client, animal and consultation details, manual systems can be developed to contain basic information using 'postcards'. Largely, these methods have been superseded with IT systems. Specifically designed to suit the requirements of veterinary practices, systems can be purchased through specialist companies 'ready to use', with 'on line' or telephone support readily available.		

Examples of filing methods

- **Alphabetical referencing** – by client surname, then initial, then address.
- **Numerical** – logically sequenced numbers to cross reference to other information.
- **Alphanumerical** – using a combination of alphabetical and numerical references – e.g. A1, G6.
- **Geographical** – clients by village or town.
- **Chronological** – date order, i.e. vaccine reminders.

It is vital that ALL filing systems and their cross referencing systems are accurately maintained. Again we are reminded of the importance of 'key skills' of spelling and problem solving that have been developed throughout life.

Certain information is of a sensitive nature and must be protected under the Data Protection Act 1998, which effectively means any sensitive or personal information relating to individuals must be securely kept. In fact some information that needs to be entered onto record cards can cause personal distress to a client; in such cases a code that is clearly established with all employees should be agreed.

Examples:

PTS = put to sleep
D&D = death and disposal
Care = animal may have behavioural problems
CFC = cash for custom (may be a bad debtor).

Disposal of records

All records must be retained for certain periods of time as they are a legal document showing events that have taken place. The length of time that this information should be stored varies dependant on the type of information stored.

Examples:

- Client records – confidentiality must be maintained under the Data Protection Act 1998 therefore incineration or shredding the documents is vital to destroy the information stored.
- There is no legal requirement to store unused records, radiographic images, laboratory results, consent forms etc.; however should a client challenge a diagnosis, the Veterinary Defence Society recommend that this evidence be retained for a two year period; the Royal College of Veterinary Surgeons actually recommend a six year period.
- Financial records such as accounting details should be stored for six years – again the information must be destroyed when disposed of.

POSTAL SERVICES

Veterinary practice relies on the postal service for a range of services. Sending and receiving information to and from clients, supplying and receiving some medicines, sending and receiving diagnostic materials and pathological samples.

Clearly, personnel involved with the service must be fully aware of the constraints and legalities involved to ensure all health and safety precautions are upheld. Concerns are particularly high in the transfer of pathological specimens and medicines.

There are a range of options to select the most appropriate method of postage – see Table 16.2.

Many clients request that a treatment be forwarded to them in the post, and indeed frequently pathological specimens are dispatched for diagnostic assessment. To comply with regulations practices should draw up guidelines and update these regularly as national guidance alters (see Table 16.3).

Franking machines

Although small practices use their local Post Office to dispatch mail, larger organisations may invest in a franking machine. An electronic machine that has prepurchased postage credits – a personalised 'frank' – is printed at speed instead of a stamp. A quick and efficient method that is cost effective for a practice that has a lot of outgoing post.

Special postage services

See Table 16.2. Some items that are dispatched can be of valuable or important nature. Selecting the appropriate method of postage for these items is vital. Insurance can be purchased through Special Delivery for the cost of valuable products being posted. More commonly used in veterinary practice, Recorded Delivery is the method of postage that ensure the recipient signs for the letter or package. Delivery does not take place unless a signature is obtained. This is suitable for the dispatch of important documents such as certificates or cheques etc.

Pathological specimens

Specimens sent to laboratories using postal services can present health hazards to postal workers under the Health and Safety at Work Act 1974, therefore guidelines set by Royal Mail are in place to reduce this hazard to a minimum. These include:

- Placing the sample in an appropriate container with a securely fitted lid.

Table 16.2 Methods of postage available

Method	Range	Delivery time	Options
First Class	Letter – up to 100g (*max 240 × 165mm – less than 5mm thick*) Large letter – up to 750g (*max 250 × 353mm – less than 25mm thick*) Packet – 1250g + (*more than 353mm long or more than 250mm wide or above 25mm in thickness*)	Next working day	Certificate of posting can be requested free of charge Discounts apply to franking and account mail customers Used for fast service not requiring a signature
Second Class	Letters, large letters and packets under 1000g in weight. Items over 1000g must be sent using another service	By the third working day	As with first class
Standard Parcels	Any weight	Within three to five days of posting	Ideal for non-urgent parcels to be delivered within the UK
Recorded (signed for)	As first and second class postage	As first or second class postage	Used for important but non-urgent items; provides proof of posting and delivery and can be traced on www.royalmail.com
Special Delivery	Items up to 10kg	Next day using either 'Special Delivery 9 am' or 'Next Day' when it will arrive by 1 pm	For valuable or urgent items; guarantees delivery the next working day or your money back. Can be traced as above

Dependent on time of posting.
The following recommendations will help to ensure that the mail is transferred quickly and safely:
Items should contain the full address including the postal code.
Items should be wrapped and packaged well.

Table 16.3 Packaging materials
The following methods of packaging are recommended:

Item for postage	Preparation	Packaging
Client correspondence	None required	White/brown envelope. Window or non window
Drugs (medicines)	Contained within a strong inner container, tablets should be 'packed' to minimise noise	Agree in advance with Royal Mail. May include padding in container with cotton wool for tablets, placing medicine container in padding – i.e. bubble wrap, sealing in padded envelope. Sender details should be clearly displayed
Pathological specimens	Suitably collected and preserved sample for purpose	Leak proof, damage proof packaging. External laboratory supply pre-printed envelopes displaying warnings. Practice should identify sender clearly. Under regular review – see text or contact Royal Mail for further details

Practices should be considerate of packaging and their origin. Suspect packages should be reported to the Police prior to opening. Senders should be advised to identify the origin on external packaging.

- Labelling the container with practice details, owner name and the date of collection.
- Padding the container with sufficient quantities of absorbent wadding such as cotton wool or thick tissue.
- Sealing the packed sample inside a plastic bag.
- Placing the fully completed laboratory form in a separate sealed plastic bag.
- Further padding the packed sample with corrugated card, wadding, bubble wrap or polystyrene pieces.
- Placing the padded sample in a rigid container such as a cardboard box.
- Sealing the box inside a padded envelope or wrapping paper.

Labelling
Include:

- Full name and postal address and post code of the laboratory.
- Full name and address of the sender (veterinary practice) on the reverse of the parcel.
- Other significant cautions SHOULD include – 'HANDLE WITH CARE', 'PATHOLOGICAL SPECIMEN'.

Posting
Pathological specimens should be dispatched to ensure arrival is not delayed. Postage may be delayed over weekends and holidays to allow correct storage of the sample prior to dispatch.

STOCK CONTROL
Ordering systems

Many veterinary practices continue to rely on manual systems for ordering supplies from their appointed wholesaler. Drug stocks should have identified MINIMUM and MAXIMUM levels to ensure that stock turn around is consistent. Goods held in stock for extended periods are unprofitable. Most wholesalers have recognised this and have regular deliveries, several times a week or even daily, to ensure that practices have no need to hold 'dead stock'.

Manual orders systems have been replaced by handheld computerised systems that hold information regarding stocking levels. The equipment can be programmed to read bar codes to speed up the ordering system; further computerised, stock levels can be constantly reviewed when outgoing and incoming systems are linked. Stock ordering can then be an administrative procedure, with a manual review to ensure that errors have not occurred.

Computerised ordering can be linked directly to the wholesaler's computer system using a modem that transfers information from the in-practice computer system to that of the wholesaler.

It is usual for the requirement of some products to change with seasonal demand. A good example of this can be antiparasitic products which are usually sold more frequently in the summer months.

Stock rotation

When locating new stock to the correct area, it is vital that both the delivered items and existing stock be checked for the 'sell by, or use by, date' to ensure that the product is still guaranteed to be active and safe for use. Existing stock usually has the shortest date and should be moved to the shelf front to ensure that it is dispensed first. Stock that has passed its 'use by date' may have diminished in its properties, or worse still undergone chemical changes and can no longer be safe to use for its original purpose.

Receipt of stock

All stock that is received by the practice should be checked as correct against the original order placed AND the delivery note that accompanies the order. The delivery note allows discrepancies to be raised and addressed prior to the invoice being raised. All stock should be checked thoroughly to include product name, pack size, quantity, sell by date; checks for damage and contamination should also take place.

Discrepancies should be recorded in writing, and reported to the wholesaler and appointed supervisor by the end of the working day of the delivery.

Storage of stock

Stock should be checked and unpacked as soon after delivery as possible to ensure that the contents are as required and the stock available immediately. Some items must be refrigerated as soon as possible to ensure their continued efficacy. The usual requirement for storage of these items is 2–8°C. Other items that require specific storage requirements should be noted and stored appropriately.

Items that are classified as Controlled Drugs should be entered into the Record Book as per the Misuse of Drugs Act 1971 and stored in an unmovable, locked cabinet in the first instance as these products must be secure under the law.

MARKETING AND RETAIL

Although in the eyes of the law a supplier has no legal obligation to supply goods or services to a buyer as long as the reasoning is not racial or sexual, most clients who request a sale must be treated respectfully and without discrimination at all times. This will involve the identification of a person's individual needs including age, disability and language barriers. Adapting the approach used with different client groups can minimise possible misunderstanding.

Customer complaints

Should complaints arise, you should be aware of the practice procedures for addressing the matter according to policy. For general guidance:

- Ascertain the nature of the complaint – internal – relating to the way in which staff members have behaved, or external – problems associated with delivery of goods.
- Determine the severity of the problem – it may be a standard situation that had been misunderstood by a client. A simple explanation may suffice.
- Invite the client if present to discuss the matter in a quiet area.
- Refer to a senior staff member such as practice manager, veterinary nurse or surgeon.
- Record the occurrence in case of repercussions.

Legalities

Sale of Goods Act 1979
The main purpose of the Act is to prevent buyers from being deceived into buying goods that are not fit to be sold.

Under the Act, goods must be:

- as described
- of merchantable quality
- fit for the purpose for which they are intended.

Trade Description Act 1968
The main purpose of this Act is to prevent the false description of goods. Vendors of products or services that are falsely described are committing an offence. This includes:

- Selling goods that are wrongly described by the manufacturer.
- Implied descriptions, i.e. using images that create a false impression.
- False descriptions of any aspect of the goods – quantity, size, compositions, method of manufacture etc.

Unfair Contract Terms Act 1977
Entry into an agreement by the buyer and seller to exchange goods or services for payment is a legally binding contract and has two elements:

- The customer's offer to purchase goods at a specified price.
- The supplier's acceptance of the order or their agreement to sell the goods.

The contract becomes binding when both parts are complete; goods cannot be returned without good reason, and the supplier cannot alter the terms of supply (cost, conditions of sale etc.).

Contracts are usually divided into three parts:

1. The offer – a customer requests to purchase certain goods at a specified cost
2. The acceptance – the seller accepts the offer
3. The consideration (not Scotland) – payment is given over.

Contracts can be brought to an end, legally by three main ways:

1. Performance – acquisition by purchase of the goods
2. Agreement – both parties agree to end the agreement
3. Breach – one party does not carry out their part of the agreement – failure to supply the goods as requested, failure to provide appropriate payment etc.

The Unfair Contract Terms Act 1977 is in place to prevent organisations evading their legal responsibilities under the law by stopping the placement of disclaimers on their products or services. Disclaimers must be proven to be fair and reasonable under this Act.

Weights and Measures Act 1985
When dispensing products for sale, this Act states that the equipment used for measuring the product must be fit for trade use.

Consumer Protection Act 1987
Further to the Trades Description Act 1968, further legislation was passed for consumer protection in general. This Act states: A person is guilty of an offence if he or she gives a misleading indication of the price at which any goods or services are available (e.g. by false comparison with other prices; by indication that the price is less than the real price – i.e. VAT is omitted from display; false comparison with a previous price – i.e. was £60 now £30).

The Act states that it is an offence to supply consumer goods that are not reasonably safe.

Promotion of products

Some veterinary practices rely on verbal marketing of products through reception, nursing and veterinary staff. However in today's competitive market of supportive sales such as pet food, anti-parasitic products, grooming tools etc. there is considerable revenue available through effective marketing of products within the veterinary practice itself. Some clients are unaware of the range of non-prescription items available in the practice, and select to shop for such items at pet supermarket chains.

Dependent upon practice policy, nursing and support staff can encourage 'counter sales' by marketing products in a range of ways. Some practices encourage this by using incentives payments to their staff!

Tools to promote awareness of product availability should be eye-catching, neat, up to date and effective to catch the eye of the customer, create awareness of possible need, encourage purchase by promoting value for money offers.

This can be achieved by:

- **Seasonal sales** – e.g. promoting awareness of prophylactic treatment against parasites in early summer, images to promote revaccination, neutering, grooming etc.
- **Special offers** – special offer prices, buy product and get something free (incentive sale)
- **Impulse buying** – positioning information that promotes a 'must buy' feel to the client
- **Impact sales techniques** – providing informative displays next to a product to ensure a significant influence on the client so they feel it imperative to purchase the goods
- **Hot spots** – positioning goods in a prime viewing location, possibly promoting special offers
- **Using promotional aids** – use of manufacturers' display units, posters, products and leaflets to promote sales.

Many products, by nature of their legal status under the Medicine Act 1968 should not be displayed unless in a locked cabinet – this would include some products that although effective prophylactics, are classified as prescription only medicine (POM), pharmacy medicine (P) or Pharmacy Merchants List (PML) products due to the nature and efficacy of their content. For value as well as health and safety these products should be securely stored.

General Sales List (GSL) products, feedstuff and pet accessories should be displayed clearly, in a logical sequence, with the display being dusted daily and changed regularly to promote interest. Many clients return several times; a dusty, unchanged display promotes a client to believe that products are rarely sold – a poor advertisement indeed! Many items for sale may have an expiry or sell-by date. At no time should products be available for general sale if they are passed or nearing the sell-by date. A product cannot be guaranteed passed this date. A client that draws this to staff attention will also raise awareness in those waiting in the waiting room.

Waiting room displays have already been identified as a good source of revenue if maintained effectively. However they can also be a great temptation for theft/pilferage. As previously identified, the use of locked cabinets is ideal for items of high value. Other methods for monitoring stock to minimise theft include:

- The use of display only items
- Positioning the display in direct view of staff
- Displaying items such as P and PML in visible but inaccessible locations
- Using locked cabinets for all products
- Using a mirror to reflect a client's actions at a stand.

Many of these methods reduce theft, but also sales as clients see difficulties associated with viewing products.

Should pilferage be suspected, it cannot be confirmed until the suspected person has left the building. This sensitive and often unpleasant circumstance should be dealt with according to individual practice policy. For general guidance it is inadvisable to make physical contact with the suspect, but to discretely follow them from the building and sensitively suggest that they have left the premises but have clearly forgotten to pay for the product they have in their possession. It may be a genuine mistake, or the accused may have acted deliberately. Where possible every opportunity should be made for return or payment of the goods. In extreme cases refer the situation to supervisory staff for further action.

Further reading

- Corsan, J. Mackay, A.R. (2001) The Veterinary Receptionist. Butterworth Heinemann, Oxford.
- Gorman, C. (2000) Clients, Pets and Vets. Threshold Press, Newbury.
- Royal Mail (April 2005) 'Keeping Our Promise'.
- Shilcock, M. Stutchfield, G. (2003) Veterinary Practice Management. Elsevier Science, Edinburgh.www.nwml.gov.uk

Multiple choice questions

Chapter 1

1. An example of a negatively charged particle is a:
   a. proton
   b. neutron
   c. electron
   d. atom

2. The function of rough endoplasmic reticulum is:
   a. synthesis of carbohydrates
   b. transport of proteins synthesised by the ribosomes
   c. production of energy
   d. disposal of unwanted cell material

3. The genetic material DNA is found in the:
   a. mitochondria
   b. Golgi body
   c. lysosomes
   d. nucleus

4. The centrosome is made up of two:
   a. centrioles
   b. centomeres
   c. chromosomes
   d. alleles

5. A property of a cell membrane is:
   a. it is impenetrable and prevents the loss of cell contents
   b. it is a semi-permeable membrane
   c. all transport across it requires energy
   d. protein channels allow the movement of any cell product out of the cell

6. A definition of osmosis is:
   a. movement of fluid from a low concentration of solute to a higher concentration through a semi-permeable membrane

   b. movement of salt particles (solute) from a low concentration of solute to a higher concentration through a semi-permeable membrane
   c. movement of fluid from a high concentration of solute to a lower concentration through a semi-permeable membrane
   d. movement of solute from a high concentration of solute to a lower concentration through a semi-permeable membrane

7. An example of endocytosis is:
   a. passive diffusion
   b. osmosis
   c. phagocytosis
   d. exocytosis

8. The fluid that surrounds the cells is called:
   a. circulating blood plasma
   b. intracellular fluid
   c. lymph fluid
   d. interstitial fluid

9. Meiosis is called reductive division because:
   a. daughter cells contain a haploid number of chromosomes
   b. daughter cells contain a diploid number of chromosomes
   c. there are fewer stages in the division process
   d. daughter cells do not contain any cell organelles

10. In a cross between two black heterozygous individuals for coat colour (Bb), what would the resultant F1 genotypes be?
    a. 3 black to 1 brown
    b. 2 black to 2 brown
    c. 1 BB to 2Bb to 1bb
    d. 2BB to 2bb

Chapter 2

1. When describing the foot of the forelimb the term PALMER describes:
   a. the front of the paw
   b. the rear of the paw
   c. closer to the middle of the body
   c. closer to the side of the body

2. Epithelial tissue that changes shape when stretched is known as:
   a. stratified squamous
   b. simple cuboidal
   c. columnar
   d. transitional

3. Examples of organs found in the MEDIASTINUM are the:
   a. heart, trachea, oesophagus
   b. heart and lungs
   c. lungs only
   d. liver, stomach and pancreas

4. Ribs are examples of:
   a. long bone
   b. short bone
   c. irregular bone
   d. flat bone

5. When the bones of a joint are moved closer together, the movement is called:
   a. extension
   b. abduction
   c. flexion
   d. pivoting

6. Tendons attach:
   a. bone to bone
   b. muscle to bone
   c. muscle to skin
   d. bone to skin

7. The QUADRICEPS FEMORIS is located on the:
   a. hindlimb
   b. neck
   c. forelimb
   d. abdomen

8. The layer of skin that contains blood vessels and nerve endings is the:
   a. epidermis
   b. dermis
   c. hypodermis
   d. hyperdermis

9. The clear front of the eye that allows light to enter is the:
   a. choroid
   b. caval foramen
   c. cornea
   d. conjunctiva

10. The part of the ear concerned with balance is the:
    a. cochlea
    b. semi-circular canal
    c. tympanic membrane
    d. round window

Chapter 3

1. The type of epithelial tissue that lines the nasal chambers is:
   a. cuboidal
   b. squamous
   c. ciliated
   d. transitional

2. The structure that does NOT lead from the pharynx is the:
   a. oral cavity
   b. right bronchus
   c. oesophagus
   d. Eustachian tube

3. Gaseous exchange occurs within the respiratory system:
   a. across the pulmonary membrane
   b. within the nasal chambers
   c. in the right and left bronchi
   d. within the bronchioles

4. The valve lying between the left atrium and the left ventricle is known as the:
   a. tricuspid
   b. mitral
   c. pulmonic
   d. aortic

5. The types of blood vessels that carry blood towards the heart are:
   a. arteries
   b. veins
   c. capillaries
   d. arterioles

6. The largest vein in the body is the:
a. hepatic vein
b. aorta
c. pulmonary vein
d. caudal vena cava

7. The cell that is NOT a granulocyte is the:
a. eosinophil
b. erythrocyte
c. neutrophil
d. basophil

8. The structure that is part of both the respiratory and digestive systems is the:
a. pharynx
b. oesophagus
c. trachea
d. stomach

9. The number of teeth the adult dog has in its permanent dentition is:
a. 20
b. 26
c. 30
d. 42

10. During digestion, proteins eaten in food are broken down into:
a. glucose
b. glycerol
c. amino acids
d. maltose

Chapter 4

1. Fertilisation of the egg occurs in the:
a. ovary
b. uterus
c. oviduct
d. fimbra

2. Implantation of the fertilised egg occurs in the:
a. uterus
b. oviduct
c. cervix
d. vagina

3. Sperm is stored in the:
a. vas deferens
b. epididymis
c. prostate gland
d. urethra

4. Testosterone is produced in the:
a. Sertoli cells
b. epididymis
c. cells of Leydig
d. scrotum

5. The bitch will allow mating to happen when she is in:
a. pro-oestrus
b. oestrus
c. metoestrus
d. anoestrus

6. Pseudopregnancy occurs in:
a. pro-oestrus
b. oestrus
c. metoestrus
d. anoestrus

7. The resting phase in the queen's oestrus cycle in the summer months is known as:
a. pro-oestrus
b. oestrus
c. inter-oestrus
d. anoestrus

8. The epithelium lining of the bladder is classed as:
a. squamous
b. transitional
c. stratified
d. cuboidal

9. Selective reabsorption in the kidney nephron occurs in the:
a. glomerulus
b. collecting duct
c. loop of Henle
d. proximal convoluted tubule

10. Prolactin is released from the:
a. anterior pituitary gland
b. ovary
c. thyroid gland
d. pancreas

11. The hormone responsible for causing ripening of the ova is:
a. prolactin
b. follicle stimulating hormone
c. oestrogen
d. luteinising hormone

12. The structure that carries impulses towards the cell body is called a/an:
a. *axon*
b. *dendrite*
c. *synapse*
d. *neuron*

Chapter 5

1. A kennel run is 2 m wide and 8 m long. The area of the run is:
a. *10 m²*
b. *16 m²*
c. *18 m²*
d. *24 m²*

2. Suitable bedding for a recumbent, incontinent dog would be:
a. *newspaper*
b. *dry-top absorbent bedding*
c. *foam*
d. *shredded paper and blankets*

3. The energy-producing nutrients are:
a. *fat, vitamins and minerals*
b. *carbohydrate, minerals and fibre*
c. *protein, carbohydrate and fat*
d. *minerals, protein and fibre*

4. The fat-soluble vitamins are:
a. *ABCD*
b. *ACEK*
c. *ADEK*
d. *ABCK*

5. The amino acid that is essential for cats, but not dogs is:
a. *taurine*
b. *arachidonic acid*
c. *lysine*
d. *linoleic acid*

6. A suitable diet for a geriatric dog with a sedentary lifestyle is:
a. *high in energy, low in fibre*
b. *high in protein, low in energy*
c. *low in energy, high in fibre*
d. *low in protein, high in energy*

7. A suitable diet for a patient with chronic renal failure is:
a. *moderate in protein, low in phosphorus*
b. *high in calcium, moderate in phosphorus*
c. *high in protein, low in calcium*
d. *low in protein, high in phosphorus*

8. Feeding a diet entirely of muscle meat could cause:
a. *blindness*
b. *skeletal deformity*
c. *infertility*
d. *skin tumours*

9. A hound glove is most suitable for a:
a. *Golden Retriever*
b. *Deerhound*
c. *Weimeraner*
d. *Border Terrier*

10. A slicker brush is most suitable for a:
a. *Samoyed*
b. *Norfolk Terrier*
c. *Bloodhound*
d. *Hungarian Vizsla*

Chapter 6

1. Should a client wish for advice on registering a litter of pedigree kittens, the organisation to contact is:
a. *The Department for Rural Affairs and the Environment*
b. *The Governing Council of the Cat Fancy*
c. *The Feline Advisory Bureau*
d. *The Kennel Club*

2. If a young puppy passes urine in an inappropriate place you should not:
a. *clean the area using a biological detergent and deodoriser*
b. *remove it immediately to a more appropriate area*
c. *rub the puppy's nose in the mess*
d. *use a cue word when it urinates outside*

3. The correct term for the stage of the reproductive cycle when the bitch or queen are most likely to accept mating is called:
a. *anoestrus*
b. *metoestrus*
c. *oestrus*
d. *pro-oestrus*

4. The correct statement is:
a. *The queen is seasonally monoestrus*
b. *The queen is seasonally polyoestrus*
c. *The bitch is seasonally polyoestrus*
d. *The bitch has many short periods of interoestrus*

5. The Alaskan Malamute is in the:
a. *Pastoral Group*
b. *Toy Group*
c. *Utility Group*
d. *Working Group*

6. The Devon Rex in is the:
a. *British Section*
b. *Foreign Section*
c. *Semi-longhaired Section*
d. *Siamese Section*

7. The best position for a cat letter tray is:
a. *at the bottom of the garden*
b. *close to a doorway well used by everyone in the house*
c. *in a quiet area*
d. *next to where the cat is fed*

8. Substances which can be used to help promote a sense of calm in hospitalised animals are:
a. *fragrant atomisers that can be plugged in to the electricity socket*
b. *herbal or perfumed sprays*
c. *lactating bitch mammary gland or feline facial pheromones*
d. *lactating bitch mammary gland of feline facial probiotics*

9. During second stage parturition what would you normally expect to see:
a. *expulsion of fetus*
b. *expulsion of fetal membranes*
c. *panting only*
d. *straining only*

10. The most appropriate restraint procedure for an aggressive brachycephalic breed of dog might include:
a. *closed muzzle and towel*
b. *holding by the scruff and using a dog catcher*
c. *holding by the scruff and applying a basket muzzle*
d. *towel around neck, collar and lead*

Chapter 7

1. The act of legislation covering cruelty to animals is the:
a. *Abandonment of Animals Act 1960*
b. *Protection of Animals Act 1911–1988*
c. *Animals Act 1971*
d. *Dog Fouling of Land Act 1996*

2. The breed not named within the Dangerous Dogs Act 1991 is the:
a. *Dogo Argentino*
b. *Japanese Tosa*
c. *English Bull Terrier*
d. *Pit Bull Terrier*

3. The Act that prohibits the breeding, selling, exchanging or parting of certain breeds of dog, often kept for fighting, is the:
a. *Protection of Animals Act 1911–1988*
b. *Control of Dogs Order 1930*
c. *Wildlife and Countryside Act 1981*
d. *Dangerous Dogs Act 1991*

4. The Act that states that dogs should wear identity discs in public is the:
a. *Abandonment of Animals Act 1960*
b. *Protection of Animals Act 1911–1988*
c. *Control of Dogs Order 1930*
d. *Wildlife and Countryside Act 1981*

5. The statement that is true regarding the Wildlife and Countryside Act 1981 is the:
a. *Schedules 1–4 cover birds only*
b. *Schedules 1–5 cover birds only*
c. *Schedules 1–4 cover animals only*
d. *Schedules 1–5 cover animals only*

6. The method of identification classed as permanent is:
a. *tattooing*
b. *micro-chipping*
c. *leg rings for birds*
d. *photographs*

7. The charity that provides free veterinary treatment for animals whose owners can genuinely not afford the fees is the:
a. *CPL*
b. *NCDL*
c. *Blue Cross*
d. *PDSA*

8. Quarantine for dogs and cats entering the UK is:
a. *6 days*
b. *6 weeks*
c. *6 calendar months*
d. *6 lunar months*

9. The Act that governs Quarantine for dogs and cats is known as:
a. *Rabies (Importation of dogs, cats and other mammals) Order 1974*
b. *Importation of Birds, Poultry and Hatching Eggs Order 1979*
c. *The Balai Directive*
d. *The Pets Travel Scheme*

10. The correct order of requirements to commence the Pets Travel Scheme are:
a. *blood testing, rabies vaccination, micro-chipping*
b. *micro-chipping, blood testing, rabies vaccination*
c. *rabies vaccination, micro-chipping, blood testing*
d. *micro-chipping, rabies vaccination, blood testing*

Chapter 8

1. Animal viruses replicate by:
a. *conjugation*
b. *utilising a host cell*
c. *binary fission*
d. *utilising a parasite*

2. An example of a fomite is a:
a. *parasite*
b. *sick animal*
c. *bacterium*
d. *food bowl*

3. An example of a bacterial disease affecting the dog is canine:
a. *leptospirosis*
b. *distemper*
c. *adenovirus*
d. *parainfluenza*

4. A symptom of canine parvovirus in a puppy is:
a. *nasal discharge*
b. *hepatitis*
c. *hardening of pads*
d. *myocarditis*

5. The acronym that describes 'cat 'flu' is:
a. *FeLv*
b. *FURD*
c. *FIV*
d. *FIE*

6. Ringworm is caused by a:
a. *fungal mould*
b. *common bacteria*
c. *protozoan parasite*
d. *enveloped virus*

7. Humans can become infected by *Toxoplasma gondii* by handling:
a. *sheep faeces*
b. *cat hair*
c. *cat faeces*
d. *sheep meat*

8. The scientific name for the canine biting louse is:
a. Lingonathus setosus
b. Psorptes cuniculi
c. Trichodectes canis
d. Ctenocephalides felis

9. *Dipylidium caninum* is the common tapeworm affecting the:
a. *canine only*
b. *rabbit only*
c. *canine and feline*
d. *feline only*

10. An example of a zoonotic ectoparasite is:
a. Trichodectes canis
b. Lingonathus setosus
c. Trixacarus caviae
d. Cheyletiella yasguri

Chapter 9

1. Surgical spirit is an example of:
a. *peroxygen compound*
b. *an alcohol*
c. *iodine*
d. *methylated spirit*

2. Which statement is true of the term disinfection?
a. *is the prevention of infection in living tissues*
b. *is the process of killing pathogens*
c. *is free from all living organisms*
d. *is a chemical that can be used on skin*

3. When using disinfectants
a. *the dilution rate is unimportant*
b. *it is not necessary to wear gloves and protective clothing*
c. *read the manufacturer's instructions*
d. *works best when mixed with other disinfectants*

4. The normal temperature for a cat is:
a. *38.0–38.5°C*
b. *38.3–38.7°C*
c. *38.5°C*
d. *38.0°C*

5. The normal pulse rate of a dog is:
a. *40–60*
b. *60–140*
c. *110–180*
d. *180–300*

6. What can cause hypothermia?
a. *convulsions*
b. *exercise*
c. *stress*
d. *shock*

7. What can cause tachycardia?
a. *sleep*
b. *low body temperature*
c. *stress*
d. *infection*

8. A 4-month-old puppy requires barrier nursing. Which statement is false?
a. *Protective clothing must be worn only for this patient*
b. *This patient can be nursed alongside other young patients*
c. *This patient should be cleaned out after other patients*
d. *Uniforms can harbour micro-organisms that can be passed on to other patients*

9. What accommodation is suitable for a budgerigar?
a. *Its own cage with perches*
b. *Its own cage with perches removed*
c. *A cage with a heat gradient*
d. *A vivarium with a hide box*

10. Which term means 'slow heart rate'?
a. *tachycardia*
b. *bradycardia*
c. *bradypnoea*
d. *hypothermia*

Chapter 10

1. The wound that is classified as an open wound is a:
a. *contusion*
b. *incised*
c. *haematoma*
d. *seroma*

2. The capillary refill time indicates:
a. *oxygenation levels*
b. *temperature range*
c. *circulatory blood volume*
d. *level of consciousness*

3. The *ideal* solution for flushing wounds is:
a. *chlorhexidine*
b. *normal saline*
c. *povidine iodine*
d. *surgical spirit*

4. Cold compresses can be in a first aid situation to help:
a. *increase the blood supply to any area*
b. *increase body temperature*
c. *decrease blood supply to an area*
d. *decrease body temperature*

5. Haemorrhage specifically from an artery can be identified by:
a. *bright red and pumping*
b. *general ooze*
c. *dark red and flowing*
d. *general flow*

6. The maximum length of time that a tourniquet can remain in one place is:
a. *15 minutes*
b. *30 minutes*
c. *1 hour*
d. *2 hours*

7. A comminuted fracture is recognised as:
a. *a fracture with no break in skin surface*
b. *a fracture with an open wound leading to fracture site*
c. *a fracture with no bone fragments*
d. *a fracture with several bone fragments*

8. Displacement of the articular surfaces of bones within a joint is known as:
a. *sprain*
b. *strain*
c. *dislocation*
d. *fracture*

9. A primary cause of unconsciousness is:
a. *cardiac failure*
b. *drug overdose*
c. *electric shock*
d. *brain trauma*

10. A normal respiratory rate range for an adult healthy cat is:
a. *0–9 breaths per minute*
b. *11–19 breaths per minute*
c. *21–29 breaths per minute*
d. *31–39 breaths per minute*

Chapter 11

1. The study of disease and its cause is termed:
a. *anatomy*
b. *histology*
c. *physiology*
d. *pathology*

2. The instrument used as a needle holder is a pair of:
a. *Allis*
b. *Doyen*
c. *Gillies*
d. *Babcocks*

3. A Jacobs chuck is an example of an instrument used in:
a. *orthopaedic surgery*
b. *ophthalmic surgery*
c. *oral surgery*
d. *obstetric surgery*

4. Spencer Wells forceps are primarily used to:
a. *dissect tissue*
b. *clamp blood vessels*
c. *retract surgical wounds*
d. *cut through bone*

5. Endotracheal tubes can be sterilised using:
a. *autoclaves*
b. *ethylene oxide*
c. *hot air ovens*
d. *boilers*

6. Bowie Dick autoclave tape indicates:
a. *change in temperature*
b. *the content of the pack*
c. *time, steam and temperature*
d. *sterility of the pack*

7. An item described as 'free from pathogens including bacterial spores' could be defined as:
a. *aseptic*
b. *cleaned*
c. *disinfected*
d. *sterilised*

8. An example of a wild patient which can be released back into the wild under the Wildlife and Countryside Act is the:
a. *common mink*
b. *little gull*
c. *grey squirrel*
d. *Canada goose*

9. Hospitalised hedgehogs should be fed a diet described as:
a. *herbivorous*
b. *carnivorous*
c. *omnivorous*
d. *insectivorous*

10. The prefix 'arthr' describes:
a. *hearing*
b. *water*
c. *clot*
d. *joint*

Chapter 12

1. A worming preparation is classified as an:
a. *anthelmintic*
b. *antibiotic*
c. *antihistamine*
d. *antitussive*

2. A 25 kg dog needs medicating with an injectable drug at a dose rate of 10 mg/kg. Each mL contains 500 mg of the drug. The dog needs:
a. *0.5 mL*
b. *2 mL*
c. *2.5 mL*
d. *5 mL*

3. When giving intravenous fluids, a standard giving set (20 drops/mL) is *most* likely to be used for a:
a. *25 kg Labrador*
b. *12-week-old Collie puppy*
c. *4 kg cat*
d. *6-year-old Pomeranian*

4. To examine the white blood cells of a stained blood smear under the microscope, the objective lens that should be used is:
a. *×4*
b. *×10*
c. *×40*
d. *×100*

5. The microscope lens that enables the light source to be focused on the specimen is the:
a. *eyepiece lens*
b. *iris diaphragm*
c. *objective lens*
d. *substage condenser*

6. COSHH stands for:
a. *Care of Substances Harmful to Health*
b. *Care of Substances Hazardous to Health*
c. *Control of Substances Harmful to Health*
d. *Control of Substances Hazardous to Health*

7. The Radiation Protection Supervisor is responsible for:
a. *giving advice about ionising radiations*
b. *giving advice about radiation protection*
c. *ensuring all radiographic procedures are carried out safely*
d. *setting the controlled area*

8. When labelling a radiograph which is to be scored under the Hip Dysplasia Scheme, the information which must NOT be shown is the:
a. *date of radiography*
b. *client's name*
c. *kennel club number*
d. *left/right marker*

9. Under the Ionising Radiations Regulations
a. *a Radiation Protection Supervisor is not always necessary*
b. *dose limits can be exceeded for designated persons*
c. *Local Rules should be displayed*
d. *the operator's hands may be in the primary beam if lead gloves are worn*

10. When positioning animals for radiography:
a. *foam wedges cannot be placed in the primary beam*
b. *limbs of conscious animals should not be tied in position*
c. *sandbags can safely be placed in the primary beam*
d. *animals should never be placed in dorsal recumbency*

Chapter 13

1. Examples of animals that carry out coprophagia are:
a. *chinchilla, hamster, rabbit*
b. *cavy, chinchilla, rabbit*
c. *cavy, rabbit, hamster*
d. *chinchilla, gerbil, mouse*

2. The dental formula of a rabbit is:
a. *{1003/1003}*
b. *{2033/1023}*
c. *{1013/1013}*
d. *{1003/1003}*

3. The type of animal that can be described as 'solitary' is the:
a. *Mongolian Gerbil*
b. *Peruvian Guinea pig*
c. *Syrian Hamster*
d. *Shaw's Jird*

4. The type of food that can cause obesity and osteoporosis if fed in high amounts to rodents is:
a. *crushed oats*
b. *flaked maize*
c. *soya bean*
d. *sunflower seeds*

5. The recommended hutch size for a 3–5 kg rabbit is (L × W × H)
a. *45 cm × 30 cm × 20 cm*
b. *60 cm × 30 cm × 23 cm*
c. *150 cm × 60 cm × 50 cm*
d. *200 cm × 100 cm × 45 cm*

6. To maintain healthy gastrointestinal tract motility and balanced gut microflora, which of the following foodstuffs is vital in the diet of a chinchilla, rabbit and guinea pig:
a. *carrots*
b. *crushed oats*
c. *sunflower seeds*
d. *hay*

7. An example of a breed of hamster is the:
a. *Abyssinian*
b. *Mongolian*
c. *Roborovski*
d. *Shaws*

8. A glass fish tank filled with a mixture of moss peat, hay and wood shavings provides ideal accommodation for a:
a. *chinchilla*
b. *gerbil*
c. *guinea pig*
d. *hamster*

9. In all herbivores the canine teeth are absent and this leaves an area in the mouth called the:
a. *appendix*
b. *caecum*
c. *diastema*
d. *glottis*

10. The animal that is classed as an induced ovulator is the:
a. chinchilla
b. rabbit
c. rat
d. hamster

Chapter 14

1. Regarding heating in a reptile vivarium the INCORRECT statement is:
a. should be connected to a thermostat
b. should have a guard around it
c. should provide a heat gradient
d. should remain constant

2. The difference between the digestive tracts of carnivores and herbivores is:
a. all herbivores have a stomach consisting of four separate compartments
b. fermentation in herbivores occurs in the caecum and colon
c. herbivores' digestive tract is longer
d. herbivores have to pass food through the system twice

3. A cloaca is found in:
a. chicken, fish, lizard
b. chicken, lizard, snake
c. fish, snake, rabbit
d. lizard, snake, rabbit

4. The statement that is FALSE when discussing the proventriculus is:
a. contains grinding plated called cuticles
b. is caudal to the crop
c. secretes a nutritive juice in some species
d. secretes gastric juice

5. The animal species that possesses a urinary bladder is the:
a. budgie
b. corn snake
c. tortoise
d. chicken

6. The best method for distinguishing the sex of a budgie is:
a. female has a brown cere
b. female has horizontal bars on the underside of the tail
c. male sings more than the female
d. male has a brown cere

7. Iodine deficiency is most commonly seen in the:
a. African gray
b. budgie
c. canary
d. cockatiel

8. The most appropriate diet for a leopard gecko is:
a. crickets and vitamin supplement
b. pinkies and waxworms
c. small locusts and crickets
d. waxworms, crickets and occasional pinkie

9. Soft shell in a young tortoise would NOT be due to:
a. hypovitaminosis D
b. lack of UV
c. parasites
d. too high quality food

10. Regarding aquaria water, the false statement is:
a. Needs a partial water change every 2–3 weeks
b. Should be tested for pH, nitrates, nitrites and ammonia
c. The quality is crucial to maintain fish health
d. Should be tested every month

Chapter 15

1. If the salutation of a letter is Dear Mrs Smith the complementary close would be:
a. Yours faithfully
b. Yours Faithfully
c. Yours sincerely
d. Yours Sincerely

2. A curriculum vitae would be used when:
a. applying for a job
b. checking a wage slip
c. terminating employment
d. completing a tax return

3. The organisation that represents veterinary nurses is:
a. BEVA
b. BVA
c. BSAVA
d. BVNA

4. The organisation that holds the list of qualified Veterinary Nurses is the:
a. BVA
b. RCVS
c. BVNA
d. RVC

5. In the sentence, 'we record our recent x-ray exposures in a black book', the adjectives are:
a. *we & our*
b. *record & exposures*
c. *recent & black*
d. *x-ray & book*

6. In English grammar the symbol that depicts a 'semi-colon' is:
a. *:*
b. *.*
c. *;*
d. *–*

7. The names that are in correct alphabetical order are:
a. *Stevens, Steven, Stephens, Stephenson*
b. *Stephens, Stephenson, Steven, Stevens*
c. *Steven, Stephenson, Stevens, Stephen*
d. *Stephenson, Stevens, Stephen, Steven*

8. The correct spelling for the term that describes liquid faeces is:
a. *diarhoea*
b. *diarrhea*
c. *diarrhoea*
d. *dihorrea*

9. Booster reminders stored in date order are filed:
a. *alphabetically*
b. *numerically*
c. *geographically*
d. *chronologically*

10. A noun:
a. *demonstrates events that will occur after the present*
b. *indicates that the action is happening now*
c. *is a word used to show action*
d. *represents an object, living thing or place*

Chapter 16

1. The method of postage that is most appropriate to send an important document of no significant value to the recipient is:
a. *Registered Post*
b. *Special Delivery*
c. *First Class*
d. *Second Class*

2. The legal category of veterinary medicines that can be left on display within the waiting room for clients to purchase as required is:
a. *Prescription only medication*
b. *Pharmaceutical Merchants List*
c. *Pharmacy*
d. *General Sales List*

3. The legislative Act that controls the sale and supply of goods is the:
a. *Consumer Protection Act*
b. *Sale of Goods Act*
c. *Trade Description Act*
d. *Data Protection Act*

4. Explain the term 'use by date' when displayed on animal feed displayed in the waiting area:
a. *date by which the product must be sold*
b. *product deteriorates after this date*
c. *date of manufacture*
d. *product undergoes change and may become unsafe after this date*

5. The term 'dead stock' in relation to ordering systems in veterinary practice is:
a. *excess quantities, unlikely to be sold quickly*
b. *maximum allowed to be stocked*
c. *products used in the euthanasia of animals*
d. *out of date products*

6. Pathological specimens should be packaged for dispatch to external laboratories:
a. *sealed in plastic, padded, with laboratory request form separately packaged*
b. *in the pre-paid envelope provided*
c. *they should always be sent by special delivery*
d. *in a cardboard box, that is sealed well with tape*

7. The labels that must be displayed when sending pathological specimens by post are the:
a. *address of sender, recipient and pathological specimen warning*
b. *addressed to laboratory, stating handle with care and pathological specimen warnings*
c. *address of sender, recipient and warnings including handle with care and pathological specimen*
d. *address of sender, handle with care and pathological specimen warnings*

8. The RCVS recommend that client records are maintained for:
    a. *2 years*
    b. *4 years*
    c. *6 years*
    d. *8 years*

9. The law that protects the identity of customers and clients is the:
    a. *Consumer Protection Act*
    b. *Consumer Credit Act*
    c. *Data Protection Act*
    d. *Sale of Goods Act*

10. Third party liability encompasses:
    a. *veterinary fees for illness*
    b. *advertising for lost pets*
    c. *transfer of the policy to new owners*
    d. *incidents affecting other people, caused by the insured pet*

Multiple choice answers

Chapter 1

1. c
2. b
3. d
4. a
5. b
6. a
7. c
8. d
9. a
10. c

Chapter 2

1. b
2. d
3. a
4. d
5. c
6. b
7. a
8. c
9. c
10. b

Chapter 3

1. c
2. b
3. a
4. b
5. b
6. d
7. b
8. a
9. d
10. c

Chapter 4

1. c
2. a
3. b
4. c
5. b
6. c
7. c
8. b
9. d
10. a
11. b
12. b

Chapter 5

1. b
2. b
3. c
4. c
5. a
6. c
7. a
8. b
9. c
10. a

Chapter 6

1. b
2. c
3. c
4. b
5. d
6. b
7. c
8. c
9. a
10. d

Chapter 7

1. b
2. c
3. d
4. c
5. a
6. d
7. d
8. c
9. a
10. d

Chapter 8

1. b
2. d
3. a
4. d
5. b
6. a
7. c
8. c
9. c
10. d

Chapter 9

1. b
2. b
3. c
4. a
5. b
6. d
7. c
8. b
9. a
10. b

Chapter 10

1. b
2. c
3. b
4. c
5. a
6. a
7. d
8. c
9. d
10. c

Chapter 11

1. d
2. c
3. a
4. b
5. b
6. a
7. d
8. b
9. c
10. d

Chapter 12

1. a
2. a
3. a
4. d
5. d
6. d
7. c
8. b
9. c
10. b

Chapter 13

1. c
2. b
3. c
4. d
5. c
6. d
7. c
8. b
9. c
10. b

Chapter 14

1. d
2. c
3. b
4. a
5. c
6. a
7. b
8. a
9. c
10. d

Chapter 15

1. c
2. a
3. d
4. b
5. c
6. c
7. b
8. c
9. d
10. d

Chapter 16

1. a
2. d
3. b
4. b
5. a
6. a
7. c
8. c
9. c
10. d

Index

Note: Page numbers in *italics* refer to figures, tables and boxes.